HANDBOOK OF
Home Health Standards
and
Documentation Guidelines for Reimbursement

HANDBOOK OF
Home Health Standards

and Documentation Guidelines for Reimbursement

Second Edition

T. M. MARRELLI, RN, MA

Home Health Care Consultant
Kent Island, Maryland

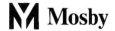 Mosby

St. Louis Baltimore Boston Chicago London Madrid
Philadelphia Sydney Toronto

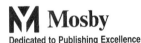
Mosby

Dedicated to Publishing Excellence

Executive Editor: N. Darlene Como
Associate Developmental Editor: Brigitte Pocta
Project Manager: Karen Edwards
Production: Spectrum Publisher Services, Inc.
Design Coordinator: Liz Fett

SECOND EDITION
Copyright © 1994 by Mosby–Year Book, Inc.

Previous editions copyrighted 1988, 1991

Printed in the United States of America

Composition by TCSystems, Inc.
Printing/binding by RR Donnelley & Sons Company

Mosby–Year Book, Inc.
11830 Westline Industrial Drive
St. Louis, Missouri 63146

NOTE TO THE READER: The author and publisher have diligently verified the nursing considerations discussed for accuracy and compatibility with officially accepted standards at the time of publication. With continual advancements in nursing practice and great variety in particular patient needs, we recommend that the reader consult the latest literature and exercise professional judgment in using the guidelines in this book. In addition, the assumption is made that the professional nurse is functioning under physician orders and adheres to other regulatory guidelines or laws.

ISBN 0-8016-7661-4

96 97   9 8 7 6 5

PREFACE

Many changes in home care have occurred since the first edition of this book was published in 1988. Based upon your comments and feedback, 18 new Clinical Guidelines have been added to this second edition.

This book contains a series of documentation guidelines for clinical problems to aid in reimbursement from third-party payers. A patient's home is often the health care setting. This trend will continue to grow as consumers are more active in their health care management. Home care continues to be the fastest growing segment of the health care industry. As the population ages, in addition to the three generations of elderly for whom the Medicare Home Health Program was initially implemented, the priority is to meet the nursing needs of these patients. This can be achieved through the nursing process. This book was written to facilitate the integration of nursing care and planning into the forms used by insurers to determine coverage. Although the Medicare Program is a medical model, it lends itself well to modern nursing practice. Home care practitioners have the clinical skills and the information to identify these needs. This book assists in the documentation process of that nursing knowledge.

These clinical guidelines communicate to the novice and the experienced professional nurse the direction and actual documentation that justifies the presence of and continuing need for home health care services. These standards can be practiced in orientation, actual home settings, and ongoing clinical case reviews. The generation of skilled reimbursable documentation is a learning process. This book integrates the documentation needed to maximize reimbursement, while listing the care needed for patients by clinical problem.

Two special devices have been included to make this book easier to use. In the clinical material, certain standard abbreviations are used throughout to simplify the descriptions of home care and to allow the reader to quickly refer to this material. If any abbreviation is confusing, check its meaning in Part Eight. The table of contents is alphabetized for the medical-surgical care sections and cross-referenced materials are found under another heading. For example, care for arthritis is actually under the heading of ''Arthritis,'' but is included in the table of contents as ''Osteoarthritis'' with the correct page number. This method should help you find material more quickly. In addition, each specific Clinical Guideline cross-refers related care guidelines to help the reader access additional information. For example, in "Depression and Other Psychiatric Home Care," the reader is also referred to "Alzheimer's Disease and Other Dementias" should that be a related problem for their patient. For a more detailed discussion of how to use this book for planning, delivering, evaluating, and documenting care, see the section "Guidelines for Use." This section details the new features of this book.

T. M. Marrelli

GUIDELINES FOR USE

As in the first edition, the goal of this book is to help the professional nurse meet reimbursement, quality and other requirements through effective documentation. The Clinical Guidelines, or topics, are organized alphabetically for easy retrieval of needed information.

There may be more than one case scenario that is appropriate for your patient. For example, when caring for a patient with diabetes mellitus and an open wound, the following scenarios could be referred to: ''Diabetes Mellitus,'' ''Wound Care,'' ''Cellulitis,'' or ''Amputation Care.'' This documentation can be used throughout the clinical record.

The following guidelines refer to the specifically numbered entries of each case:

1. **General Considerations.** Contains general information on the designated topic in relation to home health care. This diagnostic information will be utilized primarily in item nos. 11, 12, and 13 on form 485.

2. **Needs for initial visit.** This supply information will sometimes be utilized in item no. 14 of form 485, where information is requested about medical equipment and supplies.

3. **Some potential medical-surgical diagnoses and codes.** The specific ICD-9 or V-codes for the most common diagnoses are included. This information will be utilized in item nos. 11, 12, and 13 on form 485. These have been alphabetized to assist in their identification and location.

   The source for all codes was the current edition of the *ICD-9-CM* published by the Commission on Professional and Hospital Activities. The ICD-9-CM system sometimes requires secondary codes for complete description of the diagnostic entity. For example, pneumonia in the presence of AIDS is coded as both 486 (pneumonia) and 042.1 (AIDS). It is important in such instances to use all codes given, in the order given. In instances where your Regional Home Health Intermediary (RHHI) has preferred or recommended codes, those codes should be used when appropriate for your patient. These codes are usually communicated to your manager through the RHHI's newsletters.

Codes for associated operations or postoperative care are given as appropriate. These generally will follow the diagnosis code. Operation codes may be recognized by their two-digit structure. Diagnosis codes always have three digits before the decimal point, and in some cases have no decimal at all. Operation codes have only two digits before the decimal and are always followed by one or two digits following the decimal:

Diagnosis: osteomyelitis, lower leg, 715.96
Surgical procedure: S/P BKA, 84.15

V-codes are provided in the ICD-9-CM system for description of certain patient statuses. They appear in this book only to the extent that they are appropriate to home health care.

Certain essential assumptions have been made regarding home health care services. The main assumption is that services meet recognized HHA and insurer standards and are therefore justified for reimbursement. Remember that modifiers to diagnosis terms may be important. Modifiers, such as acute/ chronic, unilateral/bilateral, upper/lower, or adult/juvenile, frequently require differentiation in the ICD-9 codes. Similarly, slight variations in terminology may be significant. Please note that the ICD-9-CM system contains more than 10,000 diagnosis code categories and more than 40,000 cross-referenced diagnosis terms. We have attempted to clearly illustrate such distinctions in the text. Your intermediary may have other or additional specific ICD-9 codes they prefer for you to use. In those cases, use the intermediary's recommended codes. For further information, consult the ICD-9 code books or a qualified coder.

4. **Associated nursing diagnoses.** This section includes the approved nursing diagnoses that are related to the listed problem in the Clinical Guidelines. All the nursing diagnoses listed are approved by the North American Nursing Diagnosis Association (NANDA). These nursing diagnoses are the identified focus for intervention by the professional nurse in daily home-care practice. The nurse needs to evaluate the patient and identify those diagnoses that best address the patient's unique problems. These diagnoses are used in the

care planning record, the POC, the problem list, the daily visit record, or other documentation formats in the HHA. All or some of these diagnoses may be appropriate for the specific patient.

5. **Service skills identified.** Nursing has been placed as the first service. For those diagnoses that usually have nursing or other service needs identified, the indicated service skills have been listed. These services often use verbs in the description of care, again to clearly demonstrate the skilled service(s) provided. Both numbers 5 and 6 will be used in item no. 21 on form 485. These are examples of the orders used in home care.

6. **Other services indicated.** These services are based on the diagnosis that usually indicates the need for the ordered service(s). Both numbers 5 and 6 will be utilized on the form 485 in item no. 21. When applicable, they could also be used in item no. 16 on form 486.

7. **Associated factors based on diagnosis justifying homebound status.** For each diagnosis or clinical problem topic, the reasons listed are the most common specific to that diagnostic problem demonstrating the homebound status. Please refer to specific criteria regarding the homebound status for further clarification. These reasons are placed in item no. 17 of form 486. In item no. 18A and 18B of form 485 check what functional limitations contribute to or further explain the homebound status.

8. **Short-term goals.** These goals are based on the diagnosis. They are the daily objective goals identified by a specific service. These are utilized in the care planning record and in the narrative notes. Usually these are the goals to be placed in item no. 22 of form 485.

9. **Long-term goals.** These goals are also based on the patient's unique diagnosis. These are the realistic and measurable criteria that assist in the determination of goal achievement and discharge planning from home health care services. These patient-centered goals will be listed on form 485 in item no. 22. In addition, progress toward goals should be reflected in item no. 16 of form 486 under updated information and other clinical documentation. If stated goals have been reached and documented, the discharge process should occur, unless other problems and quantifiable goals have been identified.

10. **Discharge plans for this patient.** These are the most common plans based on the diagnosis. Clearly, this is based on the patient's prognosis and clinical course. These will be utilized in item no. 22 of form 485 and item no. 16 of form 486 as discharge is projected, based on the updated clinical information. The rehabilitation potential should assist in the formulation of goals and discharge plans. An example of a rehabilitation potential could be: *Good for partial return to prior level of functioning within 60 days, but will probably remain dependent for all ADLs.*

11. **Patient, family, and caregiver educational needs.** This **new** section addresses the educational needs of patients, their families, and caregivers in the home setting. This is particularly important because managed care and other payers often have stringent limits on the number of reimbursable visits. This places the home care nurse in the position of needing to teach multiple and complex care regimens. The most common types of information that patients need to safely remain at home are listed in this section. Please keep in mind that this is a handbook and the listing is by no means intended to be all-inclusive. Your patient's teaching needs may be as varied as their medical history. The family or caregivers will also have unique learning needs.

    Support and informational resources are listed at the end of this section to help you and your patients. For example, in "Care of the Child with Cystic Fibrosis," their national toll-free number, 1-800-FIGHT CF, is listed. Similarly, in the guideline for Alzheimer's disease, there are toll-free numbers listed for three national associations and a book resource listed for families and caregivers.

12. **Specific tips for reimbursement.** These tips are often based on diagnoses that contribute to concise, specific documentation clearly justifying reimbursement. There are specific references to the HIM-11 for those practice areas that may need further clarification. Generally, include on form 486 any new symptom or change in patient status. Often these changes alone assist in the demonstration of the patient's unstable condition.

    Remember that all services need to be based on your patient's unique medical condition and the history determined on your assessment visit and throughout the patient's length of care. For your convenience, the coverage section of the HHA manual has been included in this revised edition. In addition, the part of the HHA manual that addresses verbal orders and the correct completion of the 485 series forms has been included for easy referral.

Regardless of payer, the documentation must demonstrate the skilled care provided and the patient's response to that care. A more in-depth discussion about the level of documentation needed in home care and the many requirements that effective documentation meets is addressed in Part One.

ACKNOWLEDGMENTS

Many people have been involved at various levels in the revision of this book. I have received much feedback and many recommendations for this edition. Somehow, the information still fits in a handbook! Again, this format of Clinical Guidelines with ICD-9 codes, nursing diagnoses, interventions and, now, teaching guidelines in one place will continue to help the busy home care nurse in daily practice.

Special thanks go to the following reviewers and consultants on the next pages for their thoughtful comments and input. Their diverse areas of clinical expertise and geographic locations contributed to a broad-based, updated look at home care practice. In addition, they are some of the best managers and clinicians in the home care industry.

I am especially thankful to the following organizations: Olsten Health Care of Columbus, the very helpful staffs of the Otterbein College and The Ohio State University libraries, and the many home care nurses and managers who offered input throughout the process.

It goes without saying that without the support and dedication of Mosby's A-team of Darlene Como, executive editor; Brigitte Pocta, associate developmental editor; and Barbara Carroll, assistant editor, this needed revision would not have occurred (or at least not have occurred promptly!). Special thanks and appreciation to all of you for your perseverance, time, and effort.

Finally, thanks to Bill, Keith, and Sarah Glass for popcorn, humor, filing, and other important miscellaneous duties that families do best!

REVIEWERS

C. Taney Hamill
Vice President
Prima Care Midatlantic
Home Medical Equipment
Hanover, Maryland

Neil O. Hartman, MPH, PT
Vice President of Regulatory
  Affairs and Director of Quality
  Assessment
COMMUNI-CARE/
  PRO-REHAB, Inc.
Boone, North Carolina

Regina Hawkey, BSN, RN
Norrell Health Care
Region Contract Manager
New York, New York

Kathy Larsen, MSN, RN
President
Homebound Consultants, Inc.
Columbus, Ohio

**Dorothy R. Marshall, MA,
  RD, LD**
Consultant Dietitian
Annapolis, Maryland

**Mary Lynn McPherson,
  Pharm D, BCPS, CDE**
Assistant Professor, University
  of Maryland School of
  Pharmacy
Clinical Pharmacist Home
  Health Care/Hospice
Baltimore, Maryland

Ernani B. Morgan, RRA
Morgan and Associates
Health Information
  Management Consultants
Annapolis, Maryland

Margaret O'Brien, MS, RN
President
Margaret O'Brien Healthcare
  Consultants
Woodbine, Maryland

Muriel O'Connell, MS, RN
Director
Division of Nursing and
  Rehabilitation
The Columbus Health
  Department
Columbus, Ohio

Nancy Lee Paulson, MSN, RN
Vice President
Home Care Connection
Consulting Services
Torrance, California

Cheryl Jones Porter, BSN, RN
State Liaison for Accreditation
ABC Home Health Services, Inc.
Austin, Texas

Marcia E. Rock, RN
Home Health Nurse
Sarasota, Florida

Kathy Strunk, BSN, RN
Director of Education and
  Training
Health Care Plus
Worthington, Ohio

Sunny Sutton, BA, RN
Principal
Sutton & Colleagues
Home Health Care Consultants
Walpole, Massachusetts

**Cynthia Bowersock-Thiel,
  BSN, RN**
President and CEO
Health Care Plus
Columbus, Ohio

Carol C. Sylvester, MS, RN
President, Johns Hopkins Home
   Health Services
Baltimore, Maryland

**Sandra Martin Whittier,
   BSN, RN**
Clinical Coordinator

Whidden Memorial Hospital
   Home Care and Hospice
Everett, Massachusetts

Carol Lynne Yarletts, MS, RN
AIDS Nursing Care Specialist
The Columbus Health
   Department
Columbus, Ohio

ABOUT THE AUTHOR

T. M. Marrelli received a Bachelor's degree in Nursing from Duke University School of Nursing and a Master of Arts degree in Management and Supervision, Health Care Administration, from Central Michigan University. She is currently a student in the graduate program at The Ohio State University College of Nursing. Ms. Marrelli is the author of two other nursing books, also published by Mosby, entitled *The Nursing Documentation Handbook* and *The Nurse Manager's Survival Guide: Practical Answers to Everyday Problems.*

Ms. Marrelli has extensive experience in hospital, home health, and hospice nursing and has worked for the Health Care Financing Administration, where she received the Bureau Director's Citation. Ms. Marrelli is listed in the *World Who's Who of Women,* 1993/1994. Ms. Marrelli provides consultation services on various aspects of home care and hospice, particularly management and documentation. Correspondence, including feedback, recommendations, or suggestions about this text may be directed to the author at: T. M. Marrelli Health Care Consulting, Suite 159, 3 Church Circle, Annapolis, Maryland 21401.

CONTENTS

PART ONE

HOME CARE: A UNIQUE
NURSING SPECIALTY

A UNIQUE NURSING SPECIALTY

"This is how I thought nursing would be when I was in nursing school. I see one patient at a time, I teach, the family's involved, and I have input and can attribute outcomes almost directly to my care. What took me so long to find my niche in home care nursing?" This statement and others like it are frequently heard from nurses who have reached a comfort level of autonomous practice in the home setting.

We know home care is different. For one, the home care nurse is a guest in someone's home. And more important, from the patients' viewpoint, no one dictates visiting hours, the required age of visitors, what to wear, when to go to bed, what to eat, and myriad other details that historically have been a standard part of most health care facilities.

The term *home care* is used in the broadest sense throughout this book. It includes home health agencies (HHA), regardless of auspices; hospices who provide care as an HHA; various community programs; and other services that provide care to patients in homes.

Many changes in the external health environment have occurred that continue to make home care one of the fastest growing fields for experienced professional nurses. The nurse and patient/family interactions, the range and diversity of clinical skills employed, and the satisfaction that accompanies caring for patients in situations in which they are equal partners in care are appealing aspects to many nurses. The following list enumerates some of the characteristics common to nurses who are successful in home care practice.

SKILLS AND KNOWLEDGE NEEDED IN HOME CARE

1. **A knowledge of the basic "rules" of home care.** These consist of both administrative and clinical information and are important to being an effective home care nurse. For Medicare certified HHAs, knowledge of the following is required: (1) the Medicare Conditions of Participation, (2) the HHA Health Insurance Manual (HIM-11) provisions about home care coverage, and (3) the HIM-11 section that addresses the correct completion of the 485 series forms. These HIM-11 sections are included in Part Seven for your reference.

   Because Medicare sets many standards for home care, it is important to be familiar and up-to-date with these rules. Some other insurers also use Medicare's criteria for qualifying and/ or coverage. In addition, many insurers such as state Medicaid programs or private insurers use the HCFA 485 as the plan of care (POC).

2. **A repertoire of service-driven and patient-oriented interpersonal skills.** Community liaison and public relations activities are a part of the home care nurse's busy day.

3. **The ability to pay incredible attention to detail.** This is true both in addressing complex patient needs and in documentation. Both are equally important, and they go hand in hand.

4. **The possession of multifaceted skills, accompanied by flexibility.** It is the home care nurse who must "bend" or renegotiate to meet patient needs and achieve patient-centered goals. This flexibility usually includes visiting times and scheduling, but can also include aspects that center on accomodating patient and caregiver needs.

5. **The possession of a reliable car and safe, effective driving skills.** The home care nurse must like, or at least not mind, driving (even in inclement weather); have a good sense of direction (or a map!); and be willing to take risks.

6. **The ability to assume responsibility for the patient and the patient's POC.** True primary care or case management is possible in home care. From the initial nursing assessment

visit through the identification and use of appropriate nursing diagnoses, the home care nurse assumes the planning and follow-through of care. Sometimes, only one team member or a limited number of team members are involved in the care, depending on the patient's needs.

Because of these factors, the nurse in the community setting can directly affect the care as well as see the results of that care. Often, close communication is required between the home care nurse and the case manager from the insurance company. This total patient management function, with its associated prioritizing and complex decision making, makes the home care practice unique. It is from this aspect of home care that professional nurses may receive personal satisfaction and positive feedback from patients and their families, friends, and caregivers.

7. **Strong clinical skills and the ability to function as both a specialist and a generalist nurse.** Patients will be of all age groups, from infants to the elderly. In addition, the diagnoses and care needs of patients will vary from day to day. In home care, although there may be a wide range of clinical problems and nursing diagnoses to address, having an area of expertise for acting as a resource, teaching or orienting nurses new to home care is an important asset for the individual nurse's professional growth.

8. **Self-direction and the ability to function autonomously in a nonstructured atmosphere.** This also entails having well developed and effective time management skills to address the many aspects of home care, including visits scheduled, documentation, and detail-oriented administrative duties (e.g., completing POCs, phone calls, etc.)

9. **The desire to continue learning and to be open to new information and clinical skills.** This is particularly true as many new kinds of technologies are being used in the home setting. Dobutamine management, apnea monitoring, pain and symptom management, and ventilator care are just some of the kinds of patient care problems being addressed daily by competent home care nurses. Please refer to the ''Resources'' section at the end of this book for a list of journal articles, books, and other home care resources that may be helpful to you.

10. **A sincere appreciation of and for people.** This includes interacting positively with and being empathetic to patients, families, and caregivers, who are often in the midst of crises. Since many traditional family caregivers continue to work outside the home, professional nurses use their teaching and training skills to maintain patients safely in the home. This teaching or consulting role brings job satisfaction to home care nurses, as well as comfort and security to the families.

11. **The ability to be open and sincerely accepting of people's unique and chosen life-styles and of the associated effects that these life-styles have on their health.**

12. **The awareness and acceptance that there is a constant balance to be maintained between clinical and administrative demands.** In addition, the home care nurse must have the knowledge that both demands are equally important, but in different ways and for different reasons.

13. **The knowledge that change can be difficult.** The home care culture is very different from the structure and ''down the hall'' comraderie, supervision, and peer consultation available in the structure of other health care (e.g., hospitals, or nursing homes).

14. **The possession of a kind sense of humor that can help patients and peers get through the rough times.** This sense of humor is finally being recognized for the healing power it can convey when used appropriately.

THE HOME CARE
NURSE'S ORIENTATION

All home care nurses need an appropriate orientation period. A quality orientation is important to being successful in home care and feeling comfortable in the home care nursing role. No matter how understaffed the program may be, when possible, nurses should try to define or address their orientation (including time span and content) before accepting the position. The following list addresses some of the information that an orientation should include. Obviously, if the nurse has been in home care for some time, it may not be appropriate or necessary to review all of this information; however, it is important that all nurses have an understanding of these ''hallmarks'' of home care:

1. The HHA's orientation manual

2. The Medicare Conditions of Participation

3. The schedule of home care staff meetings

4. The HIM-11, Revision 222, the coverage of service section (see Part Seven)

5. The HHA's clinical policy and procedure manual(s)

6. An overview of the HHA's medical records, documentation system, required forms, and paper flow

7. Guidelines for home visits and what they entail

8. The opportunity to ''buddy'' with an experienced HHA nurse

9. An orientation to the HHA's required forms

10. Coverage and documentation requirements

11. Administrative details and processes

12. Equipment and supply acquisition

13. Orientation to automated clinical documentation system, where applicable

14. Continuous quality improvement (CQI) processes

15. Benefits, employee handbook, mileage, on-call process and pay, lab pickup schedules, and other miscellaneous information unique to the program

16. Occupational Safety and Health Administration (OSHA) requirements including: (1) Hepatitis B virus vaccination, (2) the HHA related policies and supplies for bloodborne pathogens, (3) universal precautions supplies, and related disposal of supplies, and (4) recordkeeping activities

THE EMPHASIS ON QUALITY IN HOME CARE

Accreditation

There is an emphasis on quality in all aspects of home care. Both the Community Health Accreditation Program (CHAP) and the Joint Commission on Accreditation of Healthcare Organizations (JCAHO) accredit home care programs of all types. HHAs have heard much discussion about "deemed" status. Hospital-based HHAs have been somewhat familiar with JCAHO because they have been involved in the process historically. If the program is accredited, this information and responsibilities regarding the standards and operational guidelines should be a part of every nurse's orientation.

Continuous Quality Improvement

Orientation and accreditation are only two factors that contribute to quality in home care. HHAs also design and implement continuous quality improvement (CQI) programs that meet the agency's unique clinical focus. Home care nurses are an integral part of an effective CQI program. HHAs traditionally track the following kinds of information: (1) readmission to hospitals within 31 days, (2) complaint logs, (3) infection surveillance and rates, (3) clinically focused studies, (4) 488 requests (the form generated to the HHA from the Medicare Regional Home Health Intermediary [RHHI] that requests additional, specific clinical information or notes), and (5) other aspects of HHA operations that have an impact on care. Part of CQI may also be monitoring physician referral sources and patient satisfaction surveys.

Certification

The educational preparation, the clinical background, and the knowledge and experience of home care nurses can be another measure of quality. This can include the orientation process, the completed proficiency skills checklist, and the experience the nurses bring to the bedside in the community. A new certification in home care is being offered by the American Nurses' Credentialing Center. This new specialty certification is a way to help ensure that nurses in home care know and practice within standard quality parameters.

MODELS OF NURSING CARE DELIVERY IN HOME CARE

Various models in home care describe how care is delivered to HHA patients. Primary nursing through assignment of client/patient care or case managers is one of the models seen in home care. It is recognized that continuity through primary nursing care promotes professional accountability and increased effectiveness in communications and outcomes. Assignments based on the nurse's preparation, experience, and capabilities promote the fullest use of skills and provide a basis for continued development and professional growth.

Regardless of the nursing model used, the home care nurse has responsibility for implementing and evaluating the ordered POC. Assigning one nurse to a patient helps ensure the quality of care by providing a mechanism for consistent rapport and communication with the patient and caregivers.

This is not to say that additional nursing staff is not also involved in the care of patients. In fact, involving another nurse, particularly in long-term patients maintained at home, can be very helpful. In some HHAs, a nurse specialist, such as an enterostomal therapist, consults with the patient and primary nurse on complex skin or wound problems needing assessment and intervention. Such a process can help ensure safe, effective, quality care. This should be the goal of all health care services, regardless of the setting. The following box describes the scope of home health nursing practice as defined by the American Nurses Association.

SCOPE OF HOME HEALTH NURSING PRACTICE

Definitions and Distinguishing Characteristics

Home health nursing refers to the practice of nursing applied to a client with a health deficit in the client's place of residence. Clients and their designated caregivers are the focus of home health nursing practice. The goal of care is to initiate, manage, and evaluate the resources needed to promote the client's optimal level of well-being. Nursing activities necessary to achieve this goal may warrant preventive, maintenance, and restorative emphases to avoid potential deficits from developing.

Home health nursing is a synthesis of community health nursing and selected technical skills from other specialty nursing practices. The health care deficits of the client determine the appropriate augmentation of other specialty skills with community health nursing practice. Community health nursing practice includes nursing care directed toward individuals, families, and groups, with the predominate responsibility for care being to the population as a whole.[3]

The practice of home health nursing is focused predominately on the care of individuals, in collaboration with the family and designated caregivers. Home health nursing stresses the holistic management of personal health practices for the treatment of disease or disability.[4] Practice activities center on secondary prevention (treatment, care, rehabilitation), assistance to families, direct treatment in a client's residence, and coordination of community resources. Home health nurses acknowledge the biopsychosocial and environmental factors affecting a client's health-illness trajectory, and support a client-focused nursing care plan addressing a comprehensive approach to goal attainment. During a client's episode of care, technically precise nursing procedures may be instituted simultaneously with demands for teaching, counseling, care management, resource coordination, and evaluative data collection.

Technical and comprehensive clinical decision-making activities and collaboration in multidisciplinary practice further strengthen both the autonomous and interdependent practice demands of home health nursing. The nursing process is the essential vehicle through which client goals are achieved.

All nursing care is based on a complete physical, psychosocial, and environmental assessment. In the home setting, the influences of family dynamics and the home environment on the physical and emotional state of the client are essential inclusions in the nursing care plan. The client, family, and caregivers are members of the health care team and will contribute to the nursing care plans and goals. Because the nurse is a guest in the home, the dynamics of the nurse-patient relationship are unique.

In addition, the client's immediate access to other health care resources in the home is limited, so that the nurse's role as a multidisciplinary care coordinator is important in facilitating the goal of care (see Fig. 1). Since the client often receives

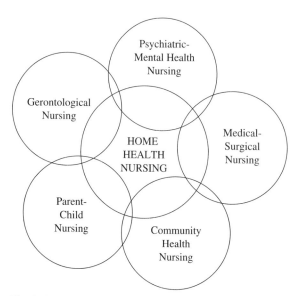

Fig. 1. A conceptual model of home health nursing. (Reprinted with permission from *A Statement on the Scope of Home Health Nursing Practice,* © 1992, American Nurses Association, Washington, DC.)

services from multiple providers and vendors, the home health nurse assumes the role of care manager in coordinating and directing all involved disciplines and caregivers to optimize client outcomes. The home health nurse shares knowledge of community health resources with the client and caregivers. This information exchange and advocacy process is used to encourage clients, families, and caregivers to plan for and seek additional services as their needs and resources dictate. Informing, supporting, and affirming client and caregiver determinism is an important adjunct to achieving the nursing care plan and client goals.

Generalist Role

The professional home health nurse practices at the generalist level in the client's home, site of residence, or appropriate community site. The focus of the nurse's practice includes the client, family, and caregivers. Responsibilities of the generalist include:

- teaching
- performing nursing activities within the nursing care plan
- managing resources needed to ensure enactment of the nursing care plan
- monitoring technical and instrumental care
- collaborating with other disciplines and providers
- supervising ancillary personnel

The use of the nursing process and advocacy skills are inherent in home health nursing practice. The generalist in home health nursing is prepared at the baccalaureate level.

All professional nurses practicing as home health nurses possess the basic knowledge and skills to carry out the following responsibilities:

- Perform holistic initial and periodic assessments of the client and family/caregiver resources to develop and support the nursing care plan.
- Identify and coordinate the community resources necessary to support optimal client outcomes.
- Use qualitative and quantitative data to evaluate client responses to care and monitor the parameters of care according to the nursing care plan.

- Educate and counsel clients, families, and caregivers to promote self-care activities.
- Initiate health promotion teaching to improve the quality of life, maintain health, and minimize disability.
- Implement the advocacy role through activities which inform, support, and affirm the client and family's self-determination.
- Promote continuity of care through discharge planning, care management, and advocacy.
- Apply the existing body of appropriate multidisciplinary knowledge to nursing practice.
- Recognize developmental and biopsychosocial changes in clients, families, and caregivers based on an understanding of psychological, cultural, social, and spiritual functioning.
- Use the *Standards of Home Health Nursing Practice*[2] and the appropriate state nursing practice act to guide nursing practice.
- Provide technical and instrumental care for the client as appropriate.
- Monitor and support caregiver participation in furthering the goals of client care.

Specialist Role

The specialist in home health nursing practice can and may be asked to perform all the functions of a generalist. In addition, the specialist possesses substantial clinical experience with individuals, families, and groups; expertise in the process of caseload management and consultation; and proficiency in planning, implementing, and evaluating programs, resources, services, and research for health care delivery to complex clients. The specialist in home health nursing is prepared at the graduate level.

All professional nurses practicing as clinical nurse specialists in home health possess advanced nursing knowledge and skills to carry out the following responsibilities:

- Provide consultation to the generalist who is participating in the delivery of care to high-risk home health clients.
- Design, monitor, and evaluate the continuous quality improvement process and risk management components of the clinical program.

- Identify and design research projects based on data generated from the continuous quality improvement program and clinical observations.
- Serve as a resource to the nurse generalist in the identification and evaluation of research findings for application to home health nursing practice.
- Educate the nurse generalists and health team members about technical, cognitive, and clinical developments emerging for care of the home health client.
- Perform direct care and documentation for select clients and caregivers who require specialist expertise.
- Manage and evaluate the care delivered by caregivers to prevent the reoccurrence of the health care deficit in complex cases.
- Design, monitor, and evaluate the caseload management system so that case mix and care demands of clients are met in an optimal manner.
- Monitor and evaluate trends and patterns of reimbursement for home health.
- Participate in developing and evaluating agency policy and procedures to promote continuity of care from preadmission to postdischarge activities.
- Facilitate a multidisciplinary and interorganizational plan of service when barriers to access and utilization are detected.
- Consult with staff and clients on ethical issues related to treatment and self-determinism.

Ethical Considerations for the Home Health Nurse

The importance of ethics in health care has dramatically increased as society grapples with the allocation of health care resources and the use of advanced technology. Advances in research and development have greatly enhanced the tools available to health care providers to extend the length, though not necessarily the quality, of life. Not only does the home health nurse deal with issues of allocation, but also with principles of autonomy, beneficence, nonmaleficence, justice, confidentiality, and truth telling.

Guided by the *Code for Nurses,*[1] the home health nurse pursues or creates a forum to deal with the myriad ethical issues confronted in practice. Such a forum allows nurses, clients, and caregivers to identify, differentiate, and clarify ethical and legal dilemmas, and begin the process of negotiating solutions that accommodate the often conflicting needs and goals that emerge.

The basic conceptualization of home health sets the tone for the nature, allocation, and range of services accessible to clients. Home health care is not merely a change in site or a version of acute care delivered at home. Home health requires a change in the definitions and structures of care so that there is a broad array of services and caregivers available to clients experiencing enduring frailty, multidimensional problems, and services outside the realm of normal or standard medical treatment.[3]

Due to the complex nature of home health services and the predominately elderly population home health serves, the ethical issues that arise pose dilemmas that will benefit from identification, discussion, and reflection by all parties. Premature discharge of clients based on expired or diminished reimbursement sources can influence the decision to provide home care. Clients who are underserved and families who are unable to successfully meet the demands of care can pose difficult problems for the health care organization and nurse. Clients, families, and caregivers may demand services that are not required or covered by insurance sources, reject reasonable and beneficial treatment and planning activities, refuse to improve environmental conditions essential to a nursing care plan, or avoid reporting abuse or neglect. Many situations in home health involve the autonomous concerns of different parties— the agency and nurse provider, the client, the family caregivers, the community, and the third-party payer.

The nature of home health care demands the mediation of values, obligations, and interests of formal and informal care providers. Home health nursing practice must include the use of formal and informal ethical structures or committees that can assist in educating, counseling, and supporting all concerned in mediating the ethical dilemmas which arise in home health nursing practice. On the health policy level, scarce resources, societal values, and allocation proposals will continue to provide difficult challenges to the practice of home health nursing.

References

1. American Nurses Association: *Code for Nurses with Interpretive Statements,* Kansas City, Missouri, 1985, American Nurses Association.
2. American Nurses Association: *Standards of Home Health Nursing Practice.*
3. Collopy B, Dubler N, Zuckerman C: The ethics of home care: autonomy and accommodation, *The Hastings Center Report* 20(2)(suppl):3, 1990.
4. Humphrey CJ: The home as a setting for care: clarifying the boundaries of practice, *Nursing Clinics of North America* 22(2):305-314, 1988.

PART TWO

AN OVERVIEW OF DOCUMENTATION

AN OVERVIEW OF DOCUMENTATION

Many changes have occurred in health care and home care since the first edition of this book published in 1988. Although not that long ago, significant events have had an impact on home care programs, thus necessitating this extensive revision.

Nurses and nursing practice in home care are described everyday to surveyors, peers, and managers through the review of clinical home care records. Nursing visit records, notes, and other information that appear in the HHA record reflect the standard of nursing care, as well as the particular care provided to a specific patient. Today, numerous third-party payers make quality and reimbursement decisions based on the care the patient received as evidenced in the medical record.

The professional home care nurse's entries in a patient's clinical record are recognized as a significant contribution that documents the standard of care provided to a patient. As the practice of nursing has become more complex, so too have the factors that influence documentation. These factors include requirements of regulatory agencies (e.g., the state health department); health insurers (e.g., Medicare, Medicaid); accreditation organizations (e.g., JCAHO, CHAP); consumers of health care; and legal entities. The home care nurse must try to satisfy these various requirements all at once, often with little time in which to accomplish the important task of documentation. Fortunately, many home care programs have integrated some of these requirements, where possible, into the HHA's policy and/or procedure manuals. In addition, the written clinical record is also the nurse's best defense against malpractice or negligence litigation.

The increased specialization of practice, the complexity of patient problems, and the new technology associated with it have contributed to multiple and varied services being provided to patients. The clinical record is the only source of written communication, and sometimes the only source of any communication, for all team members. The team members not only contribute their unique and individual assessments of interventions and outcomes, but may also actually base their subsequent actions on the events documented by another team member.

The clinical HHA record is the only document that chronicles a patient's stay from start of care through discharge. As such, the actual documentation should be completed as soon as possible. This includes beginning the form 485 (or other required forms) and the daily visit record or nursing notes as soon as possible. This documentation may include a change in the patient's condition, a description of the specific care provided, notification of the physician, and the observed patient response to interventions.

Factors Contributing To More Emphasis on Nursing Documentation

The following discussion addresses five specific areas that have increased the importance of nursing and clinical documentation.

1. **The current economics of our health care system and the emphasis on utilization management.** Patients continue to be discharged sooner or stay home while they are considerably ill. In response to spiraling health care costs, third-party payers (e.g., government, commercial, and business self-insurers) have increased their scrutiny and control of limited resources. Initially, these programs, called utilization review or utilization management, were influential in decreasing hospital lengths of stay. This review of care then moved into the outpatient and home care arenas. In addition, today, many surgeries and other procedures are provided on an outpatient-only basis. As experienced home care nurses know, the same elderly population that would have required an extensive inpatient hospital stay only 5 years ago may now have a very limited stay, if one at all, and may need extensive, skilled home care services.

   The phrase often heard to describe this phenomenon is "quicker and sicker." In general, these decreased length of hospital stays have increased home care patients' acuity levels. This often translates into increased nursing care and other needs, and is evidenced by the increase in the number of visits or hours patients are seen. In addition, some managed-care programs are decreasing their home visits while also limiting the patient's inpatient stay, which places stress on the HHA nurse to continue to provide needed care and many times, "negotiate" for the patient so that the appropriate level of safe, effective nursing care is provided. Third-party payers often need substantiating evidence—documentation—that clearly shows skilled care was provided. The information in the clinical record is the source by which third-party payers make payment or denial decisions. It is important to note that Medicare, by law, can only pay for covered care. It is nursing documentation that is the objective basis for payment determinations as these notes reflect the care provided to a home care patient.

2. **The emphasis on CQI in home care.** As quality initiatives in all health care settings have evolved, patient outcomes are being

recognized as valid indicators of care. Clinical documentation is the written record demonstrating the nursing process, based on the POC, and movement toward achieving patient-centered goals and positive outcomes.

The interdisciplinary focus on quality efforts creates an incentive for the entire health team to work together to achieve patient outcomes. The clinical documentation in the written HHA record demonstrates this collaboration in the format of team meetings, conferences, or other team activities and communications.

3. **The emphasis on standardization of care, policies, and procedures.** All patients are entitled to a certain level or standard of nursing care. As patients become more proactive consumers in their purchase of health services, patient satisfaction with the care provided is key to any HHAs reputation and ultimate survival. As patients and their families become more active consumers of health care, more are demanding to receive care in their own homes. Home care nurses, because of their healing skills and other areas of professional proficiency, are pivotal in fostering patient satisfaction. Further, the role of the home care nurse as patient advocate, listener, and teacher has become widely accepted in recent years. In general, it is also known that satisfied patients are less likely to sue.

4. **The further recognition and empowerment of the nursing profession.** Although there are more nurses in the work force than ever before, there continues to be a need for qualified professional nurses.

The nurse's notes can become the factor by which documented quality becomes demonstrated quality. All health care professions, including nursing, have recognized standards of care. As society has become litigious, the home care nurse must be aware of state practice and other accepted standards of care. These standards of care are the minimum level that any patient can expect in similar circumstances. Other standards include policies and procedures, state or federal regulations, and the published standards of the professional nursing organizations.[1] These standards necessitate keeping current and

[1] Guide GW: Legal issues in nursing: a source for practice, Norwalk, Conn, 1985, Appleton & Lange.

informed of the standards of professional nursing practice through affiliation with nursing specialty groups or other professional groups.

An example of a home health agency's nursing standard of care is as follows: Every HHA patient shall have a nursing assessment that is comprehensive, addresses specific patient needs, is performed by a registered nurse on admission, and is documented in the clinical record. Through complete, effective documentation, HHA nurses demonstrate that the standard of care has been met.

5. **The emphasis on effectiveness and efficiency in all settings in health care, particularly home care.** As home health agencies and all health care settings continue to streamline their operations, administrative tasks historically performed by nurses are being reconsidered for their effectiveness. Repetition or duplication of documentation has been an area of appropriate concern to both home care nurses and their managers. Some home care programs have moved toward automation, such as laptop or notebook computers for nurses, to help prevent the duplicative nature of much clinical and administrative information needed for effective daily HHA operations. Quality, not quantity, is now emphasized with regard to documentation.

All of the previously discussed factors have created an environment in which the home care nurse has increased responsibilities to be completed in a shorter time period.

THE IMPORTANCE OF THE MEDICAL RECORD IN HOME CARE

The importance of documentation in the medical record relates to the fact that this record is:

- The only written source for reference and communication among members of the home care team
- The primary source (written or verbal) for reference and communication among the members of the home care team
- The only text that supports insurance coverage and/or denial
- The only evidence of the basis on which patient care decisions were made
- The only legal record
- The primary foundation for the evaluation of the care provided
- The basis for staff education or other study
- The objective source for the HHA's licensing (where applicable), accreditation, and state surveyor review

Because HHA nurses often need to meet these myriad needs simultaneously, they are appropriately concerned about their ability to do so. HHA nurses in practice today can meet these needs and produce clear, effective documentation. The following points can assist in this goal.

Tips About Documentation

- Write legibly or print neatly. The record must be readable.
- Use permanent ink.
- For every entry, identify the time and date; sign the entry and include your title.
- Describe care or interventions provided and the patient's response to care.
- Write objectively when describing findings (e.g., behaviors).
- Write notes in consecutive and chronological order with no skipped lines or gaps.
- Write visit notes either at the patient's home (if safe and appropriate) or as soon as possible after care is provided.
- Be factual and specific.

- Use patient, family, or caregiver quotes.
- Use the patient's name (e.g., ''Mr. Smith'').
- Document patient complaints or needs and their resolutions. (Remember to also discuss the complaint with your manager, who may also document it in the HHA Complaint Log and note the resolution or follow-up actions taken.)
- Make sure the patient's name is listed and correct on the visit record, daily note, or other HHA form.
- Be accurate, complete, and thorough.
- Write out what you are saying if anything is questionable. (Avoid potentially confusing abbreviations.)
- Chart only the care that you provided.
- Promptly document any change in the patient's condition and the actions taken based on such a change.
- Write down the patient's, family's or caregiver's response to teaching or any other care intervention.
- To correct an error: (1) draw a line through the erroneous entry; (2) briefly describe the error (e.g., wrong date, spilled coffee on visit record); and (3) add your signature, date, and time.

Try to Avoid

- Relying on memory.
- Whiting out or erasing entries; such changes may appear to be an attempt to cover up incriminating entries.
- Crossing out words beyond recognition.
- Making assumptions, drawing conclusions, or blaming.
- Leaving blank spaces between entries and your signature.
- Waiting ''too long'' to record entries.
- Leaving gaps in documentation.
- Using abbreviations except where they are clear and appear on the HHA's list of approved, acceptable abbreviations.

HOME CARE DOCUMENTATION

It is important to remember that Medicare is a medical insurance program, and like any insurance program, there are both covered services and exclusions. For payers, documentation is the only paper trail of the care provided and of the patient's response to that care.

When admitting patients to the HHA, ensure that the patient meets the particular insurance requirements. For example, with Medicare, the patient must meet the homebound criteria, as well as other criteria. This criteria must then be reflected in the clinical documentation.

Always try to read your documentation objectively after you write. Ask yourself, does this form 485/6 or visit record reflect why the patient is homebound and how (or why) the skills of the home care nurse are needed?

When writing clinical documentation keep in mind that effective documentation simultaneously does the following:

1. Demonstrates the care provided and the patient's response to that care

2. Shows that the current standards of care are maintained

3. Meets documentation requirements for Medicare and other payers

This book is written expressly to help both new and experienced home care nurses in meeting these various requirements. The goal of this book is to help professional nurses create the specific documentation required by any payer, while factually illustrating the patient's condition and responses to teaching or other interventions.

The following box enumerates ways to ensure that quality and reimbursement requirements are being met. Remember that writing effective documentation is a learned skill and, as with any skill, improvement comes only with practice.

The Home Care Nurse's Checklist for Effective Documentation

✔ Recognize that in home care, at the first visit, the nurse initiates the process of claims payment (or denial) with the initial 485/6 forms.

✔ Try to read your documentation objectively. Ask yourself if the form 485/6 or visit record reflects why the patient is homebound (if the patient has Medicare or another insurance that has that criteria), and how or why the skills of a nurse or therapist are needed? (Many HHAs have a peer review process that significantly helps home care nurses objectively review, and create, their own documentation.)

✔ Emphasize (1) why the care was initiated, (2) what the skilled nursing interventions are, (3) where the patient's plan is going (patient-centered goals), and (4) what the plans are for discharge (rehabilitation potential).

✔ Try to complete most of your documentation as soon as possible. Patients certainly understand that there is paperwork associated with health care; allot a few minutes at the end of each visit for this important task. This is of particular importance when working with new admissions, because of all the associated forms that the patient must sign, the correct information for the completion of the 485/6 forms, and the initial and daily visit notes. It can be difficult and often, unsafe to rely on memory or rough notes after seeing many patients at the end of a long day.

✔ Remember that the POC is the most important part of the home care clinical record. All other information flows from the identified skilled needs ordered on the plan. Remember that even though the HCFA form 485 reads ''Plan of Treatment'' across the top, it is referred to as the POC. The POC must be complete and the content clear. There can be no gaps.

✔ Make sure your patients meet the HHA's and insurance program's admission criteria. Be able to clearly identify the skilled, covered service. In addition, although the patient may not meet a particular insurer's requirements, the patient may still have needs that another program can safely provide.

✔ Focus on the patient's problems in your documentation. That is why home care is being provided, and the payers must see evidence of such to justify reimbursement.

✔ Demonstrate through your documentation that the care provided is patient-centered. For example, make your patient goals quantifiable and your outcomes realistic and specific to the patient's unique problems and needs.

✔ Remember that anyone else who picks up your patient's clinical record does not have the depth of information and knowledge that you have from actually being there and seeing the patient in his or her own home setting. Because of this, document information that is objective and clearly paints a picture of the patient and his or her problems and needs, and how the care is directed for goal achievement and discharge.

✔ Remember that effective documentation does not have to be lengthy or wordy. However, it should convey to any reader (i.e., your manager, a state surveyor nurse, etc.) the status of your patient, the adherence to the ordered POC, and consistent movement toward predetermined patient-centered goals.

✔ Check that the information on the clinical record flows well and that you can tell, by objective evidence, what is happening with the patient. This includes the problems and the skilled services that are needed, again based on the clear picture presented in the documentation.

✔ Remember that the record and nursing entries need to be legible, neat, and organized consistently.

✔ Try to look at the documentation objectively. Does it tell the story of the patient's progress (or lack of progress) and the interventions implemented based on the initial assessment and POC?

✔ Make sure telephone calls and other communications with physicians, community agencies, and other team members are documented. Do they explain what occurred with the patient; what actions were ordered, modified, and implemented; and what the patient's response was to these interventions?

✔ Demonstrate the nursing process in the record. Look for the nursing diagnoses, the assessment, evidence of care planning, implementation of ordered interventions and actions, movement toward patient-centered goals, assessment of the patient's response, and continued evaluation.

✔ Document goal achievement and/or progress toward goals and outcomes. Are the goals realistic, quantifiable, and patient-centered?

✔ If progress has not occurred as planned, explain the reasons in the documentation. If a patient is too ill for a rehabilitation service or refuses the service, is there evidence of communication with the doctor about this? Has an order been made to place the service on hold or to discharge the patient from that service?

✔ Documentation should include family/caregiver teaching and their responses/demonstration of behavior and learning.

✔ Document the patient's response to care interventions and nursing actions.

✔ Modify the interventions based on the patient's response, where appropriate.

✔ Document evidence of "intradisciplinary" team conferences and discussions.

✔ The chart should show continuity of care planning goals and consistent movement toward goal achievement by all members of the health team.

✔ Generally, the record should tell the story of the patient's care, needs, and progress while he or she was receiving home care services.

✔ The nursing entries and overall information are to reflect the level of care expected by today's health care consumers and their families.

✔ Finally, the clinical documentation should demonstrate compliance with regulatory, licensure, and quality standards.

Home care is the fastest growing segment of health care. As nurses, we are acutely aware of the changes and advances in technology that have influenced the kinds of patients now seen in the home setting. The home care nurse of the present and future must be service-oriented, flexible, and strong clinically. Payers and insurers must continue to address spiraling health care costs. The historic and customary way to approach these rising costs has been to decrease authorized visits/services or to add additional review levels. It is the professional home care nurse who can validate the need for skilled care and back it up by effective documentation.

PART THREE

FREQUENCY AND LENGTH OF
SERVICE CONSIDERATIONS

FREQUENCY AND LENGTH OF SERVICE CONSIDERATIONS

The frequency of visits and the length of service are usually based on the professional nurse's assessment and ongoing evaluation of the patient's clinical status, as well as on his or her biopsychosocial and unique family system needs. The current health care environment and the increasing emphasis on quality initiatives demonstrated by positive patient outcomes identify the need for research and evaluation regarding the determination of how frequently and for how long the patient needs to be under care. The following is a discussion of the process and the knowledge that may assist in making the best determination for the frequency and duration of care needed. Throughout this discussion, remember that all visits require orders by the physician, and the nurse must maintain compliance with the Medicare Conditions of Participation, state licensure, surveyor directives, and other regulations or laws.

There are a number of considerations that help to determine the appropriate frequency of home care visits. This discussion provides a framework to assist the home care nurse in making these decisions appropriately; however, it is not to take the place of ongoing meetings with the home health care manager to determine patients' unique frequency and duration needs. Rather, this discussion is to help the home care nurse be aware of the many factors that go into making this determination.

The introduction of diagnosis-related groups (DRGs) and other prospective payment systems (PPSs) in inpatient settings has increased the scrutiny of admission, frequency, and duration of home health services. Nurses practicing in the community are acutely aware of the decreased lengths of stay in hospitals and the increased patient acuity in both the hospital and the home care setting. The increasing complexity of patient needs is demonstrated in the changing case mix of the home health nurse's case load. Early discharge and shorter lengths of stay in acute care facilities resulted in a greater number of high acuity home care patients who require services necessitating expanded skills and improved knowledge of the home health nursing staff.[1]

In addition, most health care analysts, payers, and consumers of health care realize that forms of PPSs, such as the Medicare hospice benefit, will continue to expand to other areas of health care, including home health care. The Medicare Home Care Prospective Payment

Demonstration is continuing to collate needed information on this significant change in payment to home care programs.

Experienced home care, hospice, and community health nurses know that they are in an important position to identify the patient's specific service and visit frequency needs. The objective findings, as found through the nursing assessment, are the basis for these recommendations that are made by the nurse and communicated to the physician. It is also important to note that some patients may be seen infrequently by their physician after discharge—the patient may lack adequate transportation to the physician's office, the patient may be considered ''homebound'' and, in some instances, the physician does not or will not make needed home visits. The professional nurse's judgment skills can help in making these important visit frequency decisions.

Some frequency determinations are easy; for example, when there are generally recognized medical or nursing practice standards, such as the elderly, homebound patient needing monthly nursing assessments and B-12 injections. It is known that usually these injections are given once a month, thus the nurse creates the plan with skilled nursing visits scheduled for once a month for the injection.

The HIM-11 states the following about frequency in the text addressing the completion of element 21 on the HCFA 485 form. The manual states, ''Frequency denotes the number of visits per discipline to be rendered, stated in days, weeks, or months. Duration identifies the length of time the services are to be rendered and may be expressed in days, weeks, or months.''[2] Realistically and operationally, other factors, besides recognized medical or nursing practice standards, are important to scheduling and frequency decisions. They include staffing trends, standards of practice, geographic location of patients, family and referral support systems, and the availability of qualified staff for patients with particular conditions or problems. When conflict occurs between patient needs and the agency's ability to meet those needs, other courses of action should be implemented (e.g., transferring the patient to another agency or program where the patient's needs can be safely and adequately met).

The box outlines some of the factors that are considered in the process of determining frequency and duration of care. For this discussion, *duration,* usually referred to as 60 to 62 days, is the length of stay (LOS) for which the patient is projected to need home care services in order to safely and effectively meet the patient's unique medical and other needs.

List of Patient-Related Considerations

The following is a list of the most common patient-related considerations that are evaluated by the nurse as plans are formulated and care is begun. This alphabetical list is not all-inclusive and other considerations may be as varied as the individual nurse's patient caseload. In addition, many of these factors are interrelated.

Absence of caregiver
Activities of daily living (ADLs) limitations
Adaptive or assistive devices
Affect (e.g., depression)
Behavioral or mental disorders
Caregiver support
Chemical or drug problems (e.g., alcoholism)
Chronic illness(es)
Cognitive function
Communication
Compliance/noncompliance
Disabilities
Discharge plan
Drug interactions
Educational level/barriers
Environment
Fatigue
Fire safety
Functional limitations
Goals/expected outcomes
Handicaps
History
Home medical equipment
Home setting
Independence
Instrumental activities of daily living (IADLs)
Knowledge of emergency procedures
Language
Loneliness
Loss of significant other(s)
Medical equipment or supply needs
Medications
Mobility
Motivation

Nursing assessment and reassessment findings
Nursing diagnoses
Nutritional status
Orthotic needs
Other considerations, based on patient's/family's unique needs
Pain
Parenting
Pathology
Physical assessment findings
Polypharmacy
Probability of further complications
Prognosis
Psychopathology
Reason for prior hospitalization, for referral to home care/
    hospice
Rehabilitative needs
Resources (e.g., financial, human, and other)
Risk factors
Safety
Self-care status
Skin integrity
Social factors
Social supports
Socioeconomic condition
Stability
Swallowing
Voice

A review of Section 18 (A and B) of the HCFA Form 485 "Functional Limitations" and "Activities Permitted" may also assist the nurse in the determination of frequency and duration of home care services. The nurse's rationale, experience, and, sometimes, intuition contribute to the decision-making process related to frequency and length of stay. According to Benner, "Intuitive judgment is what distinguishes expert human judgment from the decisions that might be made by a beginner or by a machine."[3] Home health and hospice are settings in which experienced professional nurses use their broad knowledge base to make effective patient care decisions, such as those determining frequency and LOS which can have a direct impact on patient outcomes. The nurse also can look to the manager for specific information, feedback, and standards of the agency or program.

Health care reform is primarily addressing three of the largest problems within the U.S. health care system—access, cost, and quality. Cost is the issue that home care and hospice programs address daily when a case management company questions or limits needed visits. As home care experts, nurses, managers, and administrators must articulate to a case manager or third-party payer the objective rationale and plan for projected visits. For example, simply because if the patient can perform the dressing or administer the injections, the nursing care is not converted to a skilled service. In fact, continuing visits for observation and assessment, teaching, and training are very often appropriate, based on the patient's unique needs. The patient may still require thorough observation and assessment of the wound, teaching about site care, monitoring of the effects of medications, venipunctures to monitor drug levels, and infection control and safety training for a period of time.

Unfortunately, when a nurse says "the patient can do her own dressing," a payer may construe that to mean that the patient is ready for discharge in an attempt to contain costs. Based on the patients' individual needs, however, this may or may not be true. Nurses must be able to communicate objectively the skills used during every visit and explain why those visits may vary, even though patients may have the same general diagnoses or problems. Nurses can do their jobs because of their education and experience.

It is the professional nurse's judgment and observational and other skills for which payment is made. Only nurses can compare that wound to the others seen in their practice experience, make a judgment regarding healing or infection, indentify dehiscence, evaluate the wound in relation to other pathology, obtain a baseline assessment and teach the patient and caregivers, and myriad other skills that are provided daily in homes to patients. It is the role and responsibility of home care and hospice professionals to educate others, including case managers, payers, consumers, and their families about the cost-effectiveness, quality, and demonstrated positive outcomes experienced by patients in home care. An emphasis on CQI and the need to define home care roles, care, and nuances of individual patient care is appropriate utilization of limited resources. As CQI focuses on the consumer of services, the industry must move toward standardizing the process, continually looking at methods to improve results (positive patient outcomes) and objectively measuring performance and demonstrated outcomes.

Research-based practice guidelines, outcome measures and standards of care are important because of the increased emphasis on cost-effective, high-quality care. These practice parameters would help home care nurses in determining patient frequency and length of service.

Some HHAs have developed their own standardized care plans based on North American Nursing Diagnosis Association (NANDA) nursing diagnoses and the nurses' experience with particular patient problems. Other home health agencies have developed or purchased automated systems that help them track and define objective findings, demonstrate goal achievement, and discharge based on outcome criteria. Nurses in practice are aware of this ongoing concern regarding provision of adequate patient care in a climate of tighter reimbursement, more limited resources, and frequent ethical dilemmas, along with an emphasis on both quality and effectiveness. This cost/quality equation must balance out in order to maintain patient satisfaction and success, productivity, and viability of health care organizations, as well as the nurses' satisfaction in the ability to meet patient need.

Home care agency managers and nurses need to be adept in articulating and quantifying patient care needs based on objective evidence and supporting documentation. The Omaha Classification System (OCS) was developed by the Visiting Nurse Association of Omaha, Nebraska. The OCS is an orderly, nursing diagnosis taxonomy listing of client problems nurses may encounter in community health settings. There are four categories, termed domains, in which each of these problems fall; they are: Environmental, Psychosocial, Physiologic, and Health Behaviors.[4] Hallmarks of this system include: (1) expected outcomes, (2) a standard terminology, and (3) the integration of the components of quality assurance initiatives into an agency's operations. Other features include (4) assigned end dates to patient's outcomes, and (5) clearly identifiable resolutions of patient problems demonstrated in the nursing documentation. As nurses identify the need to streamline and more effectively provide and demonstrate care, use of such systems will help in creating and maintaining cost- and time-effective operations and quality improvement. The use of standardized care plans as the basis for individualizing patient care helps to prioritize needs for nurses teaching patients with new or multiple health problems.

PATIENTS AND PATIENT PROBLEMS

The following are examples of some of the kinds of patients and patient problems seen in home care. These are just that, examples, and the nurses' professional judgment, recognized standards of care, and information gathered from all aspects of the patient assessment process are the cornerstones by which to identify patient services, visit frequency, and service duration needs.

1. The patient is experiencing complications of juvenile diabetes mellitus (DM), foot wound after wound debridement, impaired mobility, visual impairment, and financial concerns, and has a history of noncompliance to care regimens.

   This 78-year-old man was referred posthospitalization to the home care agency on the following medications: Cipro, Ampicillin, NPH Insulin, Viokase, and Tylenol™ with codeine for pain.

   After the nurse completed the initial assessment, the physician was called to discuss and verify the following care needs, services, and goals/outcomes identified by the nurse. The care needs were skilled nursing, instruction in diet regimen, blood glucose (BG) checking procedure, and self-observational skills, such as BG and temperature findings. Although the patient had knowledge of the aspects of DM-related care, there was a history of diabetic ketoacidosis, with three admissions to the hospital for this illness in the past year. The registered nurse (RN) was to teach the patient aspects of care for the patient with DM, teach the wound care regimen, perform the wound care, and complete dressing changes. Observation and skilled assessment of the wound would continue even though the patient started to perform some of the actual wound care himself.

   The frequency of the nursing services projected were: q day for 7 days, decrease to qod (4 times per week) for 14 days then decrease to 3 times per week for 3 weeks, two times per week for 3 weeks for a total of 9 weeks. Visit and care frequency needs, however, would actually be reevaluated at every nursing visit and, based on clinical findings, the nurse would collaborate with the physician and make POC changes, each requiring verbal order followed by written documentation.

The following goals/outcomes—stable blood glucose (BG), healed, infection-free foot wound, and return to self-care status with regular follow up by the referring physician—were identified.

This patient could perform ADLs and personal care effectively. The only other service recommended for this patient was Medical Social Services to address financial problems, particularly insufficient resources to purchase food and medications, all of which prevented effective implementation of the POC. Medical Social Worker (MSW) visits would be projected for 1 time per week for 3 weeks.

2. The patient is experiencing cellulitis of right leg, decreased sensation, hypertension, chronic obstructive pulmonary disease (COPD), leg pain, safety concerns, and has had a history of heart failure, resulting in peripheral vascular bypass surgery to increase circulation.

This 62-year-old man was referred after a hospitalization for increased edema, chest pain, and cellulitis of the leg. The patient tells the nurse the leg has been swollen for "some time." However, the admission happened when the throbbing and pain increased significantly during the previous 2 weeks. He is now on the following medications: Procardia, ASA, Persantine, Micro K supplements, Lasix, Digoxin, and Cefazolin qid IV.

The nursing skills identified by the RN are teaching and training about circulation and IV medication administration, IV maintenance, and IV therapy care to patient and family, and multiple medication changes. The RN will also draw blood every Wednesday, to obtain a complete blood count (CBC), a chemistry panel, and a sed rate. The RN will also provide skilled observation and assessment of the IV site, change the site as ordered, reinsert the peripheral line per protocol, and initially administer the IV medication by infusion pump.

The determination of visit frequency will be dependent on the information gathered and the list of patient-related considerations, which appeared previously in this part. However, if the patient or caregiver cannot or will not perform procedures safely for the administration of IV or other medications, the nurse may initially need to visit QID. This is particularly true if there are elderly caregivers or if the patient is discharged with another kind of pump than the one used for teaching in the hospital prior to discharge. In addition, the

patient may not have received training prior to discharge
or stress may have limited the patient's comprehension of the
training provided. It is important to note that there are
patients and caregivers who refuse to be involved in the patient's
care. Therefore, continued QID visits could be appropriate
as long as IV medications are ordered at that frequency.
Decrease in the frequency of the visits would depend on
changes in the physician orders and/or the caregiver or patient
becoming more involved in the provision of care.

This patient also requires home health aide services as help
with ADLs and personal care is needed. Mobility was
severely limited due to the affected leg having to be elevated
and shortness of breath on exertion. An occupational therapy
(OT) evaluation was also ordered after the nurse explained to
the physician the need for conservation of energy teaching
in the patient's home and the need for breathing exercises to
facilitate improved functioning.

The frequency of RN, HHA, and OT services would be
reevaluated as appropriate, based on the patient's or
caregiver's ability to safely and effectively manage the total
home care plan and the achievement of the identified goals/
outcomes. In this case, the goals/outcomes were the provision
and completion of IV antibiotic therapy, maintenance of
infection-free IV site and patent access, stabilized cardiac status,
decreased pain, and redness and throbbing of leg. (Note:
Remember that for Medicare patients, if the wound or other
care is daily, there must be an estimated, realistic endpoint
to the daily care ordered. See the home care definition of ''daily
care'' at the end of the book for further discussion.)

3. A patient is admitted for hospice care with the diagnosis of
cancer of the liver. The patient problems include jaundice,
ascites, and nausea.

A forty-seven year old woman is admitted for hospice care. The
hospice nurse clinical specialist who admits the patient
and family to the program explains the hospice philosophy
and the care regimen proposed, based on the needs identified.
Nursing care, home health aide care, and other components
of the interdisciplinary team are explained and care is scheduled
to begin. The frequency issue is sometimes more complex
in patients with clearly shortened life spans. Generally, patients
with an illness of a terminal nature receive more care toward
the end of their life, whereas patients with a fair or better

prognosis receive more services at the start of care and then taper down as function and independence increase.

Based on the patient's and family's unique needs, it can be very appropriate for the same amount of care to be provided throughout the hospice admission. Keep in mind that many patients are admitted to hospice at the end stages of their disease process, only after high technology interventions and cure-oriented therapies have been exhausted. As the focus changes from cure to care, the hospice takes a holistic approach to care, with the frequency determined solely on patient and family needs. For such a patient, services could consist of 3 times weekly RN visits with daily home care aides and volunteer support, or any combination of services provided by the interdisciplinary hospice team. The goals/outcomes identified were symptom-controlled death at home with hospice support and family presence.

SUMMARY

Nurses working in home care, hospice, or other community settings must be flexible and able to explain objective reasons for frequency, length of stay, or discharge decisions. These decisions and underlying rationale need to be communicated clearly to the nurse's manager or third-party payer representatives who are responsible for tracking, approving, or denying visits. As payers try to decrease the number of patient visits, we must be able to articulate the clinical and other needs of the patient. This advocacy role will assure high-quality care while the patient remains at home. This is more important now as the technology explosion continues and nurses care for patients such as those receiving dobutamine therapy, or needing management of PICC lines or ventilators in the community. Those who can explain needs based on objective information and patient findings to numerous reimbursement gatekeepers will continue to be successful in home care. The increasing complexity of patients sent home with limited resource and coverage demands these skills for safe, effective patient care.

References

1. Twardon C, Gartner MA: Strategy for growth in home care, *JONA,* 22(10):49, 1992.
2. Health and Human Services, Health Care Financing Administration: *Home Health Agency Manual,* nbr 11, Washington, DC, 1989, p.24m4f, Revision, 228.
3. Benner P, Tanner C: Clinical judgment: how expert nurses use intuition, *AJN,* January:23, 1987.
4. Weidmann J, North H: Implementing the Omaha Classification System in a public health agency, *The Nursing Clinics of North America,* 22(4):973, 1987.

PART FOUR

MEDICAL-SURGICAL CARE

ACQUIRED IMMUNE
DEFICIENCY SYNDROME

1. **General Considerations.**   Home continues to be the care setting for most patients with acquired immune deficiency syndrome (AIDS). Care is directed toward treatment of opportunistic infections, other HIV-related conditions, and prevention of further problems. Pneumocystic carinii pneumonia continues to be one of the most serious processes in the adult patient with AIDS. Comfort, support, teaching, and palliative care to patients and their caregivers is key to effective nursing care in the community.

   Please refer to ''Cancer Care,'' ''Care of the Patient with Pain,'' ''Hospice Care,'' ''IV Care,'' or ''Care of the Bedbound Patient'' should those problems be appropriate for your patient.

2. **Needs for initial visit**

   Specific initial physician orders
   Universal precautions supplies
   Other supplies or equipment, based on physician orders
   Vital signs equipment

3. **Some potential medical-surgical diagnoses and codes**

AIDS (general)	042.9
Anemia	285.9
Bacterial infections, recurrent	041.9 (and 042.9)
Candidias	112.9
Candidias, esophageal	112.84 and 042.9
Candidias, oral	112.0 and 042.9
Candidias, vaginal	112.1 and 042.9
Cervical cancer	180.9 and 042.9
Chorioretinitis	363.20 and 042.9
Cytomegalovirus	078.5 and 042.9
Cytomegalovirus retinitis	363.20 and 87.85
Dementia	289.9 and 042.9
Diarrhea	558.9 and 042.9
Encephalitis	328.8
Encephalopathy, AIDS	348.3 and 042.9
Endocarditis	424.90 and 042.9

Esophagitis	530.1 and 042.9
Herpes simplex	054
Herpes zoster	053
Histoplasmosis	115.9
HTLV III	044.9
Hyperalimentation	99.15
Kaposi's sarcoma	173.8 and 042.2
Lymphocytic interstitial pneumonia	516.8 and 042
Lymphoma	202.8 and 042.9
Malaise and fatigue	780.7
Meningitis	047.9 and 042.9
Mycobacterium avium intracellulare	031.0 and 042.9
Myocarditis	429.0 and 042.9
Neuropathy, peripheral	357.4 and 042.9
Neutropenia	288.0 and 042.9
Paraplegia	344.1
Pelvic inflammatory disease (PID) (acute)	614.3 and 042.9
Pelvic inflammatory disease (PID) (chronic)	614.4 and 042.9
Peripheral neuropathy	357.4 and 042.9
Pneumocystic carinii pneumonia	136.3 and 042.0
Pneumonia (bacterial)	482.9 and 042.9
Pneumonia (NOS)	486 and 042.1
Pneumonia (viral)	480.8 and 042.1
Polymyositis	710.4
Polyradiculopathy	729.2
Quadriplegia	344.0
Retinal detachment	361.9
Retinal hemorrhage	362.81
Seizures	780.3
Sepsis	038.9 and 042.9
Shigella	004.9 and 042.9
Shigella, dysentery	004.0 and 042.9
Thrombocytopenia	287.5 and 042.9
Total parenteral nutrition (TPN)	99.15
Toxoplasmosis	130.9 and 042.0
Tuberculosis (pulmonary)	011.9 and 042.9
Wasting syndrome	799.4 and 042.9

4. Associated nursing diagnoses

Activity intolerance
Activity intolerance, high risk for

Airway clearance, ineffective

Anxiety

Aspiration, high risk for

Body image disturbance

Body temperature, altered, high risk for

Bowel incontinence

Breathing pattern, ineffective

Cardiac output, decreased

Caregiver role strain

Caregiver role strain, high risk for

Communication, impaired verbal

Coping, ineffective family: compromised

Coping, ineffective family: disabling

Coping, ineffective individual

Diarrhea

Family processes, altered

Fatigue

Fear

Fluid volume deficit

Fluid volume deficit, high risk for

Gas exchange, impaired

Grieving, anticipatory

Home maintenance management, impaired

Incontinence, functional

Incontinence, total

Infection, potential for

Injury, potential for

Knowledge deficit (disease process and management)

Mobility, impaired physical

Nutrition, altered: less than body requirements

Oral mucous membrane, altered

Pain

Pain, chronic

Parenting, altered

Parenting, altered, high risk for

Peripheral neurovascular dysfunction, high risk for

Powerlessness

Protection, altered

Role performance, altered

Self-care deficit, bathing/hygiene

Self-care deficit, dressing/grooming

Self-care deficit, feeding

Self-care deficit, toileting

Sensory/perceptual alterations (specify) (visual, auditory, kinesthetic, gustatory, tactile, olfactory)

Sexual dysfunction

Sexuality patterns, altered

Skin integrity, impaired

Skin integrity, impaired, potential

Sleep pattern disturbance

Social isolation

Spiritual distress (distress of the human spirit)

Swallowing, impaired

Thought processes, altered

Tissue integrity, impaired

Tissue perfusion, altered (specify type) (renal, cerebral, cardiopulmonary, gastrointestinal, peripheral)

Urinary elimination, altered patterns

5. **Service skills identified**

Complete initial assessment of all systems of patient with AIDS admitted to home care for _____ (specify problem necessitating care)

Teach patient, caregiver, and family care of the patient

Weigh patient q visit, report weight loss to MD

Assess pain, other symptoms

Teach caregivers care of the bedridden patient

Instruct patient and family regarding safety and universal precautions in the home

Assist with emotional support concerning care of children and children's future

Check vital signs q visit

Assess cardiopulmonary and respiratory status, including dyspnea, change in or abnormal breath sounds, respiratory rate, sputum production and character, frequency and amount

Instruct in all aspects of home safety and use of therapy

Assess patient's nutrition and hydration status; evaluate for signs and symptoms of dehydration

Counsel patient with anorexia about diet and nutrition

Teach patient and caregiver all aspects of medications, including routes, schedules, functions, and side effects

Discuss need for guardianship or power of attorney

Discuss concepts of "living will," other advanced directives, status regarding resuscitation, other medical/technical interventions, and patient's wishes

Assist with funeral plans, if appropriate

Assess patient's spiritual needs and address plan

Assess and observe all systems and symptoms q visit and report changes, new symptoms to MD

Teach patient and caregiver all aspects of wound care, including safe disposal of dressing supplies

Weigh patient q visit and review food intake diary

Care for and assess Kaposi lesions, cleanse with _____ (specify physician orders)

Instruct regarding pet care, avoidance of cross contamination, check with MD about certain types of pets

Instruct patient about specified diet

Instruct patient and caregivers in all aspects of effective handwashing techniques, proper care of bodily fluids and bodily excretions

Encourage patient to eat small, more frequent meals of choice

Assess patient and caregiver coping skills

Provide emotional support to patient and family with chronic and/or terminal illness and associated implications

Closely monitor parenteral feeding catheter and IV therapy site for infection, other problems/complications

Assess patient for mental status and sleep disturbance problems or changes

Instruct patient and caregiver to notify RN or MD for new symptoms including fever, vomiting, diarrhea, cough, or other change

Teach site care of Hickman catheter or other venous access device

Teach pain and symptom management regimen to caregiver

Teach patient and caregiver care needed for safe, effective management at home

Address sexuality concerns and implications for safer sexual expression, including the use of condoms, abstinence, and other techniques

Instruct in the need for elevation of edematous extremities and elevation of head of bed for comfort

Implement nonpharmacologic interventions with medication schedule; may include therapeutic massage, distraction, imagery, progressive muscle relaxation, humor, biofeedback, and music therapies

Evaluate pain in relation to other symptoms, such as fatigue, confusion, diarrhea, nausea and vomiting, depression, or shortness of breath

Teach patient and caregiver other symptom relief measures

Teach patient conservation of energy techniques

Assess patient's skin and mucous membranes for problems
including bacterial infection, thrush, rashes, or other changes

Monitor patient's level of anemia

Instruct caregiver regarding need to maintain activity as
tolerated and ROM exercises to prevent loss or decrease in
mobility and to report changes to physician

Assess the patient's unique response to treatments or
interventions, and to report changes or unfavorable
responses or reactions to the physician

Management and evaluation of the patient POC

6. Other services indicated

HHA	Personal care
	Respite care
	Meal preparation
	Homemaker services
MSS	Psychosocial assessment
	Financial assessment and counseling
	Referral/linkage to community resources
	Patient/caregiver counseling and support
	Evaluate care of patient's children and future wishes of patient regarding children
OT	Evaluation
	Conservation of energy techniques
	Adaptive or assistive devices as indicated
	Muscle reeducation
	ADL training program
PT	Evaluation
	Assessment of the patient's environment for safety
	Safe transfer training
	Instruct/supervise home exercise program for conditioning and strength
	Assistive or adaptive equipment or devices
S-LP	Evaluation for swallowing problems

7. Associated factors based on diagnosis justifying homebound status

Chairbound or bedbound

Severe shortness of breath

Oxygen dependence

Pain, other symptoms, on movement
Needs assistance to ambulate
Terminal condition
Severe functional limitations, including _____ (specify)
Moderate to severe functional impairments
Needs maximum assistance for all activities
Severe immune suppression
Impaired mental status
Requires 24 hour care and supervision

8. **Short-term goals**

RN	Pain management
	Symptom management
	Adherence to POC by patient and caregivers
	Prevention of further infection
	Nutritional needs maintained/addressed
	Patient's and family's educational needs met
HHA	Effective personal care and hygiene
	ADL assistance
	Safe home environment (e.g., walking space clutter-free)
MSS	POC implementation
	Problems, resources identified
OT	Patient utilizing conservation of energy techniques or other skills taught
PT	Patient using home exercise program
	Increased endurance
S-LP	Safe swallowing
	Swallowing with decreased pain, other problems
	Recommended food list

9. **Long-term goals**

RN	Optimal nutrition and hydration for patient
	Skin dry, clear, intact, without infection
	Patient and caregivers demonstrate effective handwashing and other infection control standards taught by RN, including disposal of waste, cleaning protocols for linens, and other aspects of care at home
	Patient and caregiver integrating information and care regarding illness with life-threatening implications and the associated grieving process

Patient knowledgeable about and uses universal
precautions information behaviorally in daily care
Blood counts and electrolytes within normal range
for patient
Pain and symptom control
Caregiver able to effectively assist in
patient's care
Patient controls medical and technical
interventions

HHA Effective and safe personal hygiene
ADL assistance

MSS POC implementation
Problem and resources identified
Referral to community support groups and
resources

OT Patient using conservation of energy techniques
Optimal function maintained
Quality of life and safety improved

PT Increased function and mobility
Prevention of complications
Safe supervision of program
Caregiver able to perform exercise regimen

S-LP Swallowing improved
Patient's hydration and nutrition status improved

10. Discharge plans for this patient

Remain at home safely
Discharge when patient-centered goals achieved
Patient death with dignity
Patient pain- and other symptom-free
Patient to return to outpatient center for follow up
Patient referral to hospice
Patient remains confined to home, will need home care
through death
When caregivers are able to manage all aspects of patient's
need safely and independently, under MD supervision

11. Patient, family, and caregiver educational needs

Educational needs are the regimens that the patient or
caregiver will be managing. These include:

Symptom management
The importance of optimal nutrition and hydration

Universal precautions protocols

Home safety concerns, issues, and teaching

The avoidance of infection, whenever possible

The importance of medical follow up

Support groups in the community available to the patient, caregiver, and family

Other information based on the patient's unique needs

Some resources available are:

AIDS Clinical Trials Information Services: 1-800-TRIALS-A or 1-800-874-2572

National AIDS Hotline: 1-800-342-2437 or 1-800-342-AIDS; (Spanish): 1-800-344-7432

The CDC National AIDS Information Clearinghouse: 1-800-458-5231

Project Inform Hotline: 1-800-822-7422; In California: 1-800-334-7222

People with AIDS Coalition: 1-800-828-3280 or (212) 532-0290

HIV Nightline: (415) 668-2437

The National Gay and Lesbian Taskforce: 1-800-221-7044

The National Hemophiliac Foundation: (212) 431-8541

12. **Specific tips for reimbursement**

The patient with AIDS often has many clearly defined ''skilled care'' needs from most insurers' perspectives. However, because of the cost and chronic nature of the process, they look to the nurse's documentation to justify their coverage decision.

Remember to:

Obtain a telephone order for any change in the POC, including changing the frequency of the visits, medications, or new or changed services.

Document your care and the patient's response to your care interventions.

Document the patient's problems or changes in status, especially an exacerbation of symptoms.

Document increased sputum production, coughing, SOB, pain, diarrhea, or any change in the patient's mental status.

Document patient deterioration and improvements.

Document blood results, cultures, and treatments.

Document any increase in temperature or other objective signs that could signal a pending infection.

Document the specific teaching provided and response to teaching.

Document the patient's response to enteral or parenteral therapies.

ALZHEIMER'S DISEASE AND OTHER DEMENTIAS

1. **General Considerations.** As increasing numbers of elderly patients are cared for by their families or other caregivers in the home, the presence of Alzheimer's and other problems characterized by confusion has risen dramatically. According to the National Institute on Aging, Alzheimer's disease alone currently affects an estimated 4 million Americans. The skills of the home health nurse to both the family and the patient are important to the safety and care of these patients.

2. **Needs for initial visit**

   Specific initial physician orders
   Universal precautions supplies
   Other supplies or equipment, based on physician orders
   Vital signs equipment

3. **Some potential medical-surgical diagnoses and codes**

AIDS dementia	294.9 and 042.9
Alzheimer's disease	331.0
Amyotrophic lateral sclerosis	335.20
Anxiety state	300.00
Aphasia	784.3
Atherosclerosis	414.0
Bladder incontinence	788.30
Constipation	564.0
Creutzfeldt-Jakob disease and dementia	290.10
CVA	436
Decubitus ulcer	707.0
Dehydration	276.5
Dementia	298.9
Depressive disorder	311
Depressive psychosis	296.20
Korsakoff's dementia	294.0
Nonpsychotic brain syndrome	310.9
Organic brain syndrome	310.9
Parkinson's disease	332.0

Pernicious anemia	281.0
Pneumonia	486
Presenile dementia	290.10
Psychosis	294.9
Senile dementia	290.0
TIAs	435.9
Urinary incontinence	788.30
Urinary tract infections	599.0

4. **Associated nursing diagnoses**

Airway clearance, ineffective
Anxiety
Bowel incontinence
Caregiver role strain
Caregiver role strain, high risk for
Communication, impaired verbal
Constipation
Coping, ineffective family: compromised
Coping, ineffective, individual
Diarrhea
Fear
Health maintenance, altered
Home maintenance management, impaired
Infection, high risk for
Injury, high risk for
Knowledge deficit (related to care management)
Mobility, impaired physical
Nutrition altered: less than body requirements
Self-care deficit, bathing/hygiene
Self-care deficit, dressing/grooming
Self-care deficit, feeding
Self-care deficit, toileting
Skin integrity, impaired, high risk for
Sleep pattern disturbance
Social interaction, impaired
Spiritual distress (distress of the human spirit)
Swallowing, impaired
Thought processes, altered
Urinary elimination, altered
Violence, potential for: self-directed or directed at others

5. **Service skills identified**

Skilled assessment of the patient with dementia and family/
caregiver support/coping skills

Home safety evaluation and plan to help assure safety

Skilled observation and assessment of all systems

Teach family caregivers about disease and management

Implement and monitor bowel regimen and teach program to family

Monitor antipsychotic drug effectiveness; severe agitation, continuing psychotic behavior

RN to monitor tranquilizer effects given for severe agitation/ anxiety

Evaluate for weight loss, weigh patient q visit, and record weights

Provide emotional support to patient and family

Observation and evaluation of bladder elimination habits, management if incontinence and assess need for indwelling catheter

Monitor hydration and nutrition intake

Assist family in setting up routine patient-centered routine and stress the importance of adhering to the routine once established

Monitor patient's BP and compliance with medication regimen

Observation of skin and patient's physical status

Teach regarding importance of observation of patient's safety

RN to assess the patient's response to treatments and interventions and report changes or unfavorable responses or reactions to the physician

Management and evaluation of the patient care plan

6. Other services indicated

HHA	Personal care
	ADL assistance
MSS	Evaluation
	Psychosocial assessment of patient regarding mental status, safety, prognosis, and implications
	Assessment of health factors that have an impact on health and on the POC being successfully implemented
	Referral(s) to appropriate community resources
OT	Evaluation of patient and home setting safety
	Reality orientation
	Safety assessment of home
	Identification of need for assistive devices to help assure ADLs, safety in home

7. **Associated factors based on diagnosis justifying homebound status**

Patient with dementia cannot leave home unattended
Psychiatric problem and patient refuses to leave home
Psychiatric problem that makes it unsafe for patient to leave home unattended
Unsafe for patient without supervision
Confusion level precludes safe leaving of home without supervision
Patient needs 24-hour supervision due to mental status or confusion
Other medical problems (specify) making patient homebound

8. **Short-term goals**

RN	Patient maintained in home safely
	Adheres to medication regiment
	Caregivers being taught to care for patient effectively
	Patient's daily, consistent routine maintained
	Maintain optimal hydration and nutrition
	Maintain adequate bowel and bladder program
	Report changes, signs, symptoms of complications to MD or RN
HHA	Effective personal care
	ADL assistance
MSS	Problem identification
	Counseling begun
	Care team and patient adhering to POC
OT	Safety in home environment maintained
	Adherence to POC

9. **Long-term goals**

RN	Patient cared for safely at home
	Caregiver can manage effectively and safely with patient
HHA	Effective and safe personal care provided
	Patient clean and comfortable
MSS	Community resource identified
	Problem resolution
	Care team and patient adhering to POC

	Adjustment to long-term implications of disease process occurring
	Referral of patient and caregiver to community resources for continued support
	Caregiver/family demonstrate effective coping skills
OT	Patient and caregiver using assistive/adaptive devices or equipment
	Coping skills increased

10. Discharge plans for this patient

Patient maintained in home safely with adequate hydration, nutrition, hygiene, and other needs met by caregiver

Patient to be admitted to specialized long-term care facility when bed available

Caregivers taught to manage patient safely in home with medications regulated and under care of MD

Patient discharged to adult day-care center program

11. Patient, family and caregiver educational needs

Educational needs are the regimens that the caregiver will be managing with or for the patient. These include:

Importance of adequate hydration and nutrition

Home safety concerns, issues, and teaching

The avoidance of infection by regularly inspecting patient's skin

Multiple medications and their relationship to each other

The importance of medical follow up, including prescribed blood tests

Support groups in the community that are available to the patient and their caregivers

The need for continued family therapy

The importance of maintaining the patient's daily, consistent routines, when possible

Other information based on the patient's and family's unique needs

Please be aware that there are resources for both professional and family caregivers.

The book, *The 36-Hour Day,* by Nancy L. Mace and Peter V. Rabins, MD, addresses all aspects of the difficulties encountered by families and friends as they care for their loved ones with Alzheimer's disease or other dementias.

In addition, the National Institute of Health, National Institute on Aging, has an Alzheimer's Disease Education and Referral Center. This center has information, such as home safety booklets, available to both professionals and families caring for patients with dementias. Their number is 1-800-438-4380.

There is also the Alzheimer's Association, which can be reached at 1-800-621-0379. Another resource is a service provided through the National Association of Areas on Aging. It is called the Elder Care Locator and can be reached at 1-800-677-1116. This is a resource to locate local support services for the elderly.

12. Specific tips for reimbursement

The patient with confusion and mental status deterioration often is admitted to home care for other needs, such as a catheter or monthly B-12 injections for pernicious anemia. Consider that these patients may be very appropriate for management and evaluation of the POC to assure safety in the home and management of the overall care needs. Nurses in home care also see patients who have diabetes mellitus, cellulitis, or other problems in addition to dementia. Social work intervention may be very appropriate for these patients.

Remember that for Medicare patients, and generally for other insurers, there must be behaviors demonstrated that impede safe, effective implementation of the POC. The social work needs to be directed toward the patient, even though they are clearly meeting and communicating with the family.

AMPUTATION CARE

1. **General Considerations.**   Amputation care is associated with major body image fears that can have an impact on the patient's ability to reach program goals.

   Please refer to ''Diabetes Mellitus,'' ''Peripheral Vascular Disease,'' or ''Wound Care'' should those problems be appropriate for your patient.

2. **Needs for initial visit**

   Specific initial physician orders
   Universal precautions supplies
   Other supplies or equipment, based on physician orders
   Vital signs equipment
   Pressure bandage(s)

3. **Some potential medical-surgical diagnoses and codes**

Amputation, AKA	897.3
Amputation, BKA (right or left leg)	897.1
Amputation, toe	895.1
Angina	411.1
Arterial occlusive disease	447.1
Bilateral amputee	897.6
Debridement right or left	86.22
Deep vein thrombosis	453.8
Diabetes mellitus, with complications, adult	250.90
Diabetes mellitus, with complications, juv.	250.91
Femoral-popliteal bypass	39.29
Hypertension	401.9
Infected right or left AKA	997.62
Infected right or left BKA	997.62
Gangrene, right or left foot	785.4
Gangrene, toe	785.4
Osteomyelitis, lower leg	730.06
Peripheral vascular disease	443.9
Vasculitis	447.6

4. **Associated nursing diagnoses**

   Activity intolerance
   Activity intolerance, high risk for

Anxiety

Body image disturbance

Body temperature, altered, high risk for

Constipation

Coping, ineffective family: compromised

Coping, ineffective family: disabling

Coping, ineffective individual

Denial, ineffective

Family processes, altered

Fear

Grieving, anticipatory

Infection, high risk for

Injury, high risk for

Knowledge deficit (disease and management)

Mobility, impaired physical

Noncompliance (specify)

Pain

Pain, chronic

Role, performance, altered

Self-care deficit, bathing/hygiene

Self-care deficit, dressing/grooming

Self-care deficit, feeding

Self-care deficit, toileting

Sensory/perceptual alterations (specify) (renal, cerebral, cardiopulmonary, gastrointestinal, peripheral)

Skin integrity, impaired

Skin integrity, impaired, high risk for

Sleep pattern disturbance

Social interaction, impaired

Spiritual distress (distress of the human spirit)

Tissue integrity, impaired

Tissue perfusion, altered (specify type) (renal, cerebral, cardiopulmonary, gastrointestinal, peripheral)

5. **Service skills identified**

Observation and complete assessment of all systems with patient status/post _____ (specify) amputation

RN to monitor wound for healing and signs/symptoms of infection

Venipunctures q _____ (specify ordered frequency) for monitoring blood sugar and response to insulin dose changes

RN to teach patient and family on all aspects of care of the patient with diabetes, including foot care, signs/care of hypo/hyperglycemia, and the importance of medical follow up

Specify dressing regimen, frequency of wound changes every visit

Duration for daily wound care; requires orders with a finite and predictable endpoint date for decreasing daily services

Teach patient's family care regimen

Assess patient or caregiver coping skills

Assess and objectively document wound progress

Obtain specific wound dressing orders, including sterile or nonsterile procedure(s)

Assess safety, concerning new amputation

RN to assess the patient's response to treatments and interventions and report changes or unfavorable responses or reactions to MD

Management and evaluation of the patient's POC

6. **Other services indicated**

HHA	Personal care and ADL assistance
	Evaluation
MSS	Financial concerns and body image having an impact on patient's self-care ability
OT	Evaluation
	Stump wrapping/shrinkage
	Preprosthetic training and exercise
	Safety assessment
	Provision of adaptive equipment for independent ADLs
	Donning and doffing of prosthesis
PT	Evaluation
	Stump wrapping/shrinkage
	Home exercise regimen
	Progressive strengthening
	Preprosthetic training and exercise
	Prosthetic training
	Transfer techniques
	Donning and doffing of prosthesis
	Gait training
	Progressive ambulation to walker

7. **Associated factors based on diagnosis justifying homebound status**

Patient needs maximum assistance to ambulate, transfer

Medically restricted: leg to be wrapped and elevated
Bedbound or chairbound
Severe weakness, unsteady gait
S/P AKA/BKA or bilateral BKA/AKA
Poor endurance, limited mobility
Shortness of breath complicated by S/P amputation
Level of home on second floor with no elevator, unable to use
    stairs

8. **Short-term goals**

RN	Daily compliance with wound regimen
	Daily compliance with associated medical regimen
	Pain control
	Infection-free
HHA	Effective personal hygiene
	ADL assistance
MSS	Resources identified
	Problem compliance
OT	Daily exercise regimen compliance
	Conditioning, strengthening, and functional use of prosthesis
PT	Daily exercise regimen compliance
	Increased conditioning and strengthening
	Gait compliance
	Increased functional use

9. **Long-term goals**

RN	Patient able to self-manage skin care, ADLs, self-care, S/P amputation
	Wound healed
HHA	Effective personal hygiene
	ADL assistance
MSS	Financial situation resolved
	Body image integrated
	Return to self-care status
OT	Independent in ADLs
	Increased balance, mobility, function, and independence
PT	Safe, self-ambulation with prosthetic or other device

10. **Discharge plans for this patient**

Discharged to self-care in the community when no longer homebound, or referred to outpatient services

Continue home health visits as patient remains homebound and requires skilled care

11. **Patient, family, and caregiver educational needs**

Educational needs are the care regimens that the patient or caregiver will need to know and perform to safely care for the patient. These include:

Importance of medical follow up

Importance of an exercise program, healthy diet, decreasing or quitting smoking

Medications, their actions, effects, schedules, and relationships to each other

Support groups in the community that are available to the patient and caregivers

The need for long-term follow up on the fitting and function of prosthetic

Other teaching specific to the patient's unique medical and other identified needs

12. **Specific tips for reimbursement**

Document the wound, indicate stage, drainage amount, color, and the specific care rendered

Communicate any POC changes on the form 486

Document progress in wound healing

Document supplies used on the form 485

Take pictures of wound(s) to substantiate documentation at onset and q weeks, have patient sign release, one for the clinical record

If wound culture is obtained, document the results on the form 486

Document location of wound and size with length, depth, and width

Specify and document learning barriers, for example, arithritic hands, poor eyesight

Document the specific teaching accomplished and the behavioral outcomes of that teaching

Document patient's level of independence in care

ANEMIA (PERNICIOUS)

1. **General Considerations.** The elderly often have less efficient digestion and absorption of food and nutrients, causing anemia. Many homebound patients are deficient in iron, proteins, vitamin A, vitamin D, the B vitamins, and magnesium. Monthly B-12 injections are given to maintain adequate B-12 levels.

2. **Needs for initial visit**

   Specific initial physician orders
   Universal precautions supplies
   Other supplies or equipment, based on physician orders
   Vital signs equipment
   Injection supplies
   Vitamin B-12

3. **Some potential medical-surgical diagnoses and codes**

Alcoholic neuropathy	357.5
Anemia (pernicious)	281.0
Anemia (unspecified)	285.9
Anemia, iron deficiency	280.9
Deficiency unspecified	281.9
Epistaxis	784.7
Fish tapeworm anemia	357.5
Other B-12 deficiency	281.1

4. **Associated nursing diagnoses**

   Activity intolerance
   Breathing pattern ineffective
   Constipation
   Constipation, colonic
   Fatigue
   Fear
   Infection, high risk for
   Injury, high risk for
   Knowledge, deficit (management of anemia)
   Mobility, impaired physical
   Nutrition, altered: less than body requirements
   Pain

Skin integrity, impaired, high risk for
Tissue perfusion, altered (peripheral)

5. **Service skills identified**

Administer B-12 IM injection q month
Observe IM site(s) for adverse reaction
Venipuncture as indicated q _____
Teach patient or caregiver nutritious diet high in protein, iron,
   and vitamins
Assess for signs and symptoms: numbness, tingling of
   extremities, shortness of breath
Observation and assessment of the patient with anemia
Management and evaluation of the patient POC

6. **Other services indicated**

HHA	Personal care
	ADL assistance
	Meal preparations

7. **Associated factors based on diagnosis justifying homebound status**

Bedbound or chairbound
Needs maximum assistance to ambulate
Needs assistance for all activities
Severe arthritis
Mobility severely restricted due to _____
Weakness, dizziness
Impaired ambulation
Severe SOB on any activity
Severe functional limitations, including age

8. **Short-term goals**

RN	Anemia controlled through monthly B-12 injections
	Improved hematologic status
HHA	Effective personal hygiene
	ADL assistance

9. **Long-term goals**

RN	Optimal hematologic status
HHA	Effective personal hygiene
	ADL assistance

10. **Discharge plans for this patient**

Discharged when goals achieved
No longer homebound, referred to outpatient services
Remains homebound, needing q month B-12 injection

11. **Patient, family, and caregiver educational needs**

Educational needs are the care regimens the caregiver must know to safely care for the patient. These include:

Effective personal hygiene habits
Safety measures in the home when the patient is immobilized
The importance of medical follow up
The importance of optimal hydration and nutrition
Other teaching specific to the patient's unique medical and other identified needs

12. **Specific tips for reimbursement**

Obtain baseline hematology report, specifically a Schilling test as indicated
Document age, if appropriate, as a functional limitation
Continue to document homebound status throughout the length of stay
For Medicare patients, refer to the HIM-11 Section 205.1, page 14.15 that addresses anemias.

ANGINA

1. **General Considerations.**   Patients with any cardiac process, including angina, have appropriate safety and fear concerns. The nurse in home health care needs to be specific with the next scheduled visit date and time. In addition, reassure the patient about the 24-hour on-call system and when it would be more appropriate to contact emergency community resources.

    Please refer to ''Cardiac Care'' or ''Myocardial Infarction'' if those problems are appropriate for your patient.

2. **Needs for initial visit**

    Specific initial physician orders
    Universal precautions supplies
    Other supplies or equipment, based on physician orders
    Vital signs equipment, including a good stethoscope

3. **Some potential medical-surgical diagnoses and codes**

Angina	413.9
Angina, unstable	411.1
Atherosclerosis (coronary)	414.0
Atrial fibrillation	427.31
Atrial flutter	427.32
Cardiac dysrhythmia	427.9
Cardiomyopathy	425.4
Chronic ischemic heart disease	414.9
Congestive heart failure	428.0
COPD	496
Digoxin toxicity	995.2 and E942.1
Electrolyte and fluid imbalance	276.9
HCVD with CHF	402.91
Heart block	426.9
Hypertension with heart involvement	402.91
Left heart failure	428.1
Myocardial infarction	410.9
Pacemaker (S/P)	V45.0
Pulmonary edema with cardiac disease	428.1

Respiratory arrest (S/P)   799.1

4. **Associated nursing diagnoses**

Activity intolerance
Activity intolerance, high risk for
Anxiety
Body image disturbance
Breathing pattern, ineffective
Cardiac output, decreased
Constipation
Coping, ineffective family: compromised
Decisional conflict (treatment)
Denial, ineffective
Diversional activity deficit
Family processes, altered
Fatigue
Fear
Fluid volume excess
Gas exchange, impaired
Grieving, anticipatory
Home maintenance management, impaired
Injury, high risk for
Knowledge deficit (disease process and management)
Mobility, impaired physical
Nutrition, altered: less than body requirements
Nutrition, altered: more than body requirements
Pain
Pain, chronic
Self-care deficit (specify)
Sleep pattern disturbance
Spiritual distress (distress of the human spirit)
Tissue perfusion, altered (cardiopulmonary)

5. **Service skills identified**

Assess lungs, cardiovascular status
Measure vital signs
Assess for fluid retention
Measure lower extremities as indicated
Evaluate for fluid retention, amount, sites
Teach specified diet
Teach energy conservation techniques
Assess amount, frequency, site(s) of chest pain; report to
    physician as indicated

Weigh daily; teach family to weigh patient daily and
    document same

Teach regarding new medication regimen and side effects

Venipuncture as indicated for electrolyte or other levels

Teach patient or family to measure pulse

Assess patient for orthostatic hypotension

Assess nitroglycerin use and outcome

Observation and assessment of the patient with angina

RN to teach care and safety regarding oxygen therapy at home

RN to instruct patient and caregiver regarding multiple
    medications, including schedule, functions, and possible side
    effects

RN to assess the patient's response to treatments and
    interventions and report changes or unfavorable responses/
    reactions to the physician

Management and evaluation of the patient POC

6. **Other services indicated**

HHA	Personal care
	ADL assistance
MSS	Indicated when the patient's social problems adversely affect the response to the ordered POC
OT	Evaluation to teach conservation of energy techniques
	ADL retraining as indicated by level of cardiac restrictions
PT	Evaluation
	Endurance/general conditioning

7. **Associated factors based on diagnosis justifying
homebound status**

Bedridden

Chairbound

Needs maximum assistance to ambulate

Severe SOB

Cardiac restrictions due to chest pain

Limited energy, endurance, and dyspnea on exertion

Angina with activity

Severe functional limitations

S/P AMI

S/P unstable angina episode

Poor respiratory status
End-stage cardiac disease
Lower extremity edema impairing ambulation

8. Short-term goals

RN	Daily compliance with medication and treatment regimen
	Patient pain-free
	Blood pressure in normal for patient range
	Return to independent ADLs
	Decreased shortness of breath
HHA	Effective personal hygiene
	ADL assistance
MSS	Problems and resource identified
	POC implemented
OT	Patient practicing energy conservation techniques
PT	Increase endurance for ambulation
	Increase strength

9. Long-term goals

RN	Medications regulated
	Stable cardiovascular and respiratory status
	Vital signs in normal for patient range
	Extremity edema resolved
	Patient pain-free
	Patient awareness through verbalization of appropriate time or need to seek medical follow up
HHA	Self-care regarding ADLs
	Effective personal hygiene
MSS	Return to community
	Problem resolution
	Referred to community resources
OT	Utilization of energy conservation techniques
	Able to do ADLs
PT	Return to functional gait and independence

10. Discharge plans for this patient

Discharged, goals achieved
No longer homebound, referred to outpatient services
Continuing need for home health care because patient remains homebound and needs skilled care services
Family member taught care, patient discharged

11. **Patient, family, and caregiver educational needs**

Educational needs are the regimens that the patient or caregiver will need to safely continue to care for the patient at home. These include:

The patient's medications and their relationship to each other
The importance of compliance to the regimen
The importance of medical follow up
The symptoms that would appropriately necessitate calling
  emergency services (specify symptoms)
The need to quit or cut down on smoking
Other teaching specific to the patient and caregiver needs

12. **Specific tips for reimbursement**

Document the specific care and teaching instructions
Communicate any POC changes in documentation
Document progress toward goal
Document any abnormal laboratory values
Document the actions of your care
Obtain a telephone order for any POC change
Document any behavioral outcomes of teaching instructions
Document all episodes of angina and follow up indicated in
  the medical record
Document changes to the POC and communications with the
  physician

ARTHRITIS

1. **General Considerations.** The arthritis that may be appropriate for coverage is the acute exacerbation of osteoarthritis. These symptoms, especially in the elderly, are pain and a generalized weakened muscle condition. This deterioration can occur rapidly and usually precipitates the need for home health care services.

2. **Needs for initial visit**

   Specific initial physician orders
   Universal precautions supplies
   Other supplies or equipment, based on physician orders
   Vital signs equipment

3. **Some potential medical-surgical diagnoses and codes**

Arthritis, rheumatoid	714.04
Arthritis, spine	721.90
Cancer, lumbar spine	170.2
Laminectomy	03.09
Lumbar fracture	805.4
Lumbar stenosis	724.02
Muscular sclerosis	340
Osteoarthritis, acute exacerbation	715.98
Osteoarthritis, spine	721.9
Osteoporosis	733.00
Quadriplegia	344.0
Rheumatoid arthritis, spine	720.0
Sciatica	724.3
Sprain (strain)	848.8
Spinal cord compression	336.9
Spinal cord tumor	239.7
Spinal stenosis	724.00

4. **Associated nursing diagnoses**

   Activity intolerance
   Activity intolerance, high risk for
   Anxiety
   Body image disturbance
   Constipation

Fatigue
Fear
Home maintenance management, impaired
Infection, high risk for
Injury, high risk for
Knowledge deficit (self-care regimen)
Mobility, impaired physical
Pain
Pain, chronic
Self-care deficit, bathing/hygiene
Self-care deficit, dressing/grooming
Self-care deficit, feeding
Self-care deficit, toileting
Sleep pattern disturbance

5. **Service skills identified**

Evaluation and all systems assessment of the patient with an exacerbation of symptoms of arthritis _____ (specify symptoms necessitating skilled care)

RN to perform a comprehensive pain assessment q visit to identify pain and need for analgesic dose adjustment or other plan for relief

RN to teach patient and observe for adverse side effects of nonsteroidal anti-inflammatory drugs (NSAIDS)

RN to teach patient and family about correct positioning, body alignment, and posture

RN to monitor for side effects of gold therapy

RN to evaluate patient's bowel patterns, need for stool softeners, laxative, dietary changes/increase in fluids, develop bowel management program

RN to evaluate patient for effects of increased immobility due to pain

RN to assess the patient's response to treatments or interventions and report changes or unfavorable responses or reactions to the physician

Management and evaluation of the patient POC

6. **Other services indicated**

HHA	Personal care
	ADL assistance
OT	Evaluation
	Home safety assessment

	Evaluation for adaptive equipment or special fabrication of splints
	Training and management of adaptive devices and resting splints
	ADLs
PT	Evaluation
	Home safety assessment
	ROM
	Strengthening exercises
	Home exercise program
	Progressive exercise program
	Gait training
	Evaluate for and teach safe use of assistive devices
	Therapeutic exercise regimen
	Bed mobility exercises as tolerated
	Therapeutic massage
	Heat or cold therapy, as specified in MD orders
	Moist warm heat applications
	Teach patient and family safety and fall precautions
	Management and evaluation of the patient's care plan

7. **Associated factors based on diagnosis justifying homebound status**

Requires maximum assistance to ambulate
Unsteady gait
Pain on movement or walking
Limited mobility
Activity restricted because of pain
Braces on hips
Chairbound because of recent exacerbation of joint disease
Patient cannot safely leave home without assistive device

8. **Short-term goals**

RN	Decrease pain
	Prevent contractures
	Maintain function
HHA	Effective personal hygiene
	ADL assistance

PT	Increased mobility, strength, function

9. **Long-term goals**

RN	Pain-free with functional mobility
	Patient self-care
HHA	Effective personal hygiene
	ADL assistance
OT	Increase ADLs to functional level
	Patient using assistive, adaptive devices safely and effectively
PT	Home exercise regimen adhered to by patient and family
	Increased and safe mobility
	Teach application/use of TENS unit

10. **Discharge plans for this patient**

Discharged when patient-centered goals achieved
No longer homebound, referred to outpatient services
Self-care, under MD supervision

11. **Patient, family, and caregiver educational needs**

Educational needs are the regimens the patient or caregiver will need to know to safely care for the patient. These include:

Aspects of pain control and the analgesic regimen
The prevention of joint deformities and functional positions
The importance of optimal nutrition, hydration, rest, and home exercise program
The need for compliance to the program for optimal effectiveness
The importance of medical follow up
When to call the HHA nurse or the physician
Other information based on the patient's unique medical and other needs

One resource is the Arthritis Foundation: their national office number is (404) 872-7100. Another resource is a service provided through the National Association of Areas on Aging. It is called the Elder Care Locator and can be reached at 1-800-677-1116. This is a resource to locate local support services for the elderly.

12. **Specific tips for reimbursement**

Not all patients will need to have a nurse involved—it is
patient-dependent, based on your evaluation and objective
findings

Explain why the nurse is involved clearly in the documentation

Use "assessed," "monitored," "observed," "taught," and
other verbs that connote the care interventions provided

Remember that the patient should be discharged when the
stated patient-centered, predetermined goals have been
achieved

Remember that safety is a key factor for these patients to
remain home and sometimes alone—consider a personal
emergency response system for these patients

ASTHMA

1. **General Considerations.** In home health care the patient with asthma is usually referred after discharge from the acute care setting.

   Please refer to ''Chronic Obstructive Pulmonary Disease,'' or ''Pneumonia'' should those problems be appropriate for your patient.

2. **Needs for initial visit**

   Specific initial physician orders
   Universal precautions supplies
   Other supplies or equipment, based on physician orders
   Vital signs equipment

3. **Some potential medical-surgical diagnoses and codes**

Asthma	493.90
Asthma with status asthmaticus	493.91
Bronchitis, acute	466.0
CHF	428.0
Chronic airway obstruction	496
COPD	496
Corpulmonale	415.0
Dehydration	276.5
Emphysema	492.8
Heart failure	428.9
Hypertension	401.9
Left ventricular failure	428.1
Lung cancer	162.9
Pleural effusion (right or left)	511.9
Pneumonia	486
PVD	443.9
Trachea/bronchus disease	519.1
Tuberculosis (lung)	011.90
Ventilator, dependence on	V46.1

4. **Associated nursing diagnoses**

   Activity intolerance
   Activity intolerance, high risk for
   Airway clearance, ineffective

Anxiety
Breathing pattern, ineffective
Cardiac output, decreased
Caregiver role strain
Caregiver role strain, high risk for
Communication, impaired verbal
Coping, ineffective family: compromised
Family processes, altered
Fatigue
Fear
Fluid volume deficit, high risk for
Gas exchange, impaired
Home maintenance management, impaired
Infection, high risk for
Knowledge deficit (disease process and management)
Management of therapeutic regimen (individuals), ineffective
Noncompliance (specify)
Pain
Self-care deficit, bathing/hygiene
Self-care deficit, dressing/grooming
Self-care deficit, feeding
Self-care deficit, toileting
Sleep pattern disturbance
Spiritual distress (distress of the human spirit)
Tissue perfusion, altered (cardiopulmonary)

5. **Service skills identified**

Evaluate lung sounds, assess amount, site(s) of wheezing, rhonchi, or lung sound changes
Teach patient or caregiver new medication regimen
Teach patient or caregiver to identify and avoid specific factors that precipitate an exacerbation (attack)
Teach patient or caregiver what to do regarding an impending episode
Teach patient or caregiver how to administer injections as indicated
Teach patient or caregiver how to safely and effectively utilize aerosol inhalers or treatments at home
Teach regarding safe oxygen utilization in the home setting
Assess nutritional status
Assess hydration status
Assess for signs, symptoms of CHF
Assess vital signs

Teach ordered diet regimen of _____

Evaluate sites, amount of edema

Obtain sputum culture as indicated q _____

Venipuncture as ordered q _____

Teach energy conservation skills

Observation and complete systems assessment of the patient with asthma

Teach patient correct use and techniques of inhalers

RN to monitor respiratory rate and pattern

RN to evaluate for presence or absence of cough, frequency, character, and sputum production

Teach regarding and observe for steroid side effects

Teach use of home peak flow meter

RN to teach effective coughing and breathing exercises

RN to assess the patient's response to treatments and interventions and report changes or unfavorable responses or reactions to MD

Management and evaluation of the patient's POC

6. **Other services indicated**

HHA	Personal care
	ADL assistance
MSS	Evaluation
	Financial counseling
	Community resource referral(s)
OT	Evaluation, conservation of energy techniques
	Adaptive ADL assistive devices as indicated
PT	Evaluation, strengthening exercises
	Gait training
	Breathing exercises
	Home exercise program
	Safe use of assistive device(s)

7. **Associated factors based on diagnosis justifying homebound status**

Severe weakness

Unsteady ambulation

Frail, needs assistance to ambulate

Severe SOB

Bedridden

Wheelchair dependent

Paraplegia, paralysis, paresis

Requires maximum assistance to ambulate
Medical restriction, leg to be elevated for _____ (specify)
SOB on exertion
SOB on talking
Respiratory distress with any movement or talking
Oxygen dependence
S/P CVA, S/P TIA

8. **Short-term goals**

RN	Daily adherence to POC
	Improve oxygen exchange
	Decreased wheezing
HHA	Effective personal hygiene
	ADL assistance
MSS	POC implemented
OT	Practicing conservation of energy techniques
PT	Increased mobility
	Increased strength, endurance
	Increased breathing exercise compliance

9. **Long-term goals**

RN	Optimal oxygen exchange
	Improved color
	Adequate hydration or nutrition
	Stable respiratory status for patient
	Clear lung sounds, patient afebrile
	Patient self-care concerning care regimen
	Patient compliance to multiple drug regimen
HHA	Effective personal hygiene
	ADL assistance
MSS	Community resources identified or problem resolution
OT	Able to do ADLs with decreased SOB
	Quality of life improved
PT	Functional ambulation
	Return to mobility
	Increased strength and endurance
	Functional breathing program

10. **Discharge plans for this patient**

Discharged when patient-centered goals achieved, back to community, under MD care

No longer homebound, referred to outpatient services
Remains homebound, continues to need skilled care
Discharged, patient condition deteriorated, admitted to
   inpatient facility

11. **Patient, family, and caregiver educational needs**
Educational needs are the regimens that the patient and
caregiver will be managing need to be addressed. These
include:

The patient's medications and their relationship to each other
The avoidance of infections, stress, and other "triggers" for
   the individual patient. These can include environmental
   factors such as pollens, smoke, animals, dust, and chemicals.
The importance of optimal hydration and nutrition
The importance of medical follow up
Other teaching specific to the patient's unique medical and
   other identified needs

12. **Specific tips for reimbursement**

Document all abnormalities, such as fever, tachycardia, rales,
   wheezing, or rhonchi
Document the instability of the patient; document any edema,
   SOB, medication reaction, further acute episodes, pulse
   irregularities
Obtain a telephone order to change the visit frequency or make
   any changes to the POC
Often, these patients have other medical problems,
      specifically cardiac, that impede progress; document these
   problems also
Document medications changed or medications being regulated
   on the daily visit note or record
Document RN contacted physician regarding _____
Document new onset (any problem)
Document positive culture, patient started on _____ (specify
   medication) on _____ (date) and obtained a telephone order
   for the change

BEDBOUND (CARE OF THE PATIENT)

1. **General Considerations.** With more patients choosing to be cared for at home, the number of patients that are essentially bedridden continues to increase. While being bedridden is not a diagnosis, it is an important factor with implications for all body systems of patients. Caregivers and family are the key to these patients being cared for safely and effectively in their own home setting.

   Please refer to ''Acquired Immune Deficiency Syndrome,'' ''Cancer Care,'' ''Catheter Care,'' ''Congestive Heart Failure,'' ''Gastrostomy and Other Feeding Tube Care,'' or other specific diagnoses or problems for more in-depth discussion for these possible nursing care needs.

2. **Needs for initial visit**

   Specific initial physician orders
   Universal precautions supplies
   Other supplies or equipment, based on physician orders
   Vital signs equipment

3. **Some potential medical-surgical diagnoses and codes**

Acute myocardial infarction	410.92
AIDS	042.9
Angina	411.1
Aphasia	784.3
Attention to other artificial opening of urinary tract	V55.6
Back sprain	847.9
Bladder atony	596.4
Cancer of the lung	162.9
Cerebral vascular accident	436
Cirrhosis of the liver	571.5
Congestive heart failure	428.0
Constipation	564.0
COPD	496
Debility	799.3
Decubitus ulcer	707.0
Dehydration	276.5
Diabetes mellitus, with complications, adult	250.90
Diabetes mellitus, with complications, juv.	250.91

Fitting and adjustment of urinary devices	V53.6
Heart disease, chronic ischemic	414.9
Heart failure	428.9
Heart failure, left	428.1
Hemiplegia	342.9
Hyperalimentation	99.15
Hypertension	401.9
Ileus	560.1
Impaction	560.39
Incontinence of feces	787.6
Incontinence of urine	788.30
Lou Gehrig's disease (amyotrophic lateral sclerosis)	335.20
Multiple sclerosis	340
Muscular scoliosis	737.39
Myocardial infarction	410.92
Orthostatic hypotension	458.0
Osteoporosis	733.00
Paralysis	344.9
Paraplegia	344.1
Parkinson's disease	332.0
Pathological fracture	733.1
Pneumonia	486
Pneumonia, aspiration	507.0
Quadriplegia	344.0
Renal failure	586
Respirator, dependence on	V46.1
Septicemia	038.9
Spinal cord injury, traumatic	952.9
Spinal cord tumor	239.7
Thrombophlebitis	451.9
TPN	99.15
Transient ischemic attacks (TIAs)	435.9
Urinary incontinence	788.3
Urinary retention	788.2
Urinary tract infection	599.0
Venous thrombosis	453.8

4. **Associated nursing diagnoses**

Activity intolerance
Anxiety
Aspiration, high risk for
Body image disturbance

Body temperature, altered, high risk for
Bowel incontinence
Cardiac output, decreased
Caregiver role strain
Caregiver role strain, high risk for
Communication, impaired
Constipation
Coping, ineffective family: compromised
Coping, ineffective individual
Diarrhea
Disuse syndrome, high risk for
Diversional activity deficit
Family processes, altered
Fatigue
Fear
Fluid volume deficit, high risk for
Grieving, anticipatory
Incontinence, functional
Incontinence, total
Infection, high risk for
Injury, high risk for
Mobility, impaired physical
Nutrition, altered, less than body requirements
Nutrition, altered, more than body requirements
Oral mucous membrane, altered
Pain
Pain, chronic
Peripheral neurovascular dysfunction, high risk for
Protection, altered
Self-care deficit, bathing/hygiene
Self-care deficit, dressing/grooming
Self-care deficit, feeding
Self-care deficit, toileting
Sensory/perceptual alterations (specify) (visual, auditory,
    kinesthetic, gustatory, tactile, olfactory)
Sexuality patterns, altered
Skin integrity, impaired
Skin integrity, impaired, high risk for
Sleep pattern, disturbance
Social interaction, impaired
Spiritual distress (distress of the human spirit)
Swallowing, impaired
Thought processes, altered

Tissue perfusion, altered (specify type) (renal, cerebral, cardiopulmonary, gastrointestinal, peripheral)

Urinary elimination, altered

Urinary retention

5. **Service skills identified**

Assessment and observation of cardiovascular and other systems in bedridden patient with _____

RN to change dressing at wound site BID (remember the needed projection of a finite and predictable endpoint to daily care) using aseptic technique

Observation and assessment of wound site and healing

Teach family caregiver proper, safe wound care and signs and symptoms of infection to watch for and report to RN or MD

RN to instruct on all aspects of care of the immobilized patient

RN to instruct on all medications, including schedule, functions of specific drugs and their side effects

Monitor bowel patterns, including frequency of bowel movements and evaluate the need for a bowel regimen (e.g., stool softeners, laxatives, and dietary changes)

Check for and remove impaction per MD orders

RN to implement bladder training program

Teach caregiver importance of and all aspects of effective skin care regimens to prevent (further) breakdown. Include the need for every 1 to 2 hour position changes, pressure pads or mattresses and other measures for prevention

Observation and assessment of blood pressure and other vital signs

RN to monitor and assess for complications of new medication regimen

Teach caregiver effective and safe suctioning of patient

Teach caregiver daily catheter and equipment care and signs and symptoms of when to call RN/MD

RN to provide emotional support to patient and family in patient with a chronic illness or an illness of a terminal nature

RN to monitor patient response to medications for pain and other symptom control

RN to observe and assess patient for signs, symptoms of infection

RN to draw venipuncture for _____ as ordered

Teach caregiver effective use of turn/pull sheet to avoid friction, skin tears, or burns

RN to culture wound and urine for C and S and send to lab

Comfort measures provided to patient for pain, other symptom relief including backrub, hand massage, and soothing music of patient's choice, when possible

Antiembolus hose applied and application method taught to caregiver

RN to monitor hydration/nutrition status

RN to change catheter (specify type, size) q (specify frequency)

RN enterostomal therapist to see patient and evaluate wound for specific care needs

RN to assess the patient's response to ordered interventions and treatments and report changes or unfavorable responses or reactions to the MD as indicated

Management and evaluation of the patient care plan

6. Other services indicated

HHA	Personal care
	ADL assistance
MSS	Evaluation
	Patient assessment of emotional/social factors having an impact on POC goal achievement
	Evaluate adjustment to health problems/sexuality and diagnosis with long-term implications
	Identify eligibility for community services or benefits
	Financial counseling regarding medical regimen
	Community resource referrals
OT	Evaluation
	Teach conservation of energy techniques
	Assistive device assessment
	Splinting/positioning aids
PT	Evaluation
	Strengthening program, safe transfer training
	Teach caregiver safe home exercise regimen
	Assessment of upper body strength for trapeze or other methods to increase bed mobility
	Management and evaluation of the patient POC
	Chest physical therapy
	Bed mobility exercises
	Strengthening exercise regimen

	Teach safe use of assistive devices as indicated
	Maintenance of ROM
S-LP	Evaluation
	Swallowing assessment
	Food texture recommendations
	Speech dysphagia program
	Alternate communication program
	Establish home maintenance program

7. **Associated factors based on diagnosis justifying homebound status**

Patient needs maximum assistance to transfer safely
Patient is bedbound with _____ (specify problem)
Quadriplegia
Lower extremity hemiplegia
Severe weakness
Unsafe, unsteady gait with maximum assistance
Patient cannot leave home without maximum assistance
Severe shortness of breath
Severe arthritis
Respirator dependence
S/P CVA and needs walker
Patient is blind and cannot safely leave home unattended

8. **Short-term goals**

RN	Daily compliance to medical regimens (meds, dietary needs, catheter or wound care, others)
	Patient infection-free
	Wounds healing and infection-free
	Patient able to spend time with family and friends
	Patient, caregivers, and family experience an improved quality of life due to care interventions
	Patient cared for safely at home
HHA	Effective personal care
	ADL assistance
	Participation in mobility plan
MSS	Problem identification
	Counseling initiated
	Effective adherence to POC

OT	Daily adherence to occupational therapy POC
PT	Daily adherence to physical therapy POC
S-LP	Patient swallowing safely
	Patient beginning to be understood and communicate

9. Long-term goals

RN	Patient adheres to POC regimen
	Patient and family integrate information taught by RN about the disease process and care into their daily activities
	Patient experiences an improved quality of life due to care interventions
	Patient and caregivers are effective in care management and know when to call physician, RN, or other professionals for assistance
	Patient has input into care regimen, when possible
	Skin integrity maintained
	Wound site healed and infection-free
	Infection-free urine and patent catheter
HHA	Effective and safe personal care
	Patient clean and feels better
MSS	Community resources identified
	Problem resolution
	Team and patient able to implement and integrate care plan into patient daily care
	Appropriate adjustment to diagnosis and implications
	Referral of patient and caregiver spouse for continued support through community support services
	Patient/family demonstrate coping
OT	Patient able to use conservation of energy techniques taught in daily life activities
	Patient using adaptive or assistive devices safely and effectively
	Family caregiver using splints to maintain functional joint position
PT	Caregiver taught safe home exercise regimen including transfer techniques
	Patient practices bed exercise regimen and maintains schedule
	Patient has increased strength

Patient demonstrates or verbalizes increased
endurance
S-LP   Patient able to communicate
Patient swallowing safely

10. **Discharge plans for this patient**

Bedridden patient maintained in home, infection- and wound-
free
Caregiver, spouse able to care for patient. Discharged from
home care and under MD care.
Patient will remain in home care as long as has indwelling
catheter
Patient will remain in home care as long as wound needs
skilled care and assessment
Patient death in home with dignity and symptoms controlled
Discharge when patient goals achieved (specify patient-
centered goals)
Patient will remain in home with spouse as caregiver
providing safe care and under the supervision of the MD
Homebound patient will continue to receive home care
services as long as need for monthly B-12 injection
continues per MD orders
(If Medicare) Patient will continue to need daily wound care
by RN. The projected finite and predictable endpoint
is _____ (specify date according to the certifying
physician).

11. **Patient, family, and caregiver educational needs**

Educational needs are the regimens that the caregiver will be
managing with the patient. These include:

Skin care regimens
Catheter and wound care programs
Effective personal hygiene habits
Home exercise program, including ROM
Safety measures in the home when the patient is immobilized
The avoidance of infections
The medication program and the medication's relationships to
each other
Temperature checking and reading
The importance of medical follow up
When to call the home health agency or the physician
Other information based on the patient's unique needs

Another resource is a service provided through the National Association of Areas on Aging. It is called the Elder Care Locator and can be reached at 1-800-677-1116. This is a resource to locate local support services for the elderly.

12. **Specific tips for reimbursement**

Remember that Ensure or other nutritional solutions are usually covered by Medicare or other third-party payers when they are the *sole* source of nutrition. (They usually cannot be supplementary.) Also, they are generally covered when taken by routes other than PO, for example, enteral tube feedings.

For venipuncture, the diagnoses should correspond with the ordered test; for example, a fasting blood sugar is appropriate for patients with a diagnosis of diabetes mellitus. However, the blood test cannot be for routine screening. If the patient's MD believes the patient may have an elevated BS, communicate this in the form 485/6 so there is a clear explanation of the blood draw visit.

Many of these patients stay in home care through their death. The nurse's efforts are toward the safe and effective care of these patients with multisystem problems. There are usually many nursing "skills" involved with these patients. They include:

Observation and assessment
Wound care (hands-on teaching and assessment)
Venipuncture
Catheter care
G-tube or other feeding tube care
Management and evaluation of the patient POC
Teaching activities directed toward the caregivers
IM, IV, or SQ medication administration
Suctioning skills
Other miscellaneous skills that can only be safely and
    effectively provided by a professional nurse

BRAIN TUMOR

1. **General Considerations.** Home care nurses use all their skills in the care of patients with brain tumors. The many symptoms and problems can be overwhelming to the family and caregivers. The patient's care needs are varied based on the tumor site and type. The support and assurance that must be provided to these patients and their families can be as important as seizure control or other symptoms that can be difficult to manage at home.

   Please refer also to "Cancer Care," "Care of the Bedbound Patient," "Care of the Patient with Pain," and "Hospice Care" should those problems be appropriate for your patient.

2. **Needs for initial visit**

   Specific initial physician orders
   Universal precautions supplies
   Other supplies or equipment, based on physician orders
   Vital signs equipment

3. **Some potential medical-surgical diagnoses and codes**

Acoustic neuroma	225.1
Astrocytoma	191.9
Bone metastases	198.5
Brain tumor, recurrent	239.6
Cancer of the brain	191.9
Cerebral vascular accident	436
Depression, reactive	300.4
Glioma	191.9
Meningitis	322.9
Metastases (general)	199.1
Metastatic brain tumor	198.3
Pathological fracture	733.1
Pneumonia	486
Seizures	780.3
Radiation enteritis	558.1
Radiation myelitis	990 and 323.8
Transient ischemic attacks	435.9
Urinary tract infection	599.0

4. **Associated nursing diagnoses**

Activity intolerance
Activity intolerance, high risk for
Airway clearance, ineffective
Anxiety
Aspiration, high risk for
Body image disturbance
Body temperature, altered, high risk for
Bowel incontinence
Breathing pattern, ineffective
Caregiver role strain
Caregiver role strain, high risk for
Communication, impaired verbal
Constipation
Coping, ineffective family: compromised
Coping, ineffective family: disabling
Coping, ineffective individual
Diarrhea
Disuse syndrome, high risk for
Family processes, altered
Fatigue
Fear
Fluid volume deficit, high risk for
Fluid volume excess
Gas exchange, impaired
Grieving, anticipatory
Home maintenance management, impaired
Hopelessness
Hyperthermia
Hypothermia
Incontinence, total
Infection, high risk for
Injury, high risk for
Knowledge deficit (specify)
Mobility, impaired physical
Noncompliance (specify)
Nutrition, altered: less than body requirements
Oral mucous membrane, altered
Pain
Pain, chronic
Peripheral neurovascular dysfunction, high risk for
Powerlessness

Protection, altered
Role performance, altered
Self-care deficit, bathing/hygiene
Self-care deficit, dressing/grooming
Self-care deficit, feeding
Self-care deficit, toileting
Sensory/perceptual alterations (specify) (visual, auditory,
    kinesthetic, gustatory, tactile, olfactory)
Sexual dysfunction
Skin integrity, impaired
Skin integrity, impaired, high risk for
Sleep pattern disturbance
Social interaction, impaired
Spiritual distress (distress of the human spirit)
Swallowing, impaired
Thought processes, altered
Tissue integrity, impaired
Tissue perfusion, altered (specify type) (renal, cerebral,
    cardiopulmonary, gastrointestinal, peripheral)
Trauma, high risk for
Urinary elimination, altered
Urinary retention

5. **Service skills identified**

Assessment and observation of all systems in patient with
    brain tumor and status postsurgery
RN to instruct caregiver on all aspects of medications,
    including schedule, functions, and side effects
Monitor for signs and symptoms of infection
Monitor bowel pattern including frequency and need for stool
    softeners, laxatives, or dietary changes
Observation and assessment of patient's pain and other
    symptoms
RN to conduct neurological checks q visit, including levels of
    consciousness, pupil checks, and others as ordered
Comfort measures of back rub and hand massages
Observe for alopecia and implement management regimen
RN to monitor blood pressure and other vital signs
Teach patient radiation therapy regimen and schedule
RN to monitor patient for seizure activity, teach seizure
    precautions
Monitor patient for fluid retention
Daily weights

Teach patient and caregiver about steroid therapy and side effects to watch for

Nonpharmacologic interventions of progressive muscle relaxation imagery, positive visualization, music and humor therapy of patient's choice implemented

Teach caregiver about skin care needs including the need for frequent position changes, pressure pads and mattresses available, and the prevention of breakdown

Nutrition/hydration to be maintained by offering patient high-protein diet and foods of choice as tolerated

RN to teach caregiver daily care of catheter

Observe oral mucosa for breakdown, other problems

Assess effectiveness of pain relief program

Provide emotional support to patient and spouse with illness of a chronic (or terminal) nature

RN to assess the patient's response to treatment or interventions and report changes or unfavorable responses or reactions to the physician

Management and evaluation of the patient POC

6. **Other services indicated**

HHA	Personal care
	ADL assistance
	Home exercise program
	Meal preparation
MSS	Evaluation
	Patient assessment including adjustment to health problems and new diagnoses and its implications
	Determine factors that have an impact on the POC not being effectively implemented or followed
	Identify eligibility for services or benefits
	Community resource referral
OT	Evaluation
	Conservation of energy techniques
	Assessment of the need for adaptive or assistive devices
	Cognitive training
PT	Evaluation
	Strengthening exercise program
	Safe transfer and gait training home program
	Bed mobility exercises, as tolerated

	Instruct and supervise caregiver regarding home exercise regimen
	Teach safe use of assistive devices as indicated
	Assess gait safety
	Management and evaluation of the patient POC
	Safe transfers and positioning
S-LP	Evaluation
	Swallowing assessment and food texture recommendations
	Speech dysphagia program
	Education related to avoiding aspiration

7. **Associated factors based on diagnosis justifying homebound status**

S/P brain surgery—too weak to leave home without maximum assistance

Patient with malignant lesion is too weak to safely leave home

Patient on large doses of steroids, has meningitis in postop period—not safe to leave home

Limited mobility due to headache pain and unsafe ataxic gait

Pain and weakness

Medically restricted because of risk of infection postop

Shortness of breath on any activity

Patient up only with assistance

Patient had CVA, has right-sided weakness

Patient needs assistance in all activities

Lesion causing mental status changes, homebound for safety reasons

Comatose patient

Aphasia and lethargy due to progression of malignancy

8. **Short-term goals**

RN	Daily compliance to regimens including medications, nutrition and hydration, safety instructions, and others
	Patient able to have input and control regarding varied activities and aspects of care, when possible
	Patient able to spend time with family and friends
	Patient infection-free
	Patient seizure-free or controlled on medications
	Pain and other symptoms well controlled
	Patient cared for safely at home

	Decreased pain
HHA	Effective personal care
	ADL assistance
	Participation in home exercise program
	Adherence to safety precautions
MSS	Problem identification
	Counseling initiated
	Care team and patient able to implement care plan effectively
OT	Daily adherence to occupational therapy POC
	Use of ADL training skills
	Use of conservation of energy techniques taught
PT	Daily adherence to physical therapy POC
	Function maintained
	Patient safety maintained while transferring
	Case conference at 4 to 6 weeks into care
S-LP	Daily adherence to S-LP POC
	Safe swallowing communication

9. **Long-term goals**

RN	Pain and other symptoms well controlled
	Patient and caregiver adhere to medical regimen
	Patient and caregiver integrate information about the disease process and care into their daily activities
	Patient experiences an improved quality of life due to care interventions
	Patient and caregiver effective in care management and know when to call RN or MD for assistance
	Comfort maintained through death with dignity
	Patient without seizures or seizures controlled
	Patient infection-free and afebrile
	Patient has safe functional mobility with ambulation
	Supportive care provided to patient and family
HHA	Safe, effective personal care
	Patient clean and feels better
	ADL assistance
MSS	Community resources identified
	Problem resolution
	Care team and patient able to implement and integrate POC

	Appropriate adjustment to diagnoses and implications
	Referral of patient and spouse for continued support to community support services
	Psychosocial support
	Referral to spiritual support resources as requested by patient or family
OT	Patient using conservation of energy techniques taught
	Patient safely using adaptive or assistive devices
PT	Function maintained
	Caregiver taught home exercise regimen
	Patient practices exercise regimen and maintains schedule
	Patient has increased and safe mobility
	Patient experiences or verbalizes increased strength or endurance
S-LP	Safe swallowing
	Effective communications

10. **Discharge plans for this patient**

Patient to be cared for at home through death

Discharge from home care when patient-centered goals achieved

Patient will remain in home with trained spouse caregiver, under the care of the MD

Patient no longer homebound

Inpatient hospice bed located

Patient will remain at home long-term with indwelling catheter and management and evaluation of the POC

11. **Patient, family, and caregiver educational needs**

Educational needs are the regimens that the caregiver will be managing with the patient. These include:

Hydration/nutrition needs and any restrictions

Effective personal hygiene habits

The avoidance of infections

Pain and other symptom control measures

The patient's medications and their relationship to each other

The importance of medical follow up

Information about the disease process and seizure activity care

The importance of taking the prescribed seizure medications

The importance of the steroids

Based on patient prognosis and preference, the availability of
hospice services and support services for both the patient
and caregivers

Catheter care

Other information based on the patient's pathology from the
tumor and the patient's unique needs

The American Cancer Society has support groups such as "I
Can Cope" and other programs. To locate the chapter nearest
your patient, call 1-800-ACS-2345.

The American Cancer Society also has a "Look Good . . .
Feel Better Program" for women undergoing chemotherapy or
radiation. They can be reached at 1-800-395-LOOK.

12. **Specific tips for reimbursement**

Obtain an order for any additional service, treatment, or care
regimen provided that was not on the original POC.

If the patient's status deteriorates and the patient needs daily
or BID care, remember to obtain an order from the physician
to increase the frequency. Remember that Medicare defines
daily care as 5, 6, or 7 days a week. There needs to be a finite
and predictable endpoint that is projected at the start of daily
care. It needs to be a specific date and decided in collaboration
with the physician. It cannot state "when the patient dies." It
needs to be stated in months, weeks, or days. For example, in
2 months, 12/01/9_. For example, "Increase RN visits to
daily for 30 days for wound care (with a projected end date)
in patient with a metastatic brain tumor. The patient's personal
care needs are such that daily home care aide services for 30
days are also indicated for the safe provision of care at
home." Remember to get this initial projection extended, if
appropriate, should the patient continue to need this care past
your initial 30-day projection.

BREAST CANCER AND MASTECTOMY CARE

1. **General Considerations.**   The high incidence of breast cancer is appropriately alarming to all women. These patients appropriately need physical care and psychosocial support from their home care nurse. Home care most commonly is related to postmastectomy care, such as postoperative complications or wound care. For ongoing support, most communities have "Reach for Recovery" available to patients offering needed support and education.

    Please refer to "Cancer Care" and "Hospice Care" for further information should those needs be appropriate for your patient.

2. **Needs for initial visit**

    Specific initial physician orders
    Universal precautions supplies
    Other supplies or equipment, based on physician
       orders
    Vital signs equipment

3. **Some potential medical-surgical diagnoses and codes**

Bone marrow transplant	41.00
Bone metastases	198.5
Cancer of the breast	174.9
Fibrocystic disease	610.1
Fracture (pathological)	733.1
Lumpectomy (partial mastectomy)	85.43
Lymphedema (postmastectomy)	457.0
Mastectomy (radical)	85.45
Mastectomy (simple)	85.41
Metastatic lung cancer	197.0
Pneumonia	486
Radiation enteritis	558.1
Radiation myelitis	990 and 323.8
Secondary malignant neoplasm breast	198.81
Wound dehiscence	998.3
Wound infection	998.5

4. **Associated nursing diagnoses**

Activity intolerance
Activity intolerance, high risk for
Anxiety
Body image disturbance
Breathing pattern, ineffective
Coping, defensive
Coping, ineffective individual
Decisional conflict (e.g., treatment)
Family processes, altered
Fatigue
Fear
Fluid volume excess
Grieving, anticipatory
Home maintenance management, impaired
Infection, high risk for
Injury, high risk for
Knowledge deficit (specify)
Mobility, impaired physical
Pain
Pain, chronic
Self-care deficit, bathing/hygiene
Self-care deficit, dressing/grooming
Sexual dysfunction
Sexuality patterns, altered
Skin integrity, impaired
Sleep pattern disturbance
Tissue integrity, impaired, high risk for

5. **Service skills identified**

Assessment of the patient S/P mastectomy for diagnoses of
cancer
Rn to teach patient regarding increased risk of infection and
lymphedema in affected arm, including signs, symptoms of
cellulitis
RN to teach patient to avoid venipunctures, blood pressure
readings, etc. in that arm
Patient to elevate affected arm
RN to teach regarding compression garments or pneumatic
pumping
RN to provide skilled observation and assessment of surgical
site

RN to assess healing in reconstruction of breast site

RN to observe for signs, symptoms of infection

RN to provide emotional support to patient with significant body image change

RN to evaluate amount, type of drainage in hemovac at home

RN to instruct patient and spouse on importance of adequate hydration and nutrition needed postop for effective healing

Teach regarding pain regimen, including care for phantom sensations such as itching, tingling, or pain

Teach regarding chemotherapy regimen, if appropriate to patient's regimen

Check affected arm for edema or circulatory problems

Teach patient about need to protect arm from infection or injury

Teach patient and caregiver care related to wound including infection control measures

RN to instruct on all medications, including schedule, functions, and possible side effects

RN to evaluate for deterrents to wound healing (e.g., radiation, poor nutrition)

Teach importance of Medic Alert™ bracelet and the need not to have venipunctures, blood tests, and other procedures done on affected arm

Teach use/care of hemovac

RN to assess and monitor pain after reconstructive surgery, patient's response to interventions and effective pain, other symptom relief measures

RN to assess blood pressure, other vital signs

Monitor the patient's bowel patterns, including frequency, and evaluate the need for stool softeners, laxatives, or dietary changes

Teach patient and family safety concerns postoperatively, including no pushing, pulling, or lifting until physician approves these activities

Patient and caregiver taught regarding signs/symptoms of when they need to call MD or RN

RN to medicate patient prior to reconstruction site dressing change

RN to culture wound site and send to lab

RN to assess the patient's response to treatments and interventions and report changes or unfavorable responses or reactions to the physician

Management and evaluation of the patient POC

6. **Other services indicated**

HHA	Personal care
	ADL assistance
	Assist with home exercise program
MSS	Evaluation
	Psychosocial assessment of patient regarding disease prognosis and implications
	Assessment of factors preventing POC from being successfully implemented
	Identify eligibility for services or benefits
	Community resource referral
OT	Evaluation
	ADL assessment and home program
	Measures to improve function, body image, such as breast prosthesis
PT	Evaluation
	Home exercise/ROM regimen
	Active/resistive exercises
	Strengthening program
	Instruct and supervise patient about home program
	Passive, active, active-assistive exercise
	Pain assessment/reduction factors
	Home safety measures

7. **Associated factors based on diagnosis justifying homebound status**

Weakness and pain postoperatively

Patient on medication (specify) that are immunosuppressive; MD ordered dressing done at home for infection control

Patient has open wound site and cannot leave home without assistance

Bathroom privileges only per MD

Patient is medically restricted for 4 weeks due to extensive reconstructive surgery

Weakness due to chemotherapy or radiation treatments

8. **Short-term goals**

RN	Provide aseptic wound care
	Daily implementation of POC
	Pain, other symptom relief
	Report signs/symptoms of complications to RN or MD

HHA	Effective personal care
	ADL assistance
MSS	Problem identification
	Counseling initiated
	Care team and patient adhering to POC
OT	Beginning to use home exercise program
	ADLs and function maintained
PT	Patient adheres to exercise program
	Valuing importance of home program

9. **Long-term goals**

RN	Patient adapting appropriately to diagnosis and prognosis
	Patient understands and adheres to medical therapeutic regimen
	Wound healed
	Reconstruction physically and visually comfortable for patient
	Patient is pain-, infection-, and injury-free (no complications)
	Patient has increasing mobility
	Patient experiences or verbalizes improved strength or endurance
	Patient practices and maintains schedule of exercise programs
	Patient able to perform breast self-examination
	Patient able to resume presurgery mobility level
	Patient and family integrate information about the disease process into their daily activities
	Patient and spouse experience an improved quality of life due to nursing care interventions
	Patient and caregiver effective in self-care management and know when to contact RN or MD for professional assistance
HHA	Effective and safe personal care provided
	Patient clean and comfortable
	ADL assistance
MSS	Community resources identified
	Problem resolution
	Care team and patient able to implement and follow POC
	Adjustment to diagnoses and implications occurring

	Referral of patient and spouse/caregiver to community resources for continued support
OT	Patient able to use ADL activities taught
	Function maintained
PT	Patient has increased mobility and strength
	Patient adheres to home exercise program schedule

10. Discharge plans for this patient

Patient will remain in community under MD care

When wound healed or patient able to safely provide level of care needed

Discharge when stated patient-centered goals achieved

When patient no longer homebound, will be followed up by MD

Discharge to care of family and hospice under MD supervision

Patient discharged to hospice per patient and family request

11. Patient, family, and caregiver educational needs

Educational needs are the regimens that the caregiver will be managing with the patient. These include:

Home safety assessment and teaching

Effective personal hygiene habits

The avoidance of infections

Multiple medications and their relationship to each other

The importance of medical follow up

Self-care observational aspects of care, particularly the postop wound site

Support groups in the community that are available to your patients and their caregivers

The importance of wearing a Medic Alert™ bracelet

Other information based on your patient's unique needs

The American Cancer Society has local chapters and is a resource available for your patients. The American Cancer Society can be reached at 1-800-ACS-2345, to locate the local chapter nearest you. They also sponsor such programs as "Reach for Recovery" and "I Can Cope."

There is also a "Y-Me Hot Line" that can be reached at 1-800-221-2141. This line is for women who want to talk with other women who have breast cancer.

The ACS has a "Look Good . . . Feel Better Program" that offers support and makeover services by cosmetologists for women undergoing chemotherapy or radiation therapy. Call 1-800-395-LOOK for more information.

12. **Specific tips for reimbursement**

Although these patients have appropriate psychosocial needs, make sure that your documentation reflects what the particular third-party payer or insurer perceives as "skilled" hands-on nursing care. Be sure that in addition to the needed professional support you provide, the wound care, observation and assessment, or pain management is reflected in your notes.

CANCER CARE

1. **General Considerations.** Cancer care and the generalized care of these patients is characterized by frequent contact with health care providers over a long period of time. The documentation must clearly show that the patient is homebound and requires skilled care.

   Please refer to "Breast Cancer and Mastectomy Care," "Prostate Cancer," "Brain Tumor," "IV Care," "Ostomy Care of the Patient with Pain," or "Hospice Care" should those care needs also be appropriate for your patient.

2. **Needs for initial visit**

   Specific initial physician orders
   Universal precautions supplies
   Other supplies or equipment, based on physician orders
   Vital signs equipment

3. **Some potential medical-surgical diagnoses and codes**

Adrenal cancer	194.0
Ascites, malignant	197.6
Attention to colostomy	V55.3
Attention to ileostomy	V55.2
Bladder cancer	188.9
Bone metastases	198.5
Brain cancer	191.9
Breast cancer	174.9
Cervix, cancer of	180.9
Colon cancer	153.9
Colon lymphoma	202.83
Debility	799.3
Esophagus, cancer of the	150.9
Fitting and adjustment of urinary devices	V53.6
Fracture, pathological	733.1
Gastric cancer, metastatic	151.9 and 199.1
Gastrostomy, attention to	V55.1
Head or neck, cancer of the	195.0
Hickman catheter insertion	38.98
Leukemia, acute	208.0

Leukopenia	288.0
Liver, metastatic cancer of	197.7
Lung cancer, squamous cell	162.9
Malaise and fatigue	780.7
Mastectomy, radical	85.46
Mastectomy, simple	85.42
Metastases, general	199.1
Multiple myeloma	203.0
Nasopharyngeal	147.9
Ovarian cancer	183.0
Pancreatic cancer	157.9
Pleural effusion, right or left	197.2
Pneumonia	486
Prostate, cancer of	185
Radiation enteritis	558.1
Radiation myelitis	990 and 323.8
Rectosigmoid	154.0
Rectum, cancer of the	154.1
Renal (cancer of the kidney)	189.0
Renal cell cancer, metastatic	189.0 and 199.1
Secondary malignant neoplasm breast	198.81
Spinal cord tumor	239.7
Stomach, cancer of the	151.9
Tongue, cancer of the	141.9
Tracheostomy, attention to	V55.0
Urinary tract infection	599.0
Uterine sarcoma, metastatic	179 and 199.1
Uterus, cancer of the	179

4. **Associated nursing diagnoses**

Activity intolerance
Activity intolerance, high risk for
Adjustment, impaired
Airway clearance, ineffective
Anxiety
Aspiration, high risk for
Body image disturbance
Body temperature, altered, high risk for
Bowel incontinence
Breathing pattern, ineffective
Cardiac output, decreased
Caregiver role strain
Caregiver role strain, high risk for

Constipation
Coping, ineffective family: compromised
Decisional conflict (treatments)
Denial, ineffective
Diarrhea
Family processes, altered
Fatigue
Fear
Grieving, anticipatory
Home maintenance management, impaired
Incontinence, total
Infection, high risk for
Injury, high risk for
Knowledge deficit (disease and management)
Mobility, impaired physical
Nutrition, altered: less than body requirements
Oral mucous membrane, altered
Pain
Pain, chronic
Parenting, altered
Protection, altered
Role performance, altered
Self-care deficit (specify)
Sensory/perceptual alterations (specify) (visual, auditory,
    kinesthetic, gustatory, tactile, olfactory)
Sexual dysfunction
Skin integrity, impaired
Skin integrity, impaired, high risk for
Sleep pattern disturbance
Social interaction, impaired
Spiritual distress (distress of the human spirit)
Swallowing, impaired
Thought processes, altered
Tissue integrity, impaired
Urinary elimination, altered
Urinary retention

5. **Service skills identified**

Teach family or caregiver specific care of the patient
Assess bowel regimen and implement program as needed
Assess pain, other symptoms
Teach care of the bedridden patient
Measure vital signs

Assess cardiovascular, pulmonary, and respiratory status

Assess nutrition and hydration status

Teach new pain- or symptom-control medication regimen

Diet counseling for patient with anorexia

Rectal tube for increased flatulence

Check for and remove impaction as needed

Condom catheter or indwelling catheter as indicated

Teach feeding-tube care to family

Teach caregivers symptom control and relief measures

Assess patient and family coping skills

Assess weight as ordered

Measure abdominal girth for ascites and edema, document sites, amount

Oxygen on at _____ liters per _____ (specify orders)

Assess mental status and sleep disturbance changes

Assess disease process progression

Obtain venipuncture as ordered

Teach new medications and effects

Decubitus ulcer care as indicated

Assess for fluid and electrolyte imbalance

Administer IM or sq injection for pain control

Teach catheter care to caregiver

Teach family or caregiver signs of bleeding including hematuria, bruising, etc.

Assess amount and frequency of urinary output

Teach family regarding safety

Teach patient and family about conservation of energy techniques

Observation and complete assessment of the patient with cancer of _____ (specify site/type)

Teach and observe regarding side effects of chemotherapy including constipation, anemia, fatigue, and other actions

Venipuncture q _____ (specify ordered frequency) for monitoring platelet count

RN to teach patient regarding care of irradiated skin sites

RN to provide and teach effective oral care and comfort measures

RN to weigh patient q visit

RN to teach family reading patient's need for small, high calorie and frequent meals of patient's choice

RN to assess patient's pain or other symptoms q visit to identify need for change, addition, or other plan or dose adjustment

RN to provide emotional support to patient and family

RN to evaluate the patient's bowel patterns, need for stool softeners, laxatives, dietary adjustments, and develop bowel management plan

Assess the patient's response to treatments and interventions and report changes or unfavorable responses to the physician

RN to teach patient and caregiver regarding disease process and management

Management and evaluation of the patient POC

6. **Other services indicated**

HHA	Personal care
	ADL activities
MSS	Evaluation
	Problems evaluation
	Impeding care of plan implementation
	Financial counseling
	Community resource referral(s)
OT	Evaluation
	Adaptive assistive devices
	Energy conservation techniques
	Muscle reduction
	ADLs
PT	Evaluation
	Assess home environment of patient for safety
	Teach caregiver safe transfer
	Gait training with walker
	Home exercise program
	Teach strengthening maintenance exercise program
	Teach transfer/balance exercises
S-LP	Evaluation
	Alaryngeal speech
	Swallowing disorders
	Aphasia, other communication problems
	Food texture recommendations

7. **Associated factors based on diagnosis justifying homebound status**

Bedridden

Needs maximum assistance to ambulate

Needs assistance for all activities

Lower extremity paresis, paralysis, or paraplegia
Severe arthritis
Severe pain lower back (or other site)
Impending death, dying
Mobility severely restricted due to . . .
Weakness, dizziness
Severe SOB on any activity with oxygen dependency
Severe functional limitations, including age
Patient cannot safely leave home alone

8. **Short-term goals**

RN	POC followed as instructed by RN
	Pain, other symptom control
HHA	Effective personal hygiene
	ADL assistance
MSS	POC implementation
	Problems, resources identified
OT	Patient using adaptive devices
	Patient implementing conservation of energy program or muscle reeducation skills
PT	Strengthening/maintenance program
	Increase bed mobility
	Adherence to POC
S-LP	Able to communicate, swallow safely

9. **Long-term goals**

RN	Pain and symptom control
	Patient able to care for self
	Caregiver able to care for patient
HHA	Effective personal hygiene
	ADL assistance
MSS	Community resources identified
	Problem resolution
OT	Quality of life improved through use of adaptive devices and instructions provided
PT	Improved endurance and strength
	Increased mobility
S-LP	Patient able to communicate, swallow safely and effectively

10. **Discharge plans for this patient**

Discharged when patient-centered goals achieved

Patient death at home with symptoms controlled
No longer homebound, referred to outpatient services
Remains homebound, continues to need skilled, intermittent
care
Discharged, patient needs 24-hour care

11. **Patient, family, and caregiver educational needs**

Educational needs are the regimens that the caregiver will be
managing for or with the patient. These include:

The importance of frequent handwashing and effective hygiene
The availability of adequate pain relief measures
The need for keeping records related to and assessing for
constipation
The safe use of oxygen therapy at home
The therapeutic and palliative value of nonpharmacologic
comfort measures such as positioning, massage, progressive
muscle relaxation, and other interventions of patient choice
Multiple medications and their relationships to each other
The importance of round the clock analgesia
Patient management of hair loss
The importance of medical follow up
The availability of support and hospice programs, if
appropriate
The avoidance of infections and the signs and symptoms of
infection
Other teaching specific to the patient's unique medical and
other identified needs

The American Cancer Society has support groups such as ''I
Can Cope'' and other programs. To locate the chapter nearest
your patient call 1-800-ACS-2345.

The American Cancer Society also has a ''Look Good . . .
Feel Better Program'' for women undergoing chemotherapy or
radiation. They can be reached at 1-800-395-LOOK.

12. **Specific tips for reimbursement**

Should the patient status deteriorate and increased personal
care be needed, obtain a telephone order for the increased
service noting frequency and estimating the duration.
If a Medicare patient needs daily RN visits, obtain a projected
date that the daily care will stop. (See ''Daily Care'' in Key

Home Care Definitions for an in-depth discussion on daily nursing care.)

Obtain a telephone order for all medication and plan of care changes of the medical regimen and document these in the clinical record.

Document the problems and/or exacerbation of symptoms

Document patient deterioration if this occurs

Document dehydration, dehydrating

Document unstable, not stable

Document pain, other symptom not controlled

Document status post acute episode of _____ (specify)

Document positive urine, sputum, etc. cultue; patient started on _____ (specify drug)

Document patient impacted and impaction removed manually

Document RN in frequent communication with physician regarding _____ (specify)

Document febrile at _____ , pulse change at _____ , irr, irr

Document change noted in . . .

Document body prominences red, opening

Document RN contacted physician regarding . . .

Document any changes in the POC

Document the coordination occurring based on the POC between team members. Have the multidisciplinary conference notes and phone communications reflected in the clinical record.

If an ordered service is put on hold because a patient is "too sick," reflect this in the record and obtain an MD order for that period. Otherwise, it appears that the ordered service (i.e., PT, OT, SLP, etc.) is not making visits as specified on the POC.

CARDIAC CARE

1. **General Considerations.** Home health care patients with any cardiac process, needing cardiac care, have appropriate safety concerns. The nurse in home health care needs to be specific with the next scheduled visit date and time. In addition, reassure the patient about the 24-hour on-call system and when contacting emergency community resources would be more appropriate. Often, these patients are appropriate for a personal emergency response system.

   Please refer to ''Angina'' or ''Coronary Bypass and Other Cardiac Surgical Care'' should those problems be appropriate to your patient.

2. **Needs for initial visit**

   Specific initial physician orders
   Universal precautions supplies
   Other supplies or equipment, based on physician orders
   Vital signs equipment, including a good stethoscope

3. **Some potential medical-surgical diagnoses and codes**

Angina	413.9
Angina, unstable	411.1
Atherosclerosis (coronary)	414.0
Atrial fibrillation	427.31
Atrial flutter	427.32
Cardiac dysrhythmia	427.9
Cardiac murmurs	785.2
Cardiomyopathy	425.4
Chronic ischemic heart disease	414.9
Congestive heart failure	428.0
COPD	496
Coronary atherosclerosis	414.0
Digoxin toxicity	995.2 and E942.1
Electrolyte and fluid imbalance	276.9
HCVD with CHF	402.91
Heart block	426.9
Hypertension with heart involvement	402.91
Left heart failure	428.1
Myocardial infarction	410.9

Pacemaker (S/P)	V45.0
Pericardial disease	423.9
Peripheral vascular disease	443.9
Pulmonary edema with cardiac disease	428.1
Respiratory arrest (S/P)	799.1

4. **Associated nursing diagnoses**

Activity intolerance
Activity intolerance, high risk for
Anxiety
Body image disturbance
Breathing pattern, ineffective
Cardiac output, decreased
Caregiver role strain
Caregiver role strain, high risk for
Constipation
Coping, ineffective family: compromised
Decisional conflict (treatment)
Denial, ineffective
Diversional activity deficit
Family processes, altered
Fatigue
Fear
Fluid volume excess
Gas exchange, impaired
Grieving, anticipatory
Home maintenance management, impaired
Injury, high risk for
Knowledge, deficit (disease process and management)
Management of therapeutic regimen (individual), ineffective
Mobility, impaired physical
Nutrition, altered: less than body requirements
Nutrition, altered: more than body requirements
Pain
Pain, chronic
Self-care deficit, bathing/hygiene
Self-care deficit, dressing/grooming
Self-care deficit, feeding
Self-care deficit, toileting
Sleep pattern disturbance
Spiritual distress (distress of the human spirit)
Tissue perfusion, altered (cardiopulmonary)

5. **Service skills identified**

Measure vital signs, obtain baseline
Assess lungs, cardiovascular status, including peripheral pulses
Daily weights, family to weigh patient daily
Assess for fluid retention, amount, site(s)
Venipuncture for prothrombin time, digoxin, electrolytes as
  ordered (specify ordered frequency)
Assess hydration and nutrition status
Teach new medication regimen and side effects
Teach patient or family to take pulse
Teach signs or symptoms of digoxin toxicity
Assess for orthostatic hypotension
Implement bowel regimen
Teach low sodium or other diet as indicated
Teach patient energy conservation techniques
Teach patient signs and symptoms of pacemaker problems or
  failure
Teach patient ordered exercises addressing issues of stair
  climbing, lifting, and daily rest periods as indicated
Assess for nitroglycerin use, frequency, amount, relief patterns
Assess site, amount, frequency of chest pain episodes
Observation and complete systems assessment of the patient
  with cardiac disease _____ (specify)
RN to teach care and safety regarding oxygen therapy at home
RN to instruct patient and caregiver regarding multiple
  medications, including schedule, functions, and possible side
  effects
RN to assess the patient's response to treatments and
  interventions and report changes or unfavorable responses or
  reactions to the physician
Management and evaluation of the patient POC

6. **Other services indicated**

HHA	Personal care duties
	ADL assistance
MSS	Evaluation, indicated when the patient's social problems adversely affect the response to the POC or impede the progress toward progress goals
OT	Evaluation
	Teach energy conservation techniques
PT	Evaluation
	Cardiac rehabilitation program per protocol

7. **Associated factors based on diagnosis justifying homebound status**

    Bedridden
    Chairbound
    Poor endurance S/P AMI
    Cardiac restrictions on activity
    Not to leave home for _____ weeks
    Poor respiratory status, severe SOB
    Postsurgery new pacemaker insertion
    Frail, age _____
    Requires maximum assistance to transfer or
      ambulate
    Paralysis S/P CVA
    Severe dizziness, weakness
    Bathroom privileges only
    Limited energy and endurance; dyspnea on exertion
    Angina with activity
    Severe functional limitations
    Lower extremity edema impairing ambulation
    Cannot safely leave home without assistance

8. **Short-term goals**

RN	Daily compliance with medication and treatment regimen
HHA	Effective personal hygiene
	ADL assistance
MSS	Problem identification
OT	Follows POC regimen, using techniques taught
PT	Increased and safe mobility
	Increased endurance

9. **Long-term goals**

RN	Medications regulated
	Stable cardiovascular and respiratory status
	Vital signs and blood results normal for patient range
HHA	Effective personal hygiene
	ADL assistance
MSS	Return to community
	Referred to identified resource(s)

OT	Able to do ADLs with decreased SOB
	Quality of life improved
PT	Increased and safe mobility, endurance, and strength

10. Discharge plans for this patient

Discharge when goals achieved, return to self-care status
No longer homebound, referred to outpatient services
PT discharged, self-care, under MD supervision

11. Patient, family, and caregiver educational needs

Educational needs are the regimens that the patient or caregiver will need to safely continue to care for the patient at home. These include:

The patient's medications and their relationship to each other
The importance of compliance to the regimen
The importance of medical follow up
The application of antiembolic stockings as ordered
The symptoms that would appropriately necessitate calling emergency services (specify symptoms)
The need to quit or cut down on smoking
Other teaching specific to the patient and caregiver needs

12. Specific tips for reimbursement

Document the specific care rendered and teaching instructions
Communicate any POC changes in the record
Document progress toward goals
Document any abnormal lab values
Document any medication changes
Document the specific teaching accomplished and the behavioral outcomes of that teaching
Document any learning barriers identified
Document tachycardia, bradycardia, any pulse irregularity
Document any change in respiratory status, increased respiratory rate, SOB, and so on
Document any episodes of chest pain and note the site, characteristics, reaction, and document communication to physician
The skills used most often in cardiac care are teaching, observation and assessment, and rehabilitation-focused nursing

Document the coordination that occurs based on the POC among team members. The multidisciplinary conference notes and phone communications should reflect this in the clinical record.

If an ordered service is put on hold because a patient is ''too sick,'' this should be reflected in the record and an MD order for that period should be obtained. Otherwise, it appears that the ordered service (e.g., PT, OT, S-LP, etc.) is not making visits as specified on the POC.

CATARACT AND OPHTHALMIC CARE

1. **General Considerations.** The technology associated with cataract care has changed significantly since the first edition of this book. Today, most patients are not homebound postoperatively because of the cataract surgery. However, there are unusual instances in which it may be appropriate to provide home care to a patient postcataract surgery who is homebound for other medical reasons or has postoperative complications.

2. **Needs for initial visit**

   Specific initial physician orders
   Universal precautions supplies
   Other supplies or equipment, based on physician orders
   Vital signs equipment

3. **Some potential medical-surgical diagnoses and codes**

Cataract (acquired)	366.9
Cataract extraction or excision	13.19
(with intraocular lens implant)	13.19 and 13.71
Glaucoma	365.9
States following surgery of the eye and adnexa	V45.6

4. **Associated nursing diagnoses**

   Infection, high risk for
   Injury, high risk for
   Knowledge deficit (self-care)
   Mobility, impaired physical
   Pain
   Self-care deficit, bathing/hygiene
   Self-care deficit, dressing/grooming
   Self-care deficit, feeding
   Self-care deficit, toileting
   Sensory/perceptual alterations (visual)

5. **Service skills identified**

   Assessment of baseline vital signs

Teach regarding avoidance of movements causing ocular
  pressure
Teach regarding medication regimen
Teach administration of drops or ointment regimen
Teach regarding eye care techniques
Observation and complete systems assessment of the patient
  S/P cataract surgery and _____ (specify other complicating
  medical problems)
RN to instruct patient and caregiver regarding multiple
  medications, including schedule, functions, routes, and
  possible side effects
RN to assess the patient's response to treatments and
  interventions and report changes or unfavorable responses or
  reactions to the physician
Management and evaluation of the patient POC

6. **Other services indicated**

HHA	Personal care
	ADL assistance
MSS	Evaluation
	Home assessment
	Financial counseling
	Problems impeding POC implementation
	Community resource referral(s)

7. **Associated factors based on diagnosis justifying
homebound status**

Bedrest with BRP only S/P cataract surgery
Restricted to home for _____ weeks
Medically restricted to home S/P ophthalmologic
  surgery
Restricted activity
Blind, cannot safely leave home alone

8. **Short-term goals**

RN	Patient able to administer ointment or medication regimen
	Adherence to POC
HHA	Effective personal hygiene
	ADL assistance
MSS	Problem, resource(s) identification

9. **Long-term goals**

RN	Stable cardiac/other systems
	Infection-free
	Patient self-care
HHA	Effective personal hygiene
	ADL assistance
MSS	Problem resolution or community referral(s) as indicated

10. **Discharge plans for this patient**

Discharge, self-care, when no longer homebound or in need of further skilled services

Refer to outpatient service

Continue home care visits to patient who remains homebound due to _____ and requires skilled care

Patient discharged to self-care management under no supervision

11. **Patient, family, and caregiver educational needs**
Educational needs are the care regimens that the patient or caregiver will need to know to safely continue the care at home. These include:

The patient's medications and their relationship to each other

Patient safety concerns postop eye surgery

The importance of compliance to the medical regimens

Other teaching specific to the patient or caregiver needs

12. **Specific tips for reimbursement**

Communicate any POC changes in the clinical record and obtain orders for those changes

Decrease visit frequency as appropriate to documentation and patient status

Document the skilled service provided

Document the specific teaching accomplished and the behavioral outcomes of that teaching

Document the specific care provided

Keep in mind that for Medicare patients, page 14.16 of the HHA Manual Revision 222 states that "the administration of eye drops and topical ointments does not require the skills of a licensed nurse." This paragraph goes on to say that "this section does not eliminate coverage for skilled nursing visits for observation and assessment for the beneficiary's condition.''

Review the discussion in the HIM-11 under ''Observation and Assessment of Patient's Condition When Only the Specialized Skills of a Medical Professional Can Determine a Patient's Status.'' Example number 5 illustrates the kind of cataract patient that may be appropriate for skilled services, based on the patient's unique medical condition and other factors. This is located on pages 14.9-14.11 of Revision 222, which is located in Part Seven.

There may be other processes that occur in conjunction with the eye surgery. These may necessitate the skills of observation and assessment, management and evaluation of the POC, teaching and training activities, and other skilled nursing interventions.

If care is provided to a patient with the cataract as the principle diagnoses (i.e., the reason the care is being provided), the documentation must clearly state the other medical problems or complications that justify the care.

CATHETER CARE

1. **General Considerations.** Catheter care is routinely indicated in home care. Patients with catheters sometimes have the following problems:

   Constipation and resulting pressure on the bladder
   A urinary infection, catheter position change, or the need for a different size or kind of catheter
   Bladder spasms that can occur after catheter change
   Increased sediment, sometimes indicating need for bladder irrigation
   Catheter draining, but leaking apparent also
   Other catheter problems based on their unique history

2. **Needs for initial visit**

   Specific initial physician orders
   Universal precautions supplies
   Other supplies or equipment, based on physician orders
   Vital signs equipment
   Urinary specimen cup

3. **Some potential medical-surgical diagnoses and codes**

Attention to other artificial opening of urinary tract	V55.4
Bladder atony	596.4
Bladder repair	57.89
CVA	436
Decubitus ulcer	707.0
Fitting and adjustment of urinary devices	V53.6
Hematuria	599.7
Hypertension	401.9
Indwelling foley catheter	57.94
Neurogenic bladder	596.5
Suprapubic tube	57.19
Urinary incontinence	788.3
Urinary infection	599.0
Urinary retention	788.2

4. **Associated nursing diagnoses**

   Body image disturbance

Constipation
Constipation, perceived
Incontinence, total
Infection, high risk for
Injury, high risk for
Mobility, impaired physical
Pain
Pain, chronic
Self-care deficit, toileting
Sexual dysfunction
Sexuality patterns, altered
Skin integrity, impaired, potential
Spiritual distress (distress of the human spirit)
Urinary elimination, altered
Urinary retention

5. **Service skills identified**

Change catheter number _____ French _____ cc q month
Evaluate the patient for catheter complaints, contact physician
Obtain UA/C & S if symptoms of infection are present
Maintain hydration fluid volumes as indicated
Irrigate catheter with 30 cc NSS prn per physician order
Teach family indwelling catheter care, irrigation of catheter,
    S/S UTI, adequate hydration, skin care, change of ordinary
    drainage bag
Teach family removal of catheter with syringe, bag change,
    and care of bags
Assess amount, frequency urinary drainage, intake, and output
Maintain skin integrity, teach care of the immobilized patient
    if indicated
Teach family awareness of reason for catheter (e.g.,
    retention)
Observation and complete systems assessment of the patient
    with an indwelling catheter
RN to change catheter every 4 weeks and prn for catheter
    problems, including patient complaints, signs and symptoms
    of infection, or other factors necessitating evaluation and
    possible catheter change
RN to assess the patient's response to treatments and
    interventions and report changes or unfavorable responses or
    reactions to the physician
Management and evaluation of the patient POC

6. **Other services indicated**

    HHA   Personal care duties
                ADL assistance

7. **Associated factors based on diagnosis justifying homebound status**

Patient needs maximum assistance to ambulate, bedridden, bedbound, wheelchair bound
Quadriplegia, hemiplegia, lower extremity paresis, or paralysis
Severe weakness, unsteady gait
Poor endurance, limited mobility
Activity medically restricted
Severe SOB
Below knee amputation or above knee amputation
Needs maximum assistance to transfer
Severe arthritis
Patient cannot safely leave home without assistance

8. **Short-term goals**

    RN   Daily compliance with catheter care
                Patent catheter, no skin breakdown
                Decrease risk of urinary infection
    HHA   Effective personal hygiene
                ADL assistance

9. **Long-term goals**

    RN   Family or patient able to maintain catheter
                Patent catheter, no skin breakdown
                Infection-free
                Teach regarding complications of immobility
                Family independent to change bags, irrigation, and Foley removal
    HHA   Effective personal hygiene
                ADL assistance

10. **Discharge plans for this patient**

Home care with visits teaching the family to care for the catheter
Bladder training regimen without catheter
Catheter removal

Patient continuing to need catheter changes by home health
  nurse, as patient remains homebound
Remains home under MD care

11. **Patient, family, and caregiver educational needs**
   Educational needs are the care regimens that the family or
   caregivers need to know to safely provide care to the
   patient. These include:

   The patient's medications and their relationship to each other
   The importance of compliance to the medical regimen and
     follow up
   The symptoms of a urinary tract or other infection that
     necessitate calling the RN or MD
   Skin care and hygiene regimens in the patient with an
     indwelling catheter
   Safety issues that the caregiver needs to be aware of in safely
     caring for the homebound patient
   Other specific teaching as needed based on the patient's
     unique medical condition and the caregiver's needs

12. **Specific tips for reimbursement**

   Document the actions of your care
   On POC, specify frequency of visits and duration of
     certification period
   Obtain a telephone order for any POC change or additional
     prn visits that were needed, and specify why
   Document your catheter supplies including type and size on
     the form 485
   Document color, appearance of urine, urine C&S results in
     your clinical documentation
   Document the continuing need for personal care services of
     the home health aide
   Implement new or changed POC, teach or communicate to the
     patient or family, and document in the clinical record
   Document specific teaching needs, teaching accomplished, and
     the behavioral outcomes of that teaching
   Document any medical changes that occurred during the past
     certification period and obtain orders for these medications
   Document the last catheter insertion date, the ordered
     frequency of change (if more frequent than one time per
     month; specify why).

CELLULITIS

1. **General Considerations.** Cellulitis, often in conjunction with osteomyelitis and peripheral vascular disease, is a common diagnosis in home health care. Frequently, these patients need antibiotic therapy, as well as dressing changes and observation and assessment skills regarding the extent of the infection.

   Please refer to "Peripheral Vascular Disease," "IV Care," "Wound Care," or "Decubitis Ulcer" if those problems are also appropriate for your patient.

2. **Needs for initial visit**

   Specific initial physician orders
   Universal precautions supplies
   Other supplies or equipment, based on physician orders
   Vital signs equipment
   Dressing supplies or solution as ordered

3. **Some potential medical-surgical diagnoses and codes**

Amputation, infected right or left BKA, AKA	997.62
Amputation, transmetatarsal (right or left)	84.12
Arterial graft, S/P	39.58
Arterial insufficiency	447.1
Bullous pemphigoid	694.5
Cellulitis of the arm	682.3
Cellulitis of the trunk	682.2
Cellulitis RLE, LLE	682.6
Chronic ischemic heart disease	414.9
Congestive heart failure	428.0
Coronary artery disease	414.0
Debridement right or left BKA, AKA	86.22
Decubitus ulcer	707.0
Diabetes mellitus, with complications, adult	250.90
Diabetes mellitus, with complications, juv.	250.91
Diabetic neuropathy	250.60 and 357.2

Diabetic retinopathy	250.50 and 362.01
Femoral-popliteal bypass (right or left)	39.29
Foot abscess	682.7
Gangrene, toe	785.4
Hypertension	401.9
I and D stitch abscess	86.04 and 998.5
Leg injury	959.7
Osteomyelitis lower leg, right or left	730.06
Osteomyelitis of foot	730.07
Peripheral vascular disease	443.9
Skin eruption	782.1
Skin, excoriation of	919.8
Skin graft	86.69
Staph infection	041.1
Stasis ulcer	454.2
Stitch abscess, excision	998.5 and 86.22
Thrombophlebitis	451.9
Ulcer, heel with cellulitis	682.7
Ulcer right or left heel	707.1
Varicose leg ulcer	454.2
Vascular insufficiency	459.9
Vascular shunt bypass	32.29
Venous insufficiency	459.81
Wound, open lower leg (right or left)	891.1
Wound, open upper leg (right or left)	890.1

4. **Associated nursing diagnoses**

Activity intolerance
Activity intolerance, high risk for
Adjustment, impaired
Anxiety
Body image disturbance
Body temperature, altered, high risk for
Cardiac output, decreased
Caregiver role strain
Caregiver role strain, high risk for
Coping, ineffective individual
Fatigue
Fear
Home maintenance management, impaired
Infection, high risk for
Injury, high risk for

Knowledge deficit (care regimen)
Mobility, impaired physical
Noncompliance (self-care regimen)
Nutrition altered: less than body requirements
Nutrition altered: more than body requirements
Pain
Pain, chronic
Role performance, altered
Self-care deficit, bathing/hygiene
Self-care deficit, dressing/grooming
Self-care deficit, feeding
Self-care deficit, toileting
Sensory/perceptual alterations (tactile)
Skin integrity, impaired
Social interaction, impaired
Tissue integrity, impaired
Tissue perfusion, altered (peripheral)

5. **Service skills identified**

Dressing change _____ site, per physician orders
Wash site gently and dry
Teach new antibiotic regimen of _____
Evaluate temperature, redness of site, amount of swelling
Assess for signs of decreased circulation and report to
    physician
Evaluate healing process
To keep leg elevated at all times
To keep leg elevated when sitting
To wear Ace™ wrap or TED whenever ''up''
Skilled observation and all systems assessment of patient with
    cellulitis of _____ (specify site)
Observation and evaluation of wound, teach wound care,
    provide wound care
Assess the patient's response to treatments and interventions
    and report changes or unfavorable responses or reactions to
    the physician
Management and evaluation of the patient POC
Observe for healing, infection
Culture open wound as ordered, send for culture and
    sensitivity
Assess hydration and nutritional status
Instruct patient or caregiver on dressing change procedures
Assess peripheral circulation

Check pedal pulses

Assess amount, site(s) of edema

Medicate patient with ordered pain medication prior to dressing change

Assess pain, site, frequency, duration

Teach new medication regimen

Measure vital signs

Teach effective personal hygiene and proper handwashing techniques

Teach signs and symptoms (further) of infection

Teach sterile or prescribed dressing techniques

Teach protocol for disposal of soiled dressings and supplies

6. **Other services indicated**

HHA	Personal care
	ADL assistance
MSS	Evaluation
	Home safety assessment
	Financial counseling
	Problems with POC implementation
	Community resource referral

7. **Associated factors based on diagnosis justifying homebound status**

Weakness and no or decreased weight bearing

Limited activity due to leg wound

Medical restrictions, leg to be elevated

Heel wound, poor ambulation

Patient requires maximum assistance to ambulate

Unable to transfer without maximum assistance

Chairbound or bedbound

Pain

Open, infected wound

Surgical restriction S/P surgery

Open, draining leg lesions

Severe arthritis

Patient cannot safely leave home without assistance

Morbid obesity (specific height, weight)

Pain or other symptoms

Multiple functional limitations including _____

Poor ambulation with frequent or history of falls

8. **Short-term goals**

RN	Daily compliance with POC
	Pain control
HHA	Effective personal hygiene
	ADL assistance
MSS	Problem, resources identification

9. **Long-term goals**

RN	Return to prior self-care status
	Wound site(s) healed
	Infection-free, patient compliance with regimen(s)
HHA	Effective personal hygiene
	ADL assistance
MSS	Community referral(s), as indicated
	Returned to self-care status

10. **Discharge plans for this patient**

Discharge, self-care, when no longer homebound or in need of skilled services
Referred to outpatient services
Continue home health visits of patient who remains homebound and requires skilled care
Remain home with MD supervision

11. **Patient, family, and caregiver educational needs**

Educational needs are the regimens that the caregiver will be managing with the patient. These include:

Home safety assessment and counseling
The avoidance of injury or infection to compromised skin sites
The importance of medical follow up
Self-care observational aspects of care, particularly the affected site(s)
Signs and symptoms that necessitate calling the MD
Support groups in the community that are available to patients and caregivers
Teach patient and caregiver all aspects of care related to wound, including effective handwashing and other infection control measures
Teach patient about all medications, including schedule, route, functions, and possible side effects

Other aspects of care that are based on your patient's unique medical condition and needs

12. **Specific tips for reimbursement**

Document the wound, indicate size, drainage, color, amount, and the specific care provided

Communicate any POC changes in the documentation

Document progress in wound healing or deterioration in wound status and measure in progress notes

Document your supplies needed on the form 485 and obtain the specific orders

Decrease visit frequency as appropriate

When appropriate, take photograph(s) to substantiate documentation at onset and every 3 weeks, have patient sign release; one photograph for the clinical records

If wound culture is obtained, document the results

Document any barriers to learning

Document if patient or family member unable to do dressing (retinopathy, severity of wound, and so on)

Document the specific teaching accomplished and the behavioral outcomes of that teaching

Document patient's level of independence in care

Wound care is an area in which some managed-care companies and other payers are decreasing reimbursable visits. It is the professional nurse's responsibility to remember that it is not just the dressing change that occurs. When a nurse makes the home visit, there is an assessment of the wound healing or deterioration and teaching. These skills usually require the skills of a nurse. All of these components contribute to safe, effective wound care.

For daily wound care under Medicare, please refer to Part Seven for key home care definitions. Also, see pages 318–319.

CEREBRAL VASCULAR ACCIDENT

1. **General Considerations.** Because of the high prevalence of hypertension, cerebral vascular accident, or stroke, continues to be a leading cause of illness and death. This patient population usually has rehabilitative goals in the home setting.

    Please refer to "Care of the Bedbound Patient," "Decubitus Ulcer," "Catheter Care," or "Myocardial Infarction" should those problems be appropriate for your patient.

2. **Needs for initial visit**

    Specific initial physician orders
    Universal precautions supplies
    Other supplies or equipment, based on physician orders
    Vital signs equipment

3. **Some potential medical-surgical diagnoses and codes**

AMI	410.9
Angina	413.9
Aphasia	784.3
Atrial fibrillation	427.31
Catheter, indwelling	57.94
CHF	428.0
COPD	496
CVA	436
CVA with dysphasia	436 and 787.2
Decubitus ulcer	707.0
Diabetes mellitus, with complications, adult	250.90
Diabetes mellitus, with complications, juv.	250.91
Dysphasia	784.5
Emphysema	492.8
Heart disease, chronic ischemic	414.9
Hemiplegia or hemiparesis	436 and 342.9
Hypertension	401.9
Hypertension, accelerated	401.0
Hypertensive nephrosclerosis	403.9
Incontinence of feces	787.6
Incontinence of urine	788.3
Left heart failure	428.1

Pneumonia	486
Quadriplegia	436 and 344.0
TIA	435.9
Urinary retention	788.2
Urinary tract infection	599.0

4. **Associated nursing diagnoses**

Activity intolerance
Airway clearance, ineffective
Anxiety
Aspiration, high risk for
Body image disturbance
Body temperature, altered, high risk for
Bowel incontinence
Breathing pattern, ineffective
Cardiac output, decreased
Caregiver role strain
Caregiver role strain, high risk for
Communication, impaired verbal
Constipation
Coping, family: potential for growth
Coping, ineffective family: compromised
Coping, ineffective family: disabling
Coping, ineffective individual
Denial, ineffective
Disuse syndrome, high risk for
Diversional activity deficit
Family processes, altered
Fatigue
Fear
Fluid volume deficit, high risk for
Fluid volume excess
Gas exchange, impaired
Home maintenance management, impaired
Hopelessness
Incontinence, total
Infection, high risk for
Injury, high risk for
Knowledge deficit (care regimen)
Mobility, impaired physical
Nutrition, altered: less than body requirements
Oral mucous membrane, altered
Pain

Pain, chronic
Powerlessness
Role performance, altered
Self-care deficit, bathing/hygiene
Self-care deficit, dressing/grooming
Self-care deficit, feeding
Self-care deficit, toileting
Sensory/perceptual alterations (specify) (visual, auditory,
    kinesthetic, gustatory, tactile, olfactory)
Sexuality patterns, altered
Skin integrity, impaired
Skin integrity, impaired, high risk for
Social interaction, impaired
Spiritual distress (distress of the human spirit)
Swallowing, impaired
Thought processes, altered
Tissue integrity, impaired
Tissue perfusion, altered (specify type) (renal, cerebral,
    cardiopulmonary, gastrointestinal, peripheral)
Unilateral neglect
Urinary elimination, altered
Urinary retention

5. **Service skills identified**

Skilled assessment and observation of all systems of the
    patient S/P CVA
Evaluation
Measure vital signs
Assess nutrition and hydration status
Teach new medication regimen
Assess for side effects of new medication regimen
Teach family or caregiver care of the immobilized or
    bedridden patient
Assess neurological status
Check for and remove fecal impactions prn, per physician
    orders
Assess respiratory, cardiovascular status, other systems
Teach family or caregiver re: oxygen therapy, utilization and
    associated safety information
Implement bowel and bladder training regimen
Teach family or caregiver about feeding tubes or pumps
Venipuncture(s) as ordered q _____
Assess safety in home and counsel family re: safety

RN to change catheter (specify type, size) q _____ (specify ordered frequency)

Observe and monitor for neurological deficits

RN to assess the patient's response to ordered interventions and treatments and report changes or unfavorable responses or reactions to the MD

Management and evaluation of the patient POC

6. **Other services indicated**

HHA	Personal care
	ADL assistance
	Home exercise program assistance
MSS	Assessment of social and emotional factors
	Counseling
	Financial assistance
	Nursing home placement assistance
	Arrange for meal program(s)
	Assess home situation
	Home safety evaluation
OT	Evaluation of patient and home for safety
	ADL training program
	Muscle reeducation
	Body image training
	Increased right and left upper extremity strength
	Independent bathing or other ADLs
	Teach alternative bathing for safety
	Dressing, feeding skills
	Assistive device evaluation
	ADL retraining, especially feeding, cognitive, perceptual skills
	Teach ADL techniques
	Independent homemaking skills
	Therapeutic exercise to right or left hand to increase strength, coordination, proprioception, and sensation
PT	Evaluation
	Therapeutic exercise regimen
	Teach regarding transfer training
	Gait training with assistive device
	Teach home maintenance program
	Strengthening exercises
	Gait training with walker or other assistive device
	Chest physiotherapy program

Passive exercise regimen
Active exercise regimen
Muscle reeducation
Preprosthetic training
Proprioceptive neuromuscular facilitation (PNF)
Prosthetic training including prosthesis training
    program
Whirlpool treatment
Home exercise program for strengthening,
    endurance, and mobility
Bed mobility program
Assess home environment for safe accessibility
    with walker, wheelchair

S-LP Evaluation
Alaryngeal speech
Language processing
Speech and voice
Aural rehabilitation program
Safe swallowing evaluation
Speech dysphagia instruction program
Continue therapy to increase articulation,
    proficiency, verbal expression
Lip, tongue, and facial exercises to improve
    swallowing and vocal skills
Word fluency exercises
Food texture recommendations
Short-term memory skills
Implement functional writing skills program
Establish home maintenance program

7. **Associated factors based on diagnosis justifying
homebound status**

Residual weakness S/P CVA, AMI
Age 90, gastric tube, Foley catheter
Right or left hemiplegia or hemiparesis
Needs assistance for all activities
Requires maximum assistance to ambulate
Quadriplegia
S/P CVA with paralysis
Decubitus right buttock, nasogastric tube
Bedbound or bedridden
Wheelchair dependent
Dependent for all care S/P CVA

Total right, left hemiplegia
Poor balance, unsafe to walk
Patient unable to ambulate
Severe weakness S/P CVA
Patient also has COPD, 90° temperature outside (also high
  humidity)
Patient is nonweight bearing per physician orders
Confusion, unable to go out of home alone
Patient unable to safely leave home unassisted

8. Short-term goals

RN	Daily implementation of POC
HHA	Effective personal hygiene
	ADL assistance
MSS	Problem identification and patient or family able to implement POC
	Crisis or problem resolution
OT	Daily implementation of exercise regimen
	PT using assistive or adaptive equipment
PT	Daily implementation of POC
	Increased safe mobility
S-LP	Daily adherence to speech instruction or program
	Patient able to communicate
	Safe swallowing

9. Long-term goals

RN	Blood pressure in normal for patient range
	Bowel or bladder regimen implemented and function returns
	Adherence to nursing and medical regimen(s)
	Optimal function S/P CVA
HHA	Effective personal hygiene
	ADL assistance
MSS	Identified problem resolution
	Community resource referral(s)
OT	Patient safely using assistive devices for ADLs
	Increased strength
	Independent ADLs
	Maximum function of affected hand or extremity
PT	Ambulation, independent or with assistive device
	Optimal strength, balance, or endurance
	Patient/family using home exercises

S-LP	Functional communication
	Maximum verbal communication
	Increased short-term memory function
	Improved safe swallowing skills, speech and strength of oral-motor movements

10. Discharge plans for this patient

Discharged, no longer homebound, referred for outpatient speech-language pathology, occupational, physical therapy services

Remains homebound, in need of skilled care

Discharged to acute care facility for 24-hour care

Nursing home placement

Discharged, goals achievement

Discharged from home care, under MD supervision

11. Patient, family, and caregiver educational needs

Educational needs are the regimens that the caregiver will be managing with the patient. These include:

Catheter and wound care regimen

Effective personal hygiene, including effective handwashing techniques and safe disposal of soiled dressings/linens

Safety measures in the home

The home exercise program

The avoidance of infection

The medication program and their relationship to each other

The importance of medical follow up

When to call the home health program or the physician

The importance of and all aspects of effective skin care regimens to prevent breakdown. Include the need for frequent position changes, proper body alignment, pressure pads or mattresses, and other measures for prevention

Other information based on the patient's unique medical and other needs

12. Specific tips for reimbursement

Often the diagnosis of CVA indicates multiple identifiable nursing needs. These include: an indwelling catheter, a new medication regimen, hypertension or a gastric tube. The focus of the rehabilitative services includes PT, OT, and S-

LP. When coordinating these services, be aware of the following:

For each service, there will usually be a corresponding diagnosis: (S-LP, aphasia; PT, hemiplegia). The date of onset should be fairly recent to the home care program implementation. For example, if the patient had a CVA some months ago, this would usually not be a covered service unless documentation could clearly show the circumstances. In addition, rehabilitation is for restoring function and the implementation of a safe maintenance home exercise program.

Document that the patient continues to be homebound and why

Document conference(s) with the S-LP, OT, PT, or other services

Document the specific skill as clearly as possible

Document any change in the patient's condition

Document continued need for home health aide due to inability to do ADLs, personal hygiene

Document progress toward predetermined, patient-centered goals

When multiple services are involved, it is important to document the coordination occurring based on the POC between all team members. The multidisciplinary conference notes should reflect this in the clinical record. Also, refer to the meeting with other professional associate team members in your visit record.

If any service, such as PT, has to be put on hold because the patient is "too sick," this should be reflected in the record and an MD order for that period should be obtained. Otherwise, it appears that the PT is not making visits as ordered on the POC.

CHRONIC OBSTRUCTIVE PULMONARY DISEASE

1. **General Considerations.** In home health care, chronic obstructive pulmonary disease is a common diagnosis. Often, the acute diagnosis is emphysema, pneumonia, tuberculosis, or bronchitis.

   Please refer to ''Asthma,'' ''Cancer Care,'' or ''Pneumonia'' if those problems are appropriate for your patient.

2. **Needs for initial visit**

   Specific initial physician orders
   Universal precautions supplies, per agency protocol
   Other supplies or equipment, based on physician orders
   Vital signs equipment

3. **Some potential medical-surgical diagnoses and codes**

Airway obstruction, chronic	496
Asthma	493.90
Bronchitis	466.0
Chronic ischemic heart disease	414.9
Congestive heart failure	428.0
COPD	496
Cor pulmonale	415.0
Dehydration	276.5
Emphysema	492.8
Hemoptysis	786.3
Interstitial emphysema	770.2
Left heart failure	428.1
Lung cancer	162.9
Lung disease	518.8
Peripheral vascular disease	443.9
Pleural effusion	511.9
Pneumonia	486
Respirator, dependence	V46.1
Respiratory failure	518.81
Tracheal bronchus disease	519.1
Tuberculosis (lung)	011.90

4. **Associated nursing diagnoses**

Activity intolerance
Airway clearance, ineffective
Anxiety
Aspiration, high risk for
Body temperature, altered, high risk for
Breathing pattern, ineffective
Caregiver role strain
Caregiver role strain, high risk for
Fatigue
Fear
Fluid volume deficit, high risk for
Fluid volume excess
Gas exchange, impaired
Home maintenance management, impaired
Infection, high risk for
Injury, high risk for
Knowledge deficit (self-care management and disease process)
Management of therapeutic regimen (individuals), ineffective
Mobility, impaired physical
Noncompliance (specify)
Nutrition, altered: less than body requirements
Oral mucous membrane, altered
Pain
Pain, chronic
Self-care deficit, bathing/hygiene
Self-care deficit, dressing/grooming
Self-care deficit, feeding
Self-care deficit, toileting
Sexuality patterns, altered
Sleep pattern disturbance
Social interaction, impaired
Spiritual distress (distress of the human spirit)
Swallowing, impaired

5. **Service skills identified**

Evaluate lung sounds, assess amount, site(s) wheezing,
   rhonchi, etc.
Teach patient or caregiver new medication regimen
Teach patient or caregiver to identify and avoid specific
   factors that precipitate an exacerbation (attack)

Teach patient or caregiver what to do regarding an impending episode

Teach patient or caregiver how to administer injections as indicated

Teach patient or caregiver how to utilize aerosol inhalers or treatments at home

Teach regarding safe oxygen or nebulizer therapy utilization in the home setting

Assess nutritional status

Assess hydration status

Assess for signs, symptoms of CHF

Assess vital signs

Teach ordered diet regimen of _____

Evaluate sites, amount of edema

Obtain sputum culture as indicated

Venipuncture as ordered q _____

Assess coping skills

Assess respiratory, cardiovascular status

Teach conservation of energy measures

Assess need for chest PT

Skilled evaluation and all systems assessment of the patient with COPD

RN to teach patient conservation of energy techniques and controlled breathing exercises

Teach patient effective coughing and deep breathing, pursed lip or diaphragmatic breathing

Ongoing skilled observation and assessment of wheezing, cough, dyspnea, shortness of breath, and other symptoms

Provide emotional support to patient and family of patient with chronic illness

RN to assess patient's response to ordered treatments and interventions and report changes or unfavorable responses or reactions to the physician

Management and evaluation of the patient's POC

6. **Other services indicated**

HHA	Personal care
	ADL assistance
MSS	Evaluation
	Problem evaluation impeding POC implementation
	Financial counseling
	Community resource referral(s)

	Assess long-term needs of patient after excerbation, pulmonary rehabilitation
OT	Evaluation and ADL assessment
	Conservation of energy technique
	Adaptive assistive devices as indicated
PT	Patient evaluation
	Assess home environment for safety
	Therapeutic exercise regimen to condition and strengthen
	Safe transfers
	Gait training with assistive device
	Teach breathing exercises
	Teach postural drainage techniques

7. **Associated factors based on diagnosis justifying homebound status**

Severe weakness
Unsteady ambulation
Frail, needs assistance to ambulate
Severe SOB
Bedridden
Wheelchair dependent
Paraplegia, paralysis, paresis
Requires maximum assistance to ambulate
Medical restriction, leg to be elevated
SOB on exertion
SOB on talking
Respiratory distress with any movement or talking
Oxygen dependence
S/P CVA, S/P TIA
Patient unable to safely leave home without assistance or assistive device

8. **Short-term goals**

RN	Daily adherence to POC
	Improved oxygen exchange
	Decreased SOB
HHA	Effective personal hygiene
	ADL assistance
MSS	Crisis or problem intervention
	POC implementation
OT	Conservation of energy skills used

PT	Increased mobility, function, strength, balance
	Optimal independence

9. Long-term goals

RN	Improved oxygen exchange
	Improved color
	Adequate hydration and nutrition
	Stable respiratory status for patient
	Clear lung sounds
	Afebrile
	Patient self-care or family able to manage patient
HHA	Effective personal hygiene
	ADL assistance
MSS	Problem identification on referral(s) to community programs
OT	Functional mobility
	Safe ADLs
PT	Functional ambulation
	Return to mobility

10. Discharge plans for this patient

Discharged when goals achieved
No longer homebound, referred to outpatient services
Remains homebound, continues to need skilled care

11. Patient, family, and caregiver educational needs

Educational needs are the care regimens that the caregiver will be managing with the patient. These include:

Skin care regimens
Effective personal hygiene habits
Safety measures in the home
The avoidance of infections
The patient's medications and their relationship to each other
Temperature checking and reading
The importance of medical follow up
When to call the home health agency or the physician
Teach patient and caregiver regarding prednisone or other steroid treatment and side effects
Safe, effective inhaler or metered dose unit use
Safe, effective oxygen therapy use at home
The importance of diet, rest, and exercise

The need to decrease, or quit smoking, when possible
Other teaching specific to the patient and caregiver's unique
    medical and other identified needs

12. **Specific tips for reimbursement**

Document all medication changes on the clinical record
    medications sheet and obtain MD's orders for same
Document all abnormalities including fever, tachycardia, rales,
    wheezing, rhonchi, etc. on the next form 486
Document the instability of the patient
Document any edema, SOB, medication reaction, further acute
    episodes, pulse irregularities
Obtain a telephone order to increase the visit frequency and
    document in the clinical record
Often, these patients have other medical problems, specifically
    cardiac, that impede progress; document these problems also
Document any changes, including specific care provided
Document medications changed or medications being regulated
Document RN contacted physician regarding _____
Document new onset (any problem)
Document positive culture, patient started on _____ in the
    clinical record (specify)

CONGESTIVE HEART FAILURE

1. **General Considerations.** Patients with any cardiac process, including congestive heart failure, have appropriate safety concerns. The nurse needs to be specific with the visit, date, and time scheduled. In addition, reassure the patient about the 24-hour on-call system and when emergency community personnel would be more appropriate to be contacted. In home health, the episodes of CHF are usually an acute process or an exacerbation of CHF postacute hospitalization.

2. **Needs for initial visit**

   Specific initial physician orders
   Universal precautions supplies
   Other supplies or equipment, based on physician orders
   Vital signs equipment

3. **Some potential medical-surgical diagnoses and codes**

Angina	413.9
Angina, unstable	411.1
Aortic stenosis	424.1
Atherosclerosis (coronary)	414.0
Atrial fibrillation	427.31
Atrial flutter	427.32
Cardiac dysrhythmia	427.9
Cardiac murmurs	785.2
Cardiomyopathy	425.4
Chronic ischemic heart disease	414.9
Congestive heart failure	428.0
COPD	496
Coronary atherosclerosis	414.0
Digoxin toxicity	995.2 and E942.1
Edema	782.3
Electrolyte and fluid imbalance	276.9
HCVD with CHF	402.91
Heart block	426.9
Hypertension with heart involvement	402.91
Left heart failure	428.1
Lung edema, acute	518.4
Mitral valve prolapse	424.0
Myocardial infarction	410.9

Pacemaker (S/P)	V45.0
Pericardial disease	423.9
Peripheral vascular disease	443.9
Pleural effusion	511.9
Pneumonia	486
Pulmonary edema with cardiac disease	428.1
Respiratory arrest (S/P)	799.1

4. **Associated nursing diagnoses**

Activity intolerance
Activity intolerance, high risk for
Anxiety
Body image disturbance
Breathing pattern, ineffective
Cardiac output, decreased
Caregiver role strain
Caregiver role strain, high risk for
Constipation
Coping, ineffective family: compromised
Decisional conflict (treatment)
Denial, ineffective
Diversional activity deficit
Family processes, altered
Fatigue
Fear
Fluid volume excess
Gas exchange impaired
Grieving, anticipatory
Home maintenance management, impaired
Injury, high risk for
Knowledge deficit (disease process and management)
Mobility, impaired physical
Nutrition, altered: less than body requirements
Nutrition, altered: more than body requirements
Pain
Pain, chronic
Self-care deficit (specify)
Sexual dysfunction
Skin integrity, impaired, high risk for
Sleep pattern disturbance
Spiritual distress (distress of the human spirit)

Tissue perfusion, altered (specify type) (renal, cerebral, cardiopulmonary, gastrointestinal, peripheral)
Urinary elimination, altered

5. Service skills identified

Observation and complete systems assessment of the patient with cardiac disease _____ (specify)
Assess lungs, cardiovascular status
Measure vital signs
Assess for fluid retention, amount, site(s)
Daily weights, family to weigh patient daily
Assess hydration, nutrition status
Teach regarding new medication regimen and side effects
Venipuncture for digoxin, electrolytes, protime levels
   q _____ (specify ordered frequency)
Teach patient or family to take pulse
Assess for orthostatic hypotension
Assess for SOB, dyspnea
RN to teach care and safety regarding oxygen therapy at home
RN to instruct patient and caregiver regarding multiple medications, including schedule, functions, knowledge, compliance, and possible side effects
RN to observe for signs and symptoms dig toxicity, including GI symptoms such as vomiting or nausea, visual disturbances, headache, etc.
RN to teach conservation of energy skills
RN to monitor for presence and amount of lower leg edema
Teach patient or caregiver record keeping for daily weights and other aspects of self-observational care skills
RN to assess the patient's response to treatments and interventions and report changes or unfavorable responses or reactions to the physician
Management and evaluation of the patient POC

6. Other services indicated

HHA   Personal care duties
          ADL assistance
MSS   Indicate when the patient's social problems
          adversely impact the POC implementation

7. Associated factors based on diagnosis justifying homebound status

Bedridden
Chairbound
Needs maximum assistance to ambulate
SOB
Cardiac restrictions
Limited energy, endurance, and DOE
Angina in activity
Severe functional limitations
Weakness due to age, illness, activity
S/P AMI
Poor respiratory status, severe SOB
Lower extremity edema impairing ambulation
Oxygen dependence
Patient needs assistance to safely leave home

8. Short-term goals

RN	Daily compliance with medication and treatment regimens
	Stable cardiovascular status
HHA	Effective personal hygiene
	ADL assistance
MSS	Problems and resources identified

9. Long-term goals

RN	Medications regulated
	Stable cardiovascular and respiratory status
	Vital signs, digoxin, electrolytes in normal for patient range
HHA	Effective personal hygiene
	ADL assistance
MSS	Return to community
	Problem resolution

10. Discharge plans for this patient

Discharged when patient-centered goals achieved
No longer homebound, referred to outpatient services
Discharge to self-care, under MD supervision

11. Patient, family, and caregiver educational needs

Educational needs are the regimens that the patient or caregiver will need to safely continue to care for the patient at home. These include:

The patient's medication and their relationship to each other
The importance of compliance to the regimen
The importance of medical follow up
Effective use of oxygen, including use, liter flow, and safety
The application of antiembolic stockings as ordered
The symptoms that would appropriately necessitate calling
   emergency services (specify symptoms)
The need to quit or cut down on smoking
Other teaching specific to the patient and caregiver needs

12. **Specific tips for reimbursement**

Document the specific care and teaching instructions rendered
Communicate any treatment plan change in the documentation
Document progress toward goals
Document any abnormal lab values
Document any medication changes

CORONARY BYPASS AND OTHER CARDIAC SURGICAL CARE

1. **General Considerations.**   Recent studies show that more elderly persons die of cardiovascular problems than of any other single cause. In fact, one of every two adults over the age of 65 has heart disease, and 70% of all persons who die of cardiovascular diseases are older than 65. Many of these elderly patients have had bypass or other cardiac surgeries and are cared for at home, posthospitalization.

   Please refer to ''Cardiac Care,'' ''Peripheral Vascular Disease,'' or ''Diabetes Mellitus'' should those diagnoses be appropriate for your patient.

2. **Needs for initial visit**

   Specific initial physician orders
   Universal precautions supplies
   Other supplies or equipment, based on physician orders
   Vital signs equipment

3. **Some potential medical-surgical diagnoses and codes**

Abdominal aortic aneurysm	441.4
AMI	410.9
Anemia	285.9
Angina	413.9
Atherosclerosis	414.0
Atrial fibrillation	427.31
Atrial flutter	427.32
Cardiomyopathy	425.4
Congestive heart failure	428.0
Constipation	564.0
COPD	496
Coronary artery bypass graft surgery	
two coronary arteries	36.12
three coronary arteries	36.13
four coronary arteries	36.14
CVA	436
Diabetes mellitus, with complications, adult	250.90
Diabetes mellitus, with complications, juv.	250.91
Heart transplant	37.5

Hypertension	401.9
Hypertension with heart involvement	402.91
Mediastinitis	519.2
Obesity	278.0
Other aftercare following surgery	V58.4
Pacemaker	V45.0
Postsurgical status, aortocoronary bypass status	V45.81
Postsurgical status, presence of neuropacemaker or other electronic device (implanted automatic cardiac defibrillator)	V45.89
Substernal wound infection	998.5
Transplant, heart	37.5
Wound dehiscence	998.3
Wound infection	998.5

4. **Associated nursing diagnoses**

Activity intolerance
Activity intolerance, high risk for
Anxiety
Body image disturbance
Body temperature, altered, high risk for
Cardiac output, decreased
Caregiver role strain
Caregiver role strain, potential for
Constipation
Coping, defensive
Coping, family: potential for growth
Coping, ineffective family: compromised
Coping, ineffective family: disabling
Coping, ineffective individual
Denial, ineffective
Family processes, altered
Fatigue
Fear
Fluid volume deficit, high risk for
Fluid volume excess
Health maintenance, altered
Home maintenance management, impaired
Infection, high risk for
Injury, high risk for
Knowledge deficit (self-care management)
Mobility impaired
Nutrition altered, less than body requirements

Nutrition altered, more than body requirements
Oral mucous membrane, altered
Pain
Pain, chronic
Role performance, altered
Self-care deficit, bathing/hygiene
Self-care deficit, dressing/grooming
Self-care deficit, feeding
Self-care deficit, toileting
Sexual dysfunction
Skin integrity, impaired
Skin integrity, impaired, high risk for
Sleep pattern disturbance
Social interaction, impaired
Spiritual distress (distress of the human spirit)
Tissue integrity, impaired
Tissue perfusion, altered (specify) (renal, cerebral,
    cardiopulmonary, gastrointestinal, peripheral)

5. **Service skills identified**

Observation and complete systems assessment of the patient
    S/P cardiac surgery and admitted to home care for _____
Assessment and observation of patient's cardiopulmonary
    status postbypass (or other) cardiac surgery (e.g., lung
    sounds, peripheral edema, etc.)
Venipuncture for monitoring blood levels (specify test,
    frequency, per MD orders)
Instruct patient on how to take and record pulse
Instruct patient regarding bowel management program and the
    need to avoid constipation/straining
Teach patient about the use of stool softeners, dietary changes,
    and adequate hydration for optimal bowel function
RN to instruct patient and caregiver regarding multiple
    medications, including route, schedule, functions, and
    possible side effects
Teach patient and caregiver what symptoms necessitate calling
    the MD or nurse (or 911)
RN to assess home for safety related to oxygen use
Instruct patient in the correct use of antiembolic stockings
RN to provide skilled observation and assessment of surgical
    sites
RN to observe for signs and symptoms of infection
RN to monitor blood pressure and other vital signs

RN to instruct patient on life-style needs postsurgery;
counseling regarding the need to quit or significantly
decrease smoking, adherence to progressive exercise
rehabilitation program and low salt, low-fat diet with
increased fruits and vegetables

RN to teach pacemaker care, follow up and pacemaker checks

RN to counsel patient regarding importance of rest periods,
nutrition, and other safety information including no pulling,
lifting, or pushing during the postoperative period

RN to assess wound site, change dressing (specify dressing
orders and frequency per MD orders) and teach caregiver
about wound and infection control care

RN to culture wound site and send to lab for C & S

RN to assess and monitor patient's pain, implement ordered
pain control/relief measures and assess patient's response to
interventions—surgical or cardiac pain

RN to dress wound and care for donor site infection

Teach patient about anticoagulant therapy, schedule, and side
effects to watch for

RN to monitor intake and output, daily weights, report weight
gain of more than _____ lbs (specify), or edema noted in
ankles or other sites

RN to assess the patient's response to treatments and
interventions and report changes or unfavorable responses or
reactions to the physician

Management and evaluation of the patient POC

6. **Other services indicated**

HHA	Personal care
	ADL assistance
MSS	Evaluation
	Assessment of social and emotional factors that have an impact on health and effective POC implementation
	Identify eligibility for services or benefits
	Financial counseling
	Community resource referral
OT	Evaluation
	Conservation of energy techniques
	Home and patient evaluation for ADL or assistive devices
PT	Evaluation
	Progressive cardiac rehabilitation program
	Strengthening regimen

7. **Associated factors based on diagnosis justifying homebound status**

Patient status post-CABG surgery—on cardiac restrictions
Patient has shortness of breath and weakness S/P surgery and hospitalization that preclude leaving home safely
Patient needs walker and assistance of one to leave home
Patient with extensive, infected post-op chest wound or venous leg (right or left) site—on infection precautions. MD does not want patient exposed to hospital infections
Patient cannot safely leave home without assistance
Minimal exertion causes chest pain
Minimal ambulation due to postoperative discomfort/pain

8. **Short-term goals**

RN	Patient adhering to POC
	Support promotion of optimal cardiac function
	Patient and caregiver demonstrating understanding of care needs
HHA	Effective personal care
	ADL assistance
MSS	Problem identification
	Counseling initiated
	Care team and patient adhering to POC
OT	Conservation of energy techniques being practiced
	Identification of patient needs for assistive/ adaptive equipment
PT	Progressive exercise regimen being implemented
	Patient is gradually and safely returning to independent ADLs

9. **Long-term goals**

RN	Self-management of health care and life-style under MD supervision
	Improved, adequate cardiac output and effective tissue perfusion
	Wound infection healed, patient afebrile
	Patient has decreased anxiety
HHA	Safe, effective personal care
	Patient clean and comfortable
MSS	Community resources identified
	Problem resolution
	Financial assistance accomplished

	Effective adjustment for patient and caregiver (spouse) postsurgery
	Referrals made of patient and caregiver to community services for continued support
OT	Patient able to use assistive or adaptive devices
	Patient using conservation of energy techniques that were taught
PT	Increased mobility within limits of cardiac status
	Safe progression in resuming activity level per prescribed program
	Patient and caregiver adhering to exercise regimen

10. Discharge plans for this patient

Patient discharged to self-care management under MD supervision

Discharged from home care when patient-centered goals (specify) achieved

Discharge when patient is no longer homebound, refer to outpatient cardiac center

11. Patient, family, and caregiver educational needs

Educational needs are the regimens that the patient or caregiver will need to know and perform to care for the patient. These include:

Importance of medical follow up

Importance of correct cardiac diet, exercise regimen, decreasing or quitting smoking

The patient's medications and their relationship to each other

Support groups in the community that are available to the patient and their caregivers, including smoking cessation programs if patient (still) smokes

Pacemaker/defibrillator device for follow-up, long-term care needs

Other education and information based on patient's unique medical and other identified needs

Be aware that local chapters of the American Heart Association have resources and support available for cardiac patients. Also, many community hospitals and health centers have patient support groups.

12. Specific tips for reimbursement

The postsurgical cardiac patient has multifaceted needs for skilled care at home. With this in mind, observation and evaluation may be appropriate for longer than a 3-week period, based on the patient's past medical history, safety, and other factors. Other skills may be observation and assessment, wound care (three separate skills: hands-on wound care, observation and assessment, and teaching about the wound care), and management and evaluation of the patient POC.

Remember to document the actual care you provided, why the patient is homebound, and why the skills of a professional nurse were needed.

DECUBITUS ULCER

1. **General Considerations.** Decubitus ulcers are frequently seen in home health care because our patient population is frail, elderly, nutritionally deficient, and/or immobilized because of multiple system problems.

    Please refer to "Care of the Bedbound Patient" or "Wound Care" should those problems also be appropriate for your patient.

2. **Needs for initial visit**

    Specific initial physician orders
    Universal precautions supplies
    Other supplies or equipment, based on physician orders
    Vital signs equipment
    Dressing supplies

3. **Some potential medical-surgical diagnoses and codes**

CVA	436
Debridement	86.22
Decubitus ulcer	707.0
Diabetes mellitus, with complications, adult	250.90
Diabetes mellitus, with complications, juv.	250.91
Heel ulcer, right or left	707.1
Hypertension	401.9
Peripheral vascular disease	443.9
Quadriplegia	344.0
Stasis ulcer	454.2
Surgical wound, open	998.3
Urinary incontinence	788.3
Urinary infection	599.0
Urinary retention	788.2

4. **Associated nursing diagnoses**

    Activity intolerance
    Activity intolerance, high risk for
    Anxiety
    Body image disturbance
    Body temperature, altered, high risk for
    Cardiac output, decreased

Caregiver role strain
Caregiver role strain, high risk for
Constipation
Coping, ineffective individual
Diarrhea
Fatigue
Fear
Infection, high risk for
Injury, high risk for
Knowledge deficit (care regimen)
Mobility, impaired physical
Nutrition altered: less than body requirements
Pain
Pain, chronic
Self-care deficit, bathing/hygiene
Self-care deficit, dressing/grooming
Self-care deficit, feeding
Self-care deficit, toileting
Sensory/perceptual alterations (specify)
Skin integrity, impaired
Tissue integrity, impaired
Tissue perfusion, altered (peripheral)

5. **Service skills identified**

Measure vital signs
Observe for signs and symptoms of infection
Assess healing process
Culture wound prn
Change packing q _____ (specify)
Teach family or caregiver wound procedure and care
regimen(s)
Pack wound with _____ (specify)
Apply wet to dry dressing of _____ (specify)
Soak site with _____ (specify)
Assess peripheral circulation
Instruct patient in dressing change
Assess wound drainage and amount
Cover with sterile 4 × 4
Remove dressing using normal saline
solution
Assess hydration and nutrition status
Repack wound with _____ (specify)

Assess wound for symptoms of infection, decreased
circulation, or other problems

Elevate leg whenever sitting

TEDs or Ace™ wrap whenever up

Wash site gently with _____ (specify)

Check for impaction and remove in bedbound patient per MD
orders

Skilled observation and all systems assessment of patient with
a decubitus ulcer

Observation and evaluation of wound and surrounding skin

Evaluate patient's need for equipment, supplies to decrease
pressure; alternating pressure mattress, gel foam seat
cushion, heel, elbow protectors, etc.

Teach family to perform dressings between RN visits

RN to instruct in pain control measures and medications

Teach patient family or caregiver about proper body alignment
and positioning in bed to prevent skin tears from shearing
skin

RN to consult with enterostomal therapist nurse for evaluation
and POC, report findings, recommendations to MD

Measure the site(s) for baseline and progress, include length,
width, and depth

RN to teach infection control measures of wound care

Observation and skilled assessment of other areas for possible
breakdown including heels, hips, elbows, ankles

RN to monitor for infection, necrosis, increased exudate, or
other problems, and report to MD

Assess the patient's response to treatments and interventions
and report changes or unfavorable responses or reactions to
the physician

Management and evaluation of the patient POC

6. **Other services indicated**

HHA	Personal care
	ADL assistance
MSS	Assessment of social and emotional factors
	Counseling
	Financial assistance
	Problem impeding POC implementation and goals being achieved

7. **Associated factors based on diagnosis justifying
homebound status**

Bedridden

Unable to ambulate or transfer without maximum assistance

Requires maximum assistance to ambulate or transfer

Medical restrictions, foot to be elevated

Wheelchair dependence

Large open wound (describe size briefly)

Transfers from bed to chair only

Open skin lesions

Open wound with large amount of drainage, BRPs only

No weight bearing per physician orders

Multiple functional limitations, including _____ (specify)

Poor ambulation, fall-prone

Unsteady ambulation with cane

Level of home on _____ floor with no elevator, unable to use
stairs

Patient unable to safely leave home without maximum
assistance and effort

8. **Short-term goals**

RN	Daily compliance with wound regimen
	Wound packed per physician order
	Healing wound, infection-free
HHA	Effective personal hygiene
	ADL assistance
MSS	Problem identification
	Successful implementation of POC

9. **Long-term goals**

RN	Adequate nutrition
	Wound healing
	Vital signs normal for patient range
	Infection-free
HHA	Effective personal hygiene
	ADL assistance
MSS	Identified problem resolution
	Community resource referral(s)

10. **Discharge plans for this patient**

Discharged, goals achieved

Patient remains homebound, needing skilled care

Patient will remain in home, under MD supervision

11. **Patient, family, and caregiver educational needs**

Educational needs are the regimens that the caregiver will
be managing with the patient. These include:

Home safety assessment and counseling
The avoidance of injury or infection to compromised skin sites
The importance of medical follow up
Signs and symptoms that necessitate calling the MD
Support groups in the community that are available to your
  patient and their caregivers
Methods to help prevention another decubitus
Teach patient and caregiver all aspects of care related to
  wound, including effective handwashing, disposal of soiled
  dressings, and other infection control measures
The importance of nutrition in the healing process
Teach patient about all medications, including schedule, route,
  functions, and possible side effects
Other aspects of care that are based on your patient's unique
  medical condition and needs

12. **Specific tips for reimbursement**

Document all teaching accomplished with family or caregiver
Document progress toward goals, when identified
Document description of decubitus ulcer
Document infected area
Document any discharge, odor and amount
Document draining wound
Document homebound status
Document up only with assistance
Document can only transfer safely
Document length, width, depth of wound
Document any changes, including specific care provided
Document medication(s) changed or medication(s) being
  regulated
Document RN contacted physician regarding _____ (specify)
Document febrile, temperature _____ (specify)
Document unable to do ADLs or personal care
Document any change in the patient's status or POC
Take photograph of wound(s) to substantiate document at
  onset of q3 weeks, have patient sign release, one photograph
  for the clinical record
Specify any learning barriers, such as arthritic hands, poor
  eyesight

Document the specific teaching accomplished and the
behavioral outcomes of that teaching

Document clearly the status of the decubitus ulcer and the
clinical progress toward healing and patient-centered good
achievement

Wound care is an area in which managed-care companies
and other payers are attempting to decrease allowed numbers
of visits. It is the professional nurse's responsibility to
remember that it is not just the dressing change that occurs.
When a nurse makes the home visit, there is an assessment of
the wound healing or deterioration and teaching that occurs.
These skills usually require the skills of a nurse. All of these
components contribute to safe, effective wound care.

Remember that for Medicare patients, daily is defined as 5,
6, or 7 days. If your patient needs daily or BID ($2\times$ day)
dressing changes, obtain an order from the physician with an
estimate for the finite and predictable endpoint. This needs to
be a date, for example 10/10/9_, not ''when the decubitus
heals.'' Remember that patients who need daily home care for
the rest of their lives are usually not appropriate for Medicare.
In addition, remember that daily insulin injections (and only in
those cases in which the patient is unable or unwilling) is the
exception to daily. (This is further discussed in Diabetes
Mellitus.) Please review the HIM-11 or information from your
manager obtained from the home health intermediary for
further information.

DEPRESSION AND OTHER PSYCHIATRIC HOME CARE

1. **General Considerations.** Some home care providers have developed specialized psychiatric care programs that effectively provide care for patients in their own homes. Many of these programs are directed toward the care of homebound geriatric patients.

   Please refer to "Alzheimer's Disease and Other Dementias" should those problems be appropriate for your patient.

2. **Needs for initial visit**

   Specific initial physician orders
   Universal precautions supplies
   Other supplies or equipment, based on physician orders
   Vital signs equipment

3. **Some potential medical-surgical and psychiatric diagnoses and codes**

AIDS dementia	298.9 and 042.9
Agoraphobia	300.22
Alcoholism	303.90
Alzheimer's	331.0
Anemia	285.9
Anorexia nervosa	307.1
Anxiety state	300.0
Bipolar disorder	296.50
Bulimia	307.51
Constipation	564.0
Creutzfeldt-Jakob disease and dementia	290.10 and 046.1
Dementia	298.9
Depression, reactive	300.4
Depressive disorder	311
Depressive psychosis	296.20
Drug addiction	304.90
Hypochrondiasis	300.7
Mania	296.00
Nonpsychotic brain syndrome	310.9
Obsessive-compulsive disorder	300.3

Panic disorder	300.01
Personality disorder	301.9
Polyaddiciton	304.80
Presenile dementia	290.12
Psychosis	298.9
Schizophrenia, simple	295.00
Senile dementia	290.0
Traumatic stress disorder	308.3
Unipolar disorder	296.00

4. **Associated nursing diagnoses**

Anxiety
Body image disturbance
Caregiver role strain
Caregiver role strain, high risk for
Communication, impaired verbal
Constipation
Coping, ineffective family: disabling
Coping, ineffective individual
Decisional conflict (specify)
Family processes, altered
Fatigue
Fear
Fluid volume deficit, high risk for
Grieving, anticipatory
Grieving, dysfunctional
Hopelessness
Injury, high risk for
Knowledge deficit (self-care management)
Management of therapeutic regimen (individuals), ineffective
Mobility, impaired physical
Noncompliance
Nutrition, altered: less than body requirements
Nutrition, altered: more than body requirements
Pain
Pain, chronic
Parenting, altered
Parenting, altered, potential
Post-trauma response
Powerlessness
Rape-trauma syndrome
Rape-trauma syndrome: compound reaction
Self-care deficit (specify)

Self-esteem disturbance

Self-esteem, chronic low

Self-esteem, situational low

Sensory/perceptual alterations (specify) (visual, auditory, kinesthetic, gustatory, tactile, olfactory)

Sexual dysfunction

Sexuality patterns, altered

Sleep pattern disturbance

Social interaction, impaired

Spiritual distress (distress of the human spirit)

Thought processes, altered

Trauma, high risk for

Violence, high risk for, self-directed or directed at others

5. **Service skills identified**

Skilled assessment of the patient with _____ (specify)

RN to obtain venipuncture for liver function tests (specify frequency, type) per MD order

RN to teach regarding antidepressive medication and side effects

RN to initiate psychotherapy after acute hospitalization

RN to monitor medication regimen and compliance with lithium therapy

RN to provide emotional support to patient with severe grief reaction

RN to monitor patient's mental status for signs and symptoms of depression or _____ (specify)

Home safety evaluation and plan to help assure safety

Skilled observation and assessment of all systems

Teach patient and caregiver about disease and management

Monitor hydration and nutrition intake

RN to weigh patient (specify ordered frequency)

Observation of skin and patient's overall physical status

RN to monitor effectiveness of new antipsychotic drug for severe agitation, psychotic behavior, and suicidal thoughts or planning

RN to monitor effectiveness of new tranquilizer regimen for severe anxiety

RN to observe and assess patient's hygiene, personal care, independence with disease

RN to administer injection of psychotropic medication _____ q _____ (specify orders)

RN to evaluate behavior modification plan, including support, teaching, and evaluation of compliance

Assess the patient's response to therapeutic treatments and interventions and report any changes or unfavorable responses to the physician (i.e., extrapyramidal symptoms)

Management and evaluation of the patient's POC

6. **Other services indicated**

HHA	Personal care
	ADL assistance
MSS	Evaluation
	Crisis intervention
	Psychosocial assessment of patient's mental status and safety
	Therapeutic interventions directed toward patient's symptoms
	Assessment of both health factors and mental status having an impact on health and on the POC being effectively implemented
	Evaluation for referral to community service— day-care, postdischarge plan
OT	Assessment
	Reality orientation
	Safety assessment of home
	Identification of needed assistive devices to help assure ADLs, safety in home
	Planning, implementing, and supervising therapeutic activity program

7. **Associated factors based on diagnosis justifying homebound status**

The patient has a psychiatric problem (specify) and this illness is demonstrated in part by a refusal to leave home

The patient cannot safely leave home unattended (not oriented to time, place, person)

Patient with severe mental status deterioration cannot leave home

Unsafe for patient to be out without supervision

Confusion level precludes patient leaving home safely for needed psychotherapy

Other medical problems (specify) making patient homebound

8. **Short-term goals**

RN	Patient maintained safely in home
	Patient adheres to prescribed medications and other regimens
	Caregivers being taught to care for patient effectively
	Assessment and monitoring of patient's mental status
HHA	Effective personal care
	ADL assistance
MSS	Therapeutic interventions and counseling initiated
	Care team members and patient adhering to POC
	Patient and family counseling
OT	Identification of safety needs and assistive devices
	Home safety program being implemented

9. **Long-term goals**

RN	Patient cared for safely with home as the therapeutic environment
	Decrease in identified problem behaviors or behaviors controlled
	Caregiver able to safely and effectively care for patient in home
	Symptoms stabilized, increased or enhanced coping skills
	Caregiver able to identify acceleration of symptoms or other changes to MD
	Patient able to control and accomplish ADLs when possible and safe
HHA	Effective and safe personal care provided
	Patient clean and comfortable
MSS	Therapeutic relationship created
	Symptoms or problem behaviors addressed and stabilized
	Family and patient aware of available community resources
	Patient able to be cared for safely at home by caregiver and able to control own ADLs with support of caregiver
	Identify need for community caregiver support, self-help or support group(s)
	Crisis resolution

OT	Patient able to use assistive devices safely
	Home program adhered to by caregiver and patient

10. **Discharge plans for this patient**

Discharge to outpatient mental health setting when patient able to leave home

Discharge patient when patient-centered goals are achieved that were agreed upon by the patient with the psychiatric home care team (specify parameters)

Patient to be maintained in home setting with needs being safely addressed and under care of caregiver and MD

Patient to be admitted to long-term specialized setting when bed becomes available due to the severity and nature of symptoms and caregiver's exhaustion

Patient will develop effective coping skills

Discharge to safe care in home under MD supervision

Patient requires long-term, injectable psychotropic drugs and ongoing therapy and evaluation

11. **Patient, family, and caregiver educational needs**

Educational needs are the regimens that the caregiver will be managing with or for the patient. These include:

Importance of adherence to medical regimen, particularly safety concerns, medication compliance, and keeping psychotherapeutic appointments at the mental health center

Importance of adequate hydration and nutrition

Signs and symptoms of recurring depression or other behaviors; side effects related to drugs that necessitate seeking medical follow up

Home safety concerns and issues

The importance of medical follow up, including drug levels, if indicated, and family therapy

Support groups in the community that are available to the patient and their caregivers

Other information based on the patient's and family's unique needs

Another resource is a service provided through the National Association of Areas on Aging. It is called the Elder Care Locator and can be reached at 1-800-677-1116. This is a resource to locate local support services for the elderly.

12. Specific tips for reimbursement

For Medicare patients, the HIM-11 clearly defines the
parameters regarding nursing skilled care and psychiatric
evaluation and therapy. The nurses providing the actual
therapeutic assessments and interventions must have
specialized training or experience beyond the standard
curriculum required for an RN.

Many programs have specialized therapeutic teams that
care for this patient population especially after a discharge
from an inpatient facility for psychiatric problems. In
addition, the home health aides may also have additional in-
services or training to effectively and safely care for this
patient population in the community.

DIABETES MELLITUS

1. **General Considerations.**   Diabetes mellitus and the associated complications are frequently seen in Home Health Care. Teaching is the nursing priority for this patient population.

   Please see ''Peripheral Vascular Disease,'' ''Cellulitis,'' or ''Amputation Care'' should those problems be appropriate for your patient.

2. **Needs for initial visit**

   Specific initial physician orders
   Universal precautions supplies
   Other supplies or equipment, based on physician orders
   Vital signs equipment
   Blood glucose monitoring machine
   Venipuncture supplies
   Alcohol swabs, gauze pads
   Teaching skills
   Patience

3. **Some potential medical-surgical diagnoses and codes**

Amputee, bilateral	736.89
Angina	413.9
Arterial occlusive disease	250.70 and 447.1
BKA, S/P right or left	84.15
Cellulitis and abscess (legs)	250.80 and 682.6
Chronic ischemic heart disease	414.9
Chronic renal failure	585
COPD	496
CVA	436
Diabetes mellitus, with complications, adult	250.90
Diabetes mellitus, with complications, juv.	250.91
Diabetic neuropathy	250.60 and 357.2
Diabetic retinopathy (insulin dependent)	250.51 and 362.01
Diabetic retinopathy (noninsulin dependent)	250.50 and 362.01
Electrolyte/fluid imbalance	276.9

Femoral-popliteal bypass	39.29
Gangrene, right or left foot	250.70 and 785.4
Hyperglycemia	790.6
Hypertension	250.80 and 401.9
Hypoglycemia	251.2
Ketoacidosis, insulin dependent	250.11
Ketoacidosis, noninsulin dependent	250.10
Left heart failure	428.1
Peripheral vascular disease	250.70 and 443.9
Toe amputation	84.11
Vasculitis	250.70 and 447.6

4. **Associated nursing diagnoses**

Activity intolerance
Activity intolerance, high risk for
Adjustment, impaired
Anxiety
Body image disturbance
Body temperature, altered, high risk for
Cardiac output, decreased
Caregiver role strain
Caregiver role strain, high risk for
Coping, ineffective individual
Denial, ineffective
Family processes, altered
Fatigue
Fear
Fluid volume deficit, high risk for
Fluid volume excess
Gas exchange, impaired
Grieving, anticipatory
Infection, high risk for
Injury, high risk for
Knowledge deficit (self-care management)
Management of therapeutic regimen (individuals), ineffective
Mobility, impaired physical
Noncompliance (specify, for example, self-care regimen)
Nutrition, altered: high risk for more than body requirements
Nutrition, altered: less than body requirements
Nutrition, altered: more than body requirements
Pain
Pain, chronic
Peripheral neurovascular dysfunction, high risk for

Self-care deficit, bathing/hygiene
Self-care deficit, dressing/grooming
Self-care deficit, feeding
Self-care deficit, toileting
Sensory/perceptual alterations (specify) (visual, auditory,
   kinesthetic, gustatory, tactile, olfactory)
Sexuality patterns, altered
Skin integrity, impaired, high risk for
Sleep pattern disturbance
Social interaction, impaired
Spiritual distress (distress of the human spirit)
Tissue integrity, impaired
Tissue perfusion, altered (specify type) (renal, cerebral,
   cardiopulmonary, gastrointestinal, peripheral)
Unilateral neglect

5. **Service skills identified**

Administer _____ insulin q am
Administer additional _____ insulin before meals
Teach patient or family member to draw up and give insulin
Teach diabetes care management regimen(s)
Teach regarding diet and importance of eating at regular and
   consistent times
Glucose meter check q _____, call physician if over _____ or
   less than _____
Teach patient or family to mix insulins
Teach patient or family member safe home blood glucose
   monitoring process
Administer or teach foot care regimen
Teach signs, symptoms of hyperglycemia and hypoglycemia,
   teach emergency measures to patient and family
Venipuncture for FBS as indicated
Teach patient or family urine check procedures, as ordered
Teach regarding new insulin and medication regimen
Assess need for podiatrist for ongoing care
Teach disease process
Teach action of ordered insulin(s)
Assess for long-term ability of patient and family to comply
   with regimen
Skilled observation and all systems assessment of patient with
   diabetes mellitus
Teach use of single-site rotations for injections or other
   ordered rotation method

Ongoing monitoring and assessment of blood glucose readings and patient's management of compliance with new DM regimen

Teach patient all aspects of safe care with new SQ insulin infusion pump at home

Instruct patient in equipment and use of blood glucose monitoring program

Assess the patient's response to treatments and interventions and report changes or unfavorable responses or reactions to the physician

Management and evaluation of the patient's POC

6. Other services indicated

HHA	Personal care duties
	ADL assistance
MSS	Assessment of social and emotional factors that cause the POC not to be implemented; for example, unable to afford insulin therapy or patient has severe retinopathy resulting from disease that precludes the teaching process

7. Associated factors based on diagnosis justifying homebound status

Severe weakness
AKA, BKA
Bedbound
Needs maximum assistance to ambulate
Medically restricted for AMI (cardiac restrictions)
Paresis, paralysis from CVA
Wheelchair bound
Activity restrictions
Severe SOB
Blindness

8. Short-term goals

RN	Daily compliance to medication and insulin regimen
	Blood sugars stabilizing
HHA	Effective personal hygiene
	ADL assistance

MSS   Patient able to follow treatment regimen
            Problem identified

9. Long-term goals

RN   Patient or family will maintain self-care regarding
            diabetes mellitus with compliance to
            medication, insulin, and diet regimen and self-
            care management needs
            Stable medical status
            Blood sugar in normal for patient range
            Prevention of complications of diabetes mellitus
HHA   Effective personal hygiene
            Self-care regarding ADLs
MSS   Resources identified and patient utilizing
            community resource
            Patient able to follow POC
            Adjusting to diagnosis of chronic nature

10. Discharge plans for this patient

Discharge when blood sugars are within the normal for patient
  range
Discharge self-care
Continuing need for home health care because patient remains
  homebound and needs skilled care
No longer homebound, refer to outpatient follow up
Family member taught care, patient discharged
Discharge to self-management, under MD care

11. Patient, family, and caregiver educational needs

Educational needs are the regimens that the caregiver will
be managing with the patient. These include:

Home safety assessment and counseling
All aspects of care related to DM including self-observational
  skills such as weight, blood glucose levels, and record
  keeping
The avoidance of injury or infection
The importance of medical follow up
Signs and symptoms that necessitate calling the MD
Support groups in the community that are available to both
  patient and caregiver
Prevention and management of complications associated
  with DM

Teach patient and caregiver all aspects of safety and infection control related to needles, including effective handwashing, safe disposal of sharps, and other infection control measures

The importance of diet, exercise, and foot care

Teach patient about medications, including schedule, route, functions, and possible side effects

Other aspects of care that are based on your patient's unique medical condition and needs

The American Diabetes Association (ADA) has resources available for patients and their families. They can be reached at 1-800-232-6366. They offer literature, meal planning, videos, weight planning and management services, and patient advocates. They also have a monthly magazine entitled *Forecast* for all ADA members.

12. **Specific tips for reimbursement**

Obtain a telephone order for any POC change

Communicate any POC changes in the clinical record

Document when the patient is new to insulin therapy or the patient is newly diagnosed as having diabetes mellitus

Document abnormal blood sugar findings in the clinical record

Document initial knowledge level and progress achieved through teaching process

Document specific teaching accomplished and the behavioral outcomes of that teaching

Refer to HCFA Medicare HHA manual, Section 205.1, page 14.16, regarding insulin instructions for clarification specific to insulin therapy

Specify and document the learning barriers, for example, arthritic hands, poor eyesight and no available, able, willing caregiver

Document the specific orders, including frequency of FBS venipunctures

For Medicare patients, remember that insulin is usually self-injected by the patient or given by a family member. If you have a patient, however, who is either physically or mentally unable to self-inject insulin and there is no other person who is able and willing to inject the beneficiary, the injections would be considered a reasonable and necessary skilled nursing service. This information and an example is located on page 14.16 of Section 205.1 of the "Coverage of Services" section of the HHA manual. Please refer to Part Seven for this information.

The nurse must clearly document the patient's inability or unwillingness and the circumstances that there is no available person to inject the insulin. In addition, know that daily insulin injections are the exception to daily care; for daily insulin you usually do not need a projected finite and predictable ending date.

FRACTURE CARE
(LOWER EXTREMITY, HIP)

1. **General Considerations.**   The reduction in bone mass resulting from age and the subsequent reduction in strength causes an increase in the tendency to fracture.

    Please refer to "Osteoporosis," "Care of the Bedbound Patient," and "Care of the Patient with Pain" should those problems be appropriate for your patient.

2. **Needs for initial visit**

    Specific initial physician orders
    Universal precautions supplies
    Vital signs equipment
    Other supplies or equipment, based on physician orders

3. **Some potential medical-surgical diagnoses and codes**

Anemia	285.9
Ankle fracture, right or left	824.8
Anticoagulation	99.19
Arthritis	716.90
Arthropathy, general	716.90
Arthropathy, pelvis	716.95
Aseptic necrosis femur	733.42
Calcaneus, fracture	825.0
Closed reduction, internal fixation femur	79.15
CVA	436
Decubitus ulcer	707.0
Degenerative joint disease, hip, thigh	715.95
Degenerative joint disease, lower leg, knee	715.96
Dislocated hip	835.00
Dislocation, hip, open reduction	79.85
Dislocation, right or left hip prosthesis	996.4
Femur, fracture neck of	820.8
Fracture, pathological	733.1
Hip fracture, right or left	820.8
Hip replacement, partial	81.52
Hip replacement, revision	81.53
Hip replacement, total right or left	81.59
Humerus, fracture	812.20

Knee, degenerative arthritis	715.96
Knee replacement, total right or left	81.41
Laminectomy syndrome	722.80
Lumbar laminectomy	03.09
Lumbar stenosis	724.02
ORIF	79.35
Osteoarthritis, exacerbation, hip, thigh	715.95
Osteoarthritis, exacerbation, leg, knee	715.96
Osteomyelitis	730.05
Osteoporosis	733.09
Paralysis agitans	332.0
Partial hip replacement	81.52
Pelvic fracture	808.49
Rheumatoid arthritis	714.0
Sciatica	724.3
Sprain (acute), lumbar	847.2
Sprain (acute), lumbosacral	846.0
Sprain (acute), sacral	847.3
Stenosis, spinal	724.00
THR	81.54
Tibia, fracture	823.80
Tibia, fracture with fibula	823.82
Thrombophlebitis, deep vein	451.19
Thrombosis, deep vein	453.8

4. **Associated nursing diagnoses**

Activity intolerance
Anxiety
Constipation
Disuse syndrome, high risk for
Fatigue
Fear
Home maintenance management, impaired
Infection, high risk for
Injury, high risk for
Knowledge deficit (specify)
Mobility, impaired physical
Pain
Pain, chronic
Self-care deficit, bathing/hygiene
Self-care deficit, dressing/grooming
Self-care deficit, feeding
Self-care deficit, toileting

Sexuality patterns, altered
Skin integrity, impaired
Sleep pattern disturbance
Spiritual distress (distress of the human spirit)
Tissue perfusion, altered (peripheral)
Urinary elimination, altered

5. Service skills identified

Measure vital signs
Venipuncture for protimes q _____(specify ordered frequency)
Teach new medication regimen, side effects
Assess hydration and nutrition status
Assess lung, cardiovascular status
Teach bowel regimen to caregiver and family
Teach caregiver or family care of the bedridden; specifically
  signs and symptoms regarding decubitus, infection,
  thrombosis, pneumonia
Prn disimpaction, implement bowel management program, per
  MD orders
Skilled evaluation and systems assessment of the patient
  with _____ (specify fracture)
Ongoing observation, assessment and evaluation of patient's
  pain, and the pain management program
Teach family and caregiver proper and safe body alignment
  and positions, including total hip safety precautions
Skilled observation, assessment, and care of the incision site
Assess the patient's response to treatments and interventions
  and report changes or unfavorable responses to the physician
Management and evaluation of the patient POC

6. Other services indicated

HHA	Personal care
	ADL assistance
MSS	Assessment of social and emotional factors
	Counseling
	Financial assistance
	Nursing home placement assistance
	Arrange for meal program(s)
	Assess home situation
	Home safety evaluation
OT	Evaluation
	ADL training program

Independent homemaking skills
Home safety evaluation
Assistive device evaluation
Functional exercises
Increase right and left LE strength
Independent bathing
Other ADLs
Teach alternative bathing, dressing, feeding skills
Teach conservation of energy skills
Safety counseling regarding home for patient and caregiver

PT   Evaluation
Therapeutic exercise regimen for safe transfer training techniques with walker to increase balance, mobility, function, and independence
Establish home maintenance program
Teach hip safety precautions
Progressive gait training with assistive device
Ultrasound
ADL assessment and training
Strengthening exercises
Progressive resistive exercises
Patient and home evaluation for safety
Gait training with walker
Teach family home exercise program
Management and evaluation of the patient POC
ROM exercises
Bed mobility and trapeze
Stair climbing skills
Passive and active exercises to RLE
Passive and active exercises to LLE
Crutch walking
Care or brace placement
Transfer or mobility skills training

7. **Associated factors based on diagnosis justifying homebound status**

Needs maximum assistance to ambulate
Severely limited activity due to brace
Activity restrictions
Unsteady gait
Activity medically restricted per physician, S/P laminectomy
Braces on hips

Exacerbation of joint disease pain
Bedridden
Wheelchair bound
Severe lower back pain
Severe shortness of breath
S/P hip surgery
Age, 90, S/P fracture, Foley catheter
Patient cannot safely leave home unattended
Poor balance, unsafe to walk
Patient is nonweight bearing per physician

8. Short-term goals

RN	Daily implementation of POC
HHA	Effective personal hygiene
	ADL assistance
MSS	Problem identification
	Patient or family able to implement POC
OT	Daily implementation of ADL program
PT	Daily implementation of exercise regimen

9. Long-term goals

RN	Return to self-management of healed incision
HHA	Effective personal hygiene
	ADL assistance
MSS	Identified problem resolution
	Community resource referral(s)
OT	Increased strength
	Independent ADLs
	Maximum function of affected extremities
	Using adaptive and assistive devices safely
PT	Functional ambulation for patient, pain-free
	Increased strength, balance, and ROM

10. Discharge plans for this patient

Discharged, no longer homebound, referred to outpatient occupational and physical therapy
Remains homebound, in need of skilled care
Patient to remain in home, returned to self-care status, under MD supervision

11. **Patient, family, and caregiver educational needs**

Educational needs are the regimens that the caregiver or family should be able to safely provide between visits and after discharge from home care. These include:

The home exercise program and other regimens
Skin care and hip precautions
Safety precautions about falls and other aspects about home
    safety
The availability of personal emergency response systems in
    your community
The importance of medical follow up
When to call the physician or the home care program
Other information, based on your patient's unique medical and
    other needs

12. **Specific tips for reimbursement**

Document the progression of progress from goals identified on
    the initial assessment visit through to discharge
Document the coordination of the services rendered
Document marked progress noted since admission
Document any changes, including specific care provided
Document RN in contact with physician regarding (specify)

Document the coordination occurring among team members based on the POC. The multidisciplinary conference notes should be reflected in the clinical record. Refer to these meetings in the clinical record.

If any service, PT, for example, has to be placed on hold because the patient is "too sick," this should be reflected in the clinical documentation. Obtain an MD order for this change, otherwise it appears that the PT is not making visits as ordered on the POC.

GASTROSTOMY AND OTHER FEEDING TUBE CARE

1. **General Considerations.**   Because of the increasing number of elderly patients cared for in the home setting, gastrostomy care is becoming more common. The nursing focus of care is the nutrition and hydration goals and the associated family teaching needs.

2. **Needs for initial visit**

   Specific initial physician orders
   Universal precautions supplies
   Other supplies or equipment, based on physician orders
   Vital signs equipment
   Feeding tube
   Skin care supplies
   Nutritional supplements

3. **Some potential medical-surgical diagnoses and codes**

Attention to gastrostomy	V55.1
CVA	436
Decubitus ulcer	707.0
Dysphagia	787.2
Foley catheter	57.94
Gastrostomy (other)	43.19
Gastrostomy tube insertion	43.11
Hemipareses	342.9
Nasogastric tube feeding	96.6
Nasogastric tube insertion	96.07
Paralysis agitans (Parkinson's)	332.0
Pneumonia	486
Pneumonia, aspiration	507.0
Urinary incontinence	788.3

4. **Associated nursing diagnoses**

   Aspiration, high risk for
   Body image disturbance
   Bowel elimination, alteration in, diarrhea
   Bowel incontinence
   Caregiver role strain

Caregiver role strain, high risk for
Comfort, alteration in, pain
Diarrhea
Fluid volume deficit, high risk for
Infection, high risk for
Injury, high risk for
Knowledge deficit (care management)
Knowledge deficit, disease process
Nutrition, alteration in, actual
Nutrition, altered: less than body requirements
Nutrition, altered: more than body requirements
Oral mucous membrane, altered
Pain
Pain, chronic
Self-care deficit, feeding
Skin integrity impaired, high risk for
Skin integrity, impairment of actual, incision
Spiritual distress (distress of the human spirit)
Swallowing, impaired

5. **Service skills identified**

Measure vital signs
Teach family or caregiver about enteral feeding
Teach regarding equipment for feedings, preparation and
   storage of feeding
Skilled observation and systems assessment of patient with
   feeding tube _____ (specify type, site)
Teach patient and caregiver protocols of changing feeding
   bags and administration tubing per physician orders
RN to observe q visit for leaking, movement, discomfort, or
   other change
Instruct patient and family in jejunostomy or other tube
   feedings
Observation and assessment of the patient's bowel patterns
RN enterostomal therapist to evaluate patient and peristomal
   skin to identify nursing care needs
Teach the importance of verifying the tube's placement before
   every feeding
Teach family mouth and oral hygiene care
Teach caregiver regarding irrigation with water or per protocol
Teach family observational skills including record keeping of
   intake and output, nutritional solution or supplement, rate,
   frequency, amount, and time of ordered feedings

Monitor for complications, including diarrhea

RN to assess the patient's response to ordered interventions and treatments and report changes or unfavorable responses or reactions to the physician

Management and evaluation of the patient POC

Teach care of nasogastric feeding tube

Change nasogastric tube q _____ (specify orders)

Teach family or caregiver gastrostomy feeding

Teach family or caregiver equipment care and preparation

Teach Dobhoff tube care including _____ (specify)

Teach use of kangaroo pump to family or caregiver

Weigh daily or weekly per physician order(s)

Monitor amount, sites of edema

Teach and monitor for signs of dehydration, diarrhea

Assess hydration and nutritional status

Change and reinsert tube prn, per MD orders

Wound care to abdominal site

Assess gastric tube for proper placement, patency, teach patient or family

Cleanse gastric tube site q _____ with hydrogen peroxide and water

Teach family or caregiver care of gastric tube

Administer and teach feedings at three-fourths strength at _____ cc/hr

Assess respiratory and cardiovascular status

Gastric tube feedings of _____ in 24 hours at _____ cc/hr

Teach regarding elevated position of head in bed for safety

6. **Other services indicated**

HHA	Personal care
	ADL assistance
MSS	Evaluation
	Home safety assessment
	Financial problems impeding POC implementation
	Community resource referral
S-LP	Evaluation
	Swallowing disorder assessment
	Aphasia, dysphasia treatment
	Dysphagia treatment

7. **Associated factors based on diagnosis justifying homebound status**

Bedridden or chairbound

Hemiplegia S/P CVA

Foley catheter, incontinence of bowel and bladder, frail, elderly

Decubitus ulcer(s), Foley catheter, gastric tube

Unresponsive, needs maximum assistance to transfer to chair

Multiple functional limitations, including _____

Poor ambulation with frequent falls

Gastrostomy tube S/P abdominal surgery

Patient unable to leave home with assistance

8. Short-term goals

RN	Daily compliance with hydration, nutrition regimen
	Patent tube
HHA	Effective personal hygiene
	ADL assistance
MSS	Problem, resource identification
	POC able to be implemented
S-LP	Able to communicate
	Improved swallowing

9. Long-term goals

RN	Safe administration of nutrition and medications
	Patient is nourished, hydrated
	Patent tube(s) infection-free
	Patient and family compliant with medications and tube feeding schedules and routines
	Caregiver or family able to care for patient
	Skin care optimal for patient
HHA	Effective personal hygiene
	ADL assistance
MSS	Community resources identified
	Problem resolution
S-LP	Maximum potential reached with swallowing and speech articulation or other communication

10. Discharge plans for this patient

Discharge to 24-hour care facility

Continue home health care visits on patient who remains homebound and requires skilled care

Remain in own home under family care and MD supervision

11. **Patient, family, and caregiver educational needs**

Educational needs are the regimens that the caregiver will be managing with the patient. These include:

Peristomal skin site care routines
The importance of medical follow up
When to call the home care program or the physician
Teach caregiver all aspects of the particular tube (e.g., teach care of percutaneous gastrostomy tube)
Teach regarding continuous infusion or other ordered method of administration
All aspects of safe enteral feeding preparation and delivery
Teach effective handwashing and infection control techniques, including safe storage of feedings and care and changing of supplies
Other information that this patient and family needs to know to function safely and effectively between visits and after discharge, based on their unique medical and other needs

12. **Specific tips for reimbursement**

Document the gastrostomy site wound, indicate color, any drainage, amount, and the specific care rendered
Communicate any POC changes
Document the reason for the tube feeding and the type of tube chosen
Document progress in wound healing or deterioration in wound status in the clinical documentation
Document the supplies needed on the form 485 and obtain MD orders for all supplies or equipment
Obtain a telephone order for any additional visits not projected on the original form 485 and state why (e.g., RN to visit $\times 1$ to reinsert tube). Better yet, obtain prn orders for tube dislodgement (e.g., prn $\times 3$), patient complaint, or other tube problem needing evaluation
If a wound culture is obtained, document the results on the form 486
Document if patient, family, or caregiver is unable to do dressing (retinopathy, severity of wound, etc.)
Document any learning barriers
Document the specific care and teaching accomplished and the behavioral and objective outcomes of that teaching
Document patient's level of independence in care

Document that the nutritional solutions are the patient's sole source of nutrition, when appropriate. Medicare and many other insurers will pay only if it is the *sole* source of nutrition (e.g., Ensure)

Document any problems with the skin site surrounding the tube and care provided

Document the specific type and size of tube on the 485. Specify the insertion date and site, the ordered feeding schedule, and teaching needs identified and accomplished.

HYPERTENSION

1. **General Considerations.**   Hypertension is one of the most frequent diagnoses in home health care. Often, fear of the disease and treatment and the lack of symptoms contribute to noncompliance.

    Please refer to "Care of the Bedbound Patient," "Cerebral Vascular Accident," "Decubitus Ulcer," or "Renal Failure" should those problems be appropriate for your patient.

2. **Needs for initial visit**

    Specific initial physician orders
    Universal precautions supplies
    Other supplies or equipment, based on physician orders
    Vital signs equipment

3. **Some potential medical-surgical diagnoses and codes**

AMI	410.9
Angina	413.9
Aphasia	784.3
Atrial fibrillation	427.31
Catheter, indwelling	57.94
CHF	428.0
COPD	496
Cor pulmonale	415.0
CVA	436
CVA with dysphasia	436 and 787.2
Decubitus ulcer	707.0
Diabetes mellitus, with complications, adult	250.90
Diabetes mellitus, with complications, juv.	250.91
Dysphasia	784.5
Emphysema	492.8
Fluid and electrolyte imbalance	267.9
Heart disease, chronic ischemic	414.9
Hemiplegia or hemiparesis	436 and 342.9
Hypertension	401.9
Hypertension, accelerated	401.0
Hypertensive nephrosclerosis	403.9
Incontinence of feces	787.6

Incontinence of urine	788.3
Left heart failure	428.1
Obesity	278.0
Pneumonia	486
Quadriplegia	436 and 344.0
TIA	435.9
Urinary retention	788.2
Urinary tract infection	599.0

4. **Associated nursing diagnoses**

Activity intolerance
Anxiety
Cardiac output, decreased
Communication, impaired verbal
Coping, family: potential for growth
Coping, ineffective family: compromised
Coping, ineffective family: disabling
Coping, ineffective individual
Denial, ineffective
Fatigue
Fear
Knowledge deficit (disease process and self-care regimens)
Management of therapeutic regimen (individuals), ineffective
Nutrition, altered: more than body requirements
Oral mucous membrane, altered
Sexuality patterns, altered
Spiritual distress (distress of the human spirit)
Thought processes, altered
Tissue perfusion, altered (specify type) (renal, cerebral,
    cardiopulmonary, gastrointestinal, peripheral)

5. **Service skills identified**

Evaluation, measure baseline vital signs, especially blood
    pressure, cardiovascular assessment, assess lung sounds,
    obtain weights per ordered frequency, assess patient activity
    levels
Teach patient, family, and caregiver regarding signs and
    symptoms of potassium loss
Venipuncture as ordered for sodium, BUN, other electrolytes
    q _____ (specify MD orders)
Teach patient, family, or caregiver regarding foods high in
    potassium including dry fruits, orange juice, bananas, fish,
    leafy green vegetables when applicable

Check for orthostatic BP changes in patient, teach regarding postural hypotension, safety implications

Teach patient, family, and caregiver regarding stress factors

Teach patient, family, and caregiver new medication regimen

Teach patient, family, and caregiver new medication, desired effect and adverse effects

Teach patient, family, and caregiver importance of diet and exercise regimens

Teach patient, family, and caregiver reasons for compliance to treatment regimen

Teach patient, family, and caregiver urinary frequency pattern changes caused by treatment

Teach patient, family, and caregiver low sodium diet and decreased caffeine

Measure lower extremities as indicated, note site and amount of edema

Skilled evaluation and assessment of all systems in the patient with hypertension

Observe and monitor for neurological deficits or changes

RN to observe for signs, symptoms, dehydration, low K, fatigue, and other adverse effects based on specific drug therapies

RN to assess the patient's response to ordered interventions and treatments and report changes or unfavorable responses or reactions to the MD

Management and evaluation of the patient's POC

6. **Other services indicated**

HHA	Personal care
	ADL assistance
MSS	Evaluation
	Economic and socioeconomic factors which have an impact on noncompliance to the POC
	Resource identification and referral to community programs

7. **Associated factors based on diagnosis justifying homebound status**

Status after CVA with paresis, paralysis

Status post below the knee amputation

SOB on any exertion

Medical restriction due to hypertension, BRPs only

Severe weakness caused by new medication regimen
Orthostatic hypotension
S/P TIAs
Patient cannot safely leave home without assistance

8. **Short-term goals**

   Patient taking medication regimen every day
   BP in normal range

9. **Long-term goals**

   Compliance with treatment regimen
   Blood pressure is in normal for patient range
   Vision remains normal for patient
   Teaching understood and integrated into daily living

10. **Discharge plans for this patient**

    Remains homebound, needing skilled care
    No longer homebound, referred to outpatient service(s)
    Needs a more acute level of care, discharged to acute hospital
      setting
    Returned to self-care, under MD supervision

11. **Patient, family, and caregiver educational needs**

    Educational needs are regimens that the caregiver will be
    managing with the patient. These include:

    Safety measures in the home
    The importance of nutrition, exercise, relaxation, and weight
      loss in the management of hypertension
    The need to decrease significantly or quit smoking
    The patient's medications and their relationship to each other
    The importance of medical follow up, even when there are no
      symptoms or problems apparent to the patient
    When to call the home health program or the physician
    Other information based on the patient's unique medical and
      other needs

12. **Specific tips for reimbursement**

    Document any abnormal blood pressure
    Document progress toward goal
    Document any medication change

Document physician contact regarding _____ (specify)
Document dehydration, side effects
Document orthostatic hypotension
Document medication(s) being regulated or adjusted
Document all changes in the nursing visit record

IMPACTION

1. **General Considerations.**   Impactions are seen in the homebound elderly because of multiple factors, including poor nutrition or hydration status, decreased gastrointestinal motility, and increased immobility.

2. **Needs for initial visit**

    Specific initial physician orders
    Universal supplies precautions
    Other supplies or equipment, based on physician orders
    Vital signs equipment
    Lubricant
    Gloves

3. **Some potential medical-surgical diagnoses and codes**

Bowel impaction	560.30
Cancer, colon	153.9
Cancer, rectosigmoid	154.0
Constipation	564.0
Dehydration	276.5

4. **Associated nursing diagnoses**

    Constipation
    Fluid volume deficit, high risk for
    Management of therapeutic regimen (individuals), ineffective
    Pain

5. **Service skills identified**

    Skilled observation on assessment of the patient with an
       impaction
    Evaluation, check for, and manual removal of, fecal impaction
    Assess hydration and nutritional status
    Teach new bowel training regimen
    Teach regarding needed increase in fiber, fruit, and fluid diet
    Administer enema per order
    Teach suppository administration
    Assess bowel sounds, all four quadrants
    Management and evaluation of the patient POC

6. **Other services indicated**

    HHA   Personal care
                 ADL assistance

7. **Associated factors based on diagnosis justifying homebound status**

Needs assistance to ambulate
Bedbound or wheelchair bound
Cardiac restriction (history of AMI)
Extreme weakness, no weight bearing
Unsteady gait
Patient cannot safely leave home without assistance

8. **Short-term goals**

    RN   Daily compliance with increased fluid, fiber, and
                 fruit diet
                 Impaction removed
                 New bowel regimen being implemented
    HHA   Effective personal hygiene
                 ADL assistance

9. **Long-term goals**

    RN   Regular bowel movements or disimpaction when
                 needed
                 Increased comfort
                 Optimal hydration
    HHA   Effective personal hygiene
                 ADL assistance

10. **Discharge plans for this patient**

Impaction removed, then infrequent, yet intermittent visits for follow up, new diet and bowel training regimen or disimpaction, based on findings by RN

11. **Patient, family, and caregiver educational needs**

The importance of adequate hydration and nutrition
The bowel training regimen and schedule
The need to call the home care program should the patient experience discomfort and need to be disimpacted
The importance of medical follow up

Any other information based on the patient's unique medical condition and needs

12. **Specific tips for reimbursement**

The manual removal of fecal impaction(s) and bowel training are covered services, see HCFA HHA manual for specific guidelines; located in Section 205.1 p. 15.1, in Part Seven

Document the last bowel movement (if known) before RN visit

Document distention noted, as indicated

Document actual removal of fecal material

Document family and caregiver teaching, regarding bowel training program

Document family and caregiver teaching, regarding new diet regimen

Be aware that these patients are considered intermittent and, as such, can stay home care patients while receiving infrequent RN visits for occasional disimpactions

INTRAVENOUS THERAPY AND OTHER LINE CARE

1. **General Considerations.**   As more patients want to be home and with reimbursement emphasis on decreasing inpatient length of stay, intravenous therapy is a viable program that integrates home nursing care with medical treatment at home. The reasons for home IV therapy are varied and include pain management, hydration, TPN, antibiotic therapy, and chemotherapy.

   Please see "Cancer Care," "Cellulitis," or "Wound Care" should these problems be appropriate for your patient.

2. **Needs for initial visit**

   Specific initial physician orders, including solution ordered, rate, site change frequency, and so on
   Universal precautions supplies
   Other supplies or equipment, based on physician orders
   Vital signs equipment
   Solution
   Tubing
   Catheter(s)
   Pump
   Tape
   Tourniquet
   $2 \times 2s$
   Alcohol swabs
   Other equipment as directed per agency protocol(s)
   Anaphylaxis kit

3. **Some potential medical-surgical diagnoses and codes**

AIDS	042.2
Amputation, infected stump	997.62
Appendix abscess	540.1
Bone, aseptic necrosis	733.40
Breast cancer	174.9
Cellulitis, right or left lower leg	682.6
Cervix, cancer of	180.9
Colon cancer	153.9
Congestive heart failure	428.0

Dysphagia	787.2
CVA	436
Dehydration	276.5
Diabetes mellitus, with complications, adult	250.90
Diabetes mellitus, with complications, juv.	250.91
Esophagus, cancer of	150.9
Fluid and electrolyte imbalance	276.9
Foot abscess	682.7
Head or neck, cancer of the	195.0
Hickman catheter insertion	39.98
Hypertension	401.9
Osteomyelitis	730.00
Osteomyelitis, ankle	730.07
Osteomyelitis, foot	730.07
Osteomyelitis, leg	730.26
Ovarian cancer	183.0
Pancreatic cancer	157.9
Pericarditis, acute	420.90
Pneumonia	486
Pneumonia, aspiration	507.0
Staph infection	041.1
Urinary tract infection	599.0
Venous thrombosis	453.8
Wound infection	

4. **Associated nursing diagnoses**

Anxiety
Cardiac output, decreased
Caregiver role strain
Caregiver role strain, high risk for
Fear
Fluid volume deficit
Fluid volume excess
Infection, high risk for
Injury, high risk for
Knowledge deficit (self-care management)
Pain
Pain, chronic
Protection, altered
Skin integrity, impaired
Skin integrity, impaired, high risk for
Tissue perfusion, altered (specify type) (renal, cerebral,
   cardiopulmonary, gastrointestinal, olfactory)

5. **Service skills indicated**

Observation and complete systems assessment of the patient
with an IV for _____ (specify)

Provide IV site care, IV therapy program implementation

Assess needle, supplies, site for contamination

Teach patient, family, and caregiver effective handwashing
techniques

Teach signs and symptoms of infiltration, home safety

Teach signs and symptoms of impeded or rapid flow of
medication solution

Teach accurate calculation of milliliters per minute

Teach care of heparin lock for intermittent antibiotic
medications

Teach flush of heparin with NS solution techniques to ensure
patency of heparin lock and use of line for ordered
medications

RN to change tubing and filters q _____, per agency protocol

Teach family or caregiver to document date and time for all
infusions started and completed

Teach patient, family, and caregiver regarding position of site
with IV

Assess urinary elimination changes related to hydration,
change, and status

Teach patient, family, and caregiver signs and symptoms of
infection, phlebitis

Teach patient, family, and caregiver when to contact on-call
RN or physician

RN to instruct patient and caregiver regarding multiple
medications, including schedule, route, functions, and
possible side effects

RN to obtain blood for _____ (specify test and frequency)
from central venous catheter per protocol

Teach patient and family signs and symptoms of phlebitis,
occlusion, displacement, infection, and other possible
problems

Observation and assessment of patient with a peripherally
inserted central catheter (PICC) for long-term therapy

RN to monitor patient for evidence of infection, metabolic
problems, or other complications in patient on TPN

Teach self-observational and record keeping skills to
patient and caregiver for documenting response to
_____ therapy

Perform sterile IV dressing change and site care
q _____ (specify)
RN to restart peripheral IV q _____ (specify orders)
RN to teach patient and caregiver in correct operation and care
related to safe use of PCA pump for pain management
RN to assess the patient's response to treatments or
interventions and report changes or unfavorable responses or
reactions to the physician
Management and evaluation of the patient's POC

6. Other services indicated

HHA	Personal hygiene
	ADL assistance
MSS	Evaluation of emotional and social factors
	affecting POC implementation
	Home assessment
	Financial counseling
	Problems with treatment plan implementation
OT	Evaluation
	Safety assessment of home
	Adaptive equipment assessment
	ADL retraining
	Conservation of energy techniques

7. Associated factors based on diagnosis justifying homebound status

Immunosuppressed due to disease/chemotherapy
Leg to be elevated
Antibiotic therapy at home
Reverse isolation
Severe SOB
Patient cannot safely leave home without assistance

8. Short-term goals

RN	Patient receives ordered solutions and medications without complication
	Patent IV site, without induration, other problems at site
	Patient, family, and caregiver able to support care at home
	Pain management

HHA	Effective personal hygiene
	ADL assistance
MSS	Problem identification
	Care team and patient adhering to POC
OT	Daily adherence to OT POC
	Concentration on immediate ADL needs in eating, dressing, bathing, personal hygiene

9. Long-term goals

RN	Vital signs normal
	Infection resolved
	Adequate hydration achieved
	Fluid and electrolyte status within normal limits for patient
	Safe, effective TPN administration
	IV antibiotic course completed
	IV discontinued
	Wound healed
	Safe delivery of ordered medications
	Pain management
HHA	Effective personal hygiene
	ADL assistance
MSS	Community resources identified
	Problem resolution
	Care team and patient able to implement and follow POC
OT	Return to independent functional living skills

10. Discharge plans for this patient

Discharged when antibiotic regimen completed
No longer homebound, refer to outpatient service(s)
Remains homebound, requiring skilled care
Patient will require TPN for rest of life
Therapy no longer indicated
Patient demonstrates effective PICC (or other line) care and can self-manage safely
When no further need for ongoing blood draws
Line no longer needed for hydration or _____ (specify)
Patient will need long-term IV care

11. Patient, family, and caregiver educational needs

Educational needs are the regimens the patient and

caregiver will need to know to safely and effectively provide care to the patient between visits or after discharge. These include:

The patient's medications and their relationship to each other

Simple IV troubleshooting techniques and problem resolution

Care of the groshong (or other catheter) and all aspects of care related to the safe delivery of the therapy, includes teaching catheter function, potential problems, self-observational skills, safety, and site care

The importance of compliance to the regimen

The importance of medical follow up

Effective handwashing techniques and other infection control measures

Safe disposal of needles and other sharps in the home

The symptoms that would appropriately necessitate calling emergency services

Other teaching specific to the patient and caregiver's needs based on the patient's unique medical condition

12. **Specific tips for reimbursement**

Teaching, training, observation, assessment, venipunctures, and IV line care are usually covered by most insurers on a case-by-case basis and with clear documentation. Page 14.15 of the HHA manual in Part Seven addresses specific IV skills

Document positive outcomes regarding teaching

Consider adding prn to your nursing frequency and duration orders for catheter site changes, removal, change of catheters, and complaints necessitating an additional visit

Document type of catheter used and purpose

Document dates of insertion or site changes

Document frequency of site change or site care given

Document specific orders for site care and the frequency of that care

Document schedule and rate of infusion

Document any schedule for flushing and these specific procedures or protocols

Document progress noted since admission

Document infected area site(s), symptoms

Document exacerbation of any symptoms, side effects of antibiotic, chemotherapeutic drug, or other therapy

Document dehydration symptoms

Document not stable, unstable

Document if patient unable to do ADLs, personal care

Document discharge projected less than _____ days (if patient is on a fixed protocol)

Document any medication and solution change

Document any rate and frequency of therapy changes

Document the last date of catheter insertion and the site care provided

KNEE REPLACEMENT

1. **General Considerations.**   Home health care patients having knee replacement surgery may have no skilled nursing needs identified. The physical therapy may be the skilled service. Other medical problems or an infected surgical wound site may necessitate skilled nursing services.

2. **Needs for initial visit**

   Specific initial physician orders
   Universal precautions supplies
   Other supplies or equipment, based on physician orders
   Vital signs equipment

3. **Some potential medical-surgical diagnoses and codes**

Arthritis	716.96
Arthritis, degenerative	715.96
Knee replacement, right or left	81.41
Osteoarthritis, leg	715.16
Osteomyelitis	730.05

4. **Associated nursing diagnoses**

   Activity intolerance
   Activity intolerance, high risk for
   Fatigue
   Fear
   Infection, high risk for
   Injury, high risk for
   Knowledge deficit (safety restrictions and self-care)
   Mobility, impaired physical
   Pain
   Pain, chronic

5. **Service skills identified**

   Observation and all systems assessment of the patient S/P total knee replacement
   RN to teach fall and safety precautions concerning knee replacement
   Venipuncture for pro-time q _____ (specify ordered frequency)

Wound care to surgical incision site, observation and
assessment for increased pain, edema, drainage, and other
signs of infection

Pain management of patient with arthritis in all joints
post-op TKR

RN to teach patient and caregiver regarding medication
regimen including schedule, functions, and possible side
effects

RN to assess the patient's response to treatments or
interventions

Report changes or unfavorable responses or reactions to MD

Management and evaluation of the patient POC

6. **Other services indicated**

HHA	Personal care
	ADL assistance
MSS	Evaluation
	Home assessment
	Financial counseling
	Problems with treatment plan implementation
	Community resource referral
PT	Evaluation
	Therapeutic exercise
	Gait training
	Home exercise program
	ADL training
	CPM immobilizer use
	Strengthening exercises
	ROM to lower extremities
	Transfer techniques
	Increased muscle strength to lower extremities
	Use of crutches as indicated

7. **Associated factors based on diagnosis justifying
homebound status**

Knee safety precautions
No weight bearing
Needs assistance to transfer or ambulate
Frail, elderly, S/P LE joint replacement
Decreased weight bearing, weakness
Medically restricted activity S/P LE surgery
Chairbound or bedbound

Patient cannot safely leave home alone without assistance
device

8. **Short-term goals**

RN	Incision healing
	Medication requested
	Stable CVP systems
	Patient can self-manage
	Pain control
HHA	Effective personal hygiene
	ADL assistance
MSS	Problems, resources identified
PT	Patient practices home exercise regimen safely
	Gait training with assistive device with
	progressive weight bearing as tolerated

9. **Long-term goals**

RN	Healed incision
	Infection-free
	Safe ambulation with assistive device
HHA	Effective personal hygiene
	ADL assistance
MSS	Community resource referral(s) as indicated
	Return to self-care status
PT	Increased joint function, strength, ROM
	Optimal mobility

10. **Discharge plans for this patient**

Discharge, self-care when no longer homebound or in need of
skilled services, refer to outpatient services
Discharge, under MD supervision, back to self-care status
Continue home health care visits for patient who remains
homebound and requires skilled care

11. **Patient, family, and caregiver educational needs**

Educational needs are the regimens that the patient or
caregiver will need to safely continue care after discharge
or provide between skilled visits. These include:

The importance of compliance to the regimen and medical
follow up

The patient's medications and their doses, functions, schedule,
and relationship to other medications

Safety aspects of care post-op total knee replacement

Other teaching specific to the patient's unique medical
condition and needs

12. **Specific tips for reimbursement**

For physical therapy services documentation, show that the
physical therapy is restorative; also, the patient should have
good or fair rehabilitation potential for identified goals, even
when indicated for safety or to set up a maintenance PT
home exercise program

Document the continued homebound status and specify why

Document any POC changes on the next form 486

Document any learning barriers identified

Remember that these patients may be appropriate for
management and evaluation of the patient POC by either
nursing or physical therapy.

LAMINECTOMY CARE

1. **General Considerations.**   In home health care, patients needing laminectomy care often have nursing needs related to pain control and physical therapy needs focused on rehabilitation of optimal function.

2. **Needs for initial visit**

   Specific initial physician orders
   Universal precautions supplies
   Other supplies or equipment, based on physician orders
   Vital signs equipment

3. **Some potential medical-surgical diagnoses and codes**

Arthritis spine	721.90
Cancer, lumbar spine	170.2
Laminectomy	03.09
Lumbar fracture	805.4
Lumbar stenosis	724.02
Osteoarthritis, spine	721.9
Quadriplegia	344.0
Rheumatoid arthritis, spine	720.0
Sciatica	724.3
Spinal cord compression	336.9
Spinal cord tumor	239.7
Spinal stenosis	724.00

4. **Associated nursing diagnoses**

   Activity intolerance
   Anxiety
   Constipation
   Fatigue
   Fear
   Home maintenance management, impaired
   Infection, high risk for
   Injury, high risk for
   Knowledge deficit (self-care regimen)
   Mobility, impaired physical
   Pain
   Pain, chronic

Self-care deficit, bathing/hygiene
Self-care deficit, dressing/grooming
Self-care deficit, feeding
Self-care deficit, toileting
Sleep pattern disturbance

5. **Service skills identified**

Evaluation and systems assessment of the patient S/P
laminectomy
RN to assess patient's pain q visit to identify pain and need
for analgesic dose adjustment or other plan for relief post-op
RN to evaluate patient's bowel patterns, need for stool
softeners, laxative, dietary changes/increase in fluids;
develop bowel management program
RN to assess the patient's response to treatments or
interventions and report changes or unfavorable responses or
reactions to the physician
Management and evaluation of the patient POC

6. **Other services indicated**

HHA	Personal care
	ADL assistance
MSS	Evaluation
	Counseling of problem(s) impeding POC implementation
	Financial resources assessment
	Nursing home placement
	Community resource referral(s)
OT	Evaluation
	Home safety assessment
	Increased upper or lower extremity strength
	Increase coordination
	Instruction in therapeutic tasks and exercises
	ADL retraining
PT	Evaluation
	Assess home environment for accessibility and with walker or other assistive device
	Therapeutic exercises
	Strengthening exercises
	Gait training with assistive device
	Home exercise program
	Stair climbing

Program to condition and strengthen
Active ROM
Teach patient use, application of TENS unit,
  ultrasound
Safe transfer mobility
Moist heat pack

7. **Associated factors based on diagnosis justifying homebound status**

Bedridden
Chair dependent
Bed rest
Paralysis
Paresis
Postoperative 1 week
Pain on movement
Quadriplegia
Frail, needs assistance to transfer or ambulate
Severe pain
Unsteady gait S/P surgery
Activity medically restricted
Patient unable to safely leave home without assistance

8. **Short-term goals**

RN	Pain control
	Safe mobility
HHA	Effective personal care
	ADL assistance
MSS	Problem identification
OT	Daily adherence to occupational therapy POC regimen
PT	Daily adherence to physical therapy POC and home exercise program
	Gait training implemented

9. **Long-term goals**

RN	Pain relief
	Increased safe mobility
HHA	Effective personal care
	ADL assistance
MSS	Community resources identified or problem resolution

OT	Independent ADLs
	Increased coordination, strength
PT	Functional ambulation
	Return to mobility
	Optimal function and mobility, independence

10. Discharge plans for this patient

Discharged when patient-centered goals achieved
No longer homebound, referred to outpatient services
Remain homebound, continues to need skilled care
Discharge under MD supervision and caregiver able to safely
provide care

11. Patient, family, and caregiver educational needs

Educational needs are the regimens the patient and caregiver
will need to know to safely and effectively provide care to the
patient between visits or after discharge. These include:

All the aspects of pain control
The importance of optimal nutrition, hydration, rest, and home
exercise program
The importance of medical follow up
Other information based on the patient's unique medical and
other needs

12. Specific tips for reimbursement

In rehabilitative therapy, documentation should show that the
services are restorative. Document the continued homebound
status and specify why.

Remember that these patients may need nursing skills of
observation and assessment, management and evaluation of the
patient POC, and care of the immobilized patient.

LARYNGECTOMY

1. **General Considerations.** Functional communication is a major priority in this patient population. Laryngectomy patients often need support for their underlying pathophysiology that indicated the need for this surgery.

2. **Needs for initial visit**

   Specific initial physician orders
   Universal precautions supplies
   Other supplies or equipment, based on physician orders
   Vital signs equipment
   Tracheostomy care supplies

3. **Some potential medical-surgical diagnoses and codes**

Airway obstruction, chronic	496
Attention to tracheostomy	V55.1
Bronchitis, acute	466.0
Cancer of the esophagus	150.9
Cancer of the larynx	161.9
Cancer of the pharynx	149.0
Cancer of the tongue	141.9
Cancer of the trachea	162.0
Laryngectomy	30.4
Tracheitis, acute	464.10
Tracheostomy closure	31.72
Tracheostomy permanent	31.29

4. **Associated nursing diagnoses**

   Airway clearance, ineffective
   Anxiety
   Body image disturbance
   Caregiver role strain
   Caregiver role strain, high risk for
   Communication, impaired verbal
   Fear
   Gas exchange, impaired
   Home maintenance management
   Infection, high risk for
   Injury, high risk for

Knowledge deficit (self-care management)
Nutrition altered: less than body requirements
Pain
Pain, chronic
Skin integrity, impaired
Swallowing, impaired

5. **Service skills identified**

Skilled observation and assessment of the patient with a
  laryngectomy due to _____ (specify)
Assess pulmonary status
Assessment of respiratory status, including amount and
  character of secretions
Suction per physician orders
Assess vital signs
Teach patient, family, and caregiver suction procedure(s) with
  return demonstration
Measure weight
Assess hydration and nutrition status
Teach patient, family, and caregiver site care
Teach patient, family, and caregiver oxygen utilization and
  safety concerns
Teach patient, family, and caregiver environmental safety
  concerns
Implement and teach respiratory therapy program
Teach care of tracheostomy
Provide care of tracheostomy
Teach signs and symptoms of URI and infection at site
Teach CPR with tracheostomy
Management and evaluation of the patient POC

6. **Other services indicated**

HHA	Personal care
	ADL assistance
S-LP	Evaluation
	Comprehension
	Alaryngeal speech
	Esophageal speech
	Assess and teach use of electrolarynx
	Teach swallowing skills
	Alternative communication skills

7. **Associated factors based on diagnosis justifying homebound status**

Limited mobility or pain
Needs maximum assistance to ambulate
Severe SOB
Unsteady on walking
90° heat and humidity, postlaryngectomy with SOB
Weakness after surgery
Shortness of breath
Bedbound
Pain or weakness
Weakness after surgery
Medically restricted because of the risk of infection after
   surgery
Dyspnea on exertion requiring oxygen continuously
Patient cannot safely leave home unattended

8. **Short-term goals**

RN	Daily adherence to care regimens, patent airway
HHA	Effective personal hygiene
	ADL assistance
S-LP	Patient able to communicate

9. **Long-term goals**

RN	Patent airway
	Stable respiratory status
	Dyspnea decreased or absent
	Self-care with medical regimen, able to perform care
	Patient infection-free
HHA	Effective personal care
	ADL assistance
S-LP	Functional communications
	Patient able to be understood

10. **Discharge plans for this patient**

Discharge when patient-centered goals achieved
Remains on service, in need of skilled care, remains
   homebound
Patient remains in home, self-care, under MD supervision

11. **Patient, family, and caregiver educational needs**

Educational needs are the regimens that the caregiver will be
managing with or for the patient. These include:

Importance of adequate hydration, optimal nutrition, and rest
for healing and recovery

Effective handwashing techniques, the avoidance of infection
and, particularly, respiratory irritants such as smoking

All aspects of stoma site care include self-observational skills,
cleansing routines, need for humidity, hygiene measures,
and safety care related to stoma

Referral to a local support group for patients with
laryngectomies

The importance of continuing S-LP services on an outpatient
basis when the patient is no longer homebound

Other information based on the patient's unique medical
history and other identified needs

The American Cancer Society (ACS) has support groups
such as "I Can Cope" and other programs. To locate the
chapter nearest your patient, call 1-800-ACS-2345.

The ACS has a "Look Good . . . Feel Better Program"
that offers support and makeover services by cosmetologists
for women undergoing chemotherapy or radiation therapy. Call
1-800-395-LOOK for more information.

12. **Specific tips for reimbursement**

Document all care provided and the responses to treatments,
interventions

Document the outcomes of the nursing care

Document the continuing homebound status

Document any change in the POC and obtain MD orders for
any changes

Document amount, character of secretions

Document any respiratory changes

Document any increased temperature or other vital sign
changes

Communicate to the MD any changes and document these
discussions in the clinical record

LUMBAR STENOSIS

1. **General Considerations.**   Home health care patients who have lumbar stenosis often have nursing needs related to pain control and physical therapy needs focused on restoring functional mobility.

2. **Needs for initial visit**

   Specific initial physician orders
   Universal precautions supplies, per agency protocol
   Other supplies or equipment, based on physician orders
   Vital signs equipment

3. **Some potential medical-surgical diagnoses and codes**

Arthritis, spine	721.90
Cancer of the lumbar spine	170.2
Laminectomy	03.09
Lumbar fracture	805.4
Lumbar stenosis	724.02
Osteoarthritis, spine	721.90
Quadriplegia	334.0
Rheumatoid arthritis, spine	20.0
Sciatica	724.3
Spinal cord compression	336.9
Spinal cord tumor	239.7
Spinal stenosis	724.00

4. **Associated nursing diagnoses**

   Activity, intolerance
   Anxiety
   Constipation
   Fatigue
   Fear
   Home maintenance management, impaired
   Injury, high risk for
   Knowledge deficit (self-care management)
   Mobility, impaired physical
   Pain
   Pain, chronic
   Self-care deficit, bathing/hygiene

Self-care deficit, dressing/grooming
Self-care deficit, feeding
Self-care deficit, toileting
Sleep pattern disturbance

5. **Service skills identified**

Skilled systems assessment of the patient with lumbar stenosis
RN to monitor patient's bowel habits and assess need for
    bowel management program
Assessment of patient's pain and relief with analgesia other
    pain relief measures
Management and evaluation of the patient POC

6. **Other services indicated**

MSS	Evaluation
	Counseling of problem(s) impeding POC implementation
	Financial resources assessment
	Nursing home placement
	Community resource referral(s)
OT	Evaluation
	Increased upper or lower extremity strength
	Increase coordination
	Instruction in therapeutic tasks and exercises
	ADL retraining
PT	Evaluation
	Assess home environment for safety and accessibility with walker or other assistive device
	Therapeutic exercises
	Strengthening exercises
	Gait training with assistive device
	Home exercise program
	Stair climbing
	Active ROM
	Teach patient use, application of TENS unit
	Ultrasound to _____
	Transfer mobility
	Moist heat pack
	Teach patient and family safety precautions as appropriate

7. **Associated factors based on diagnosis justifying homebound status**

Bedridden
Bed rest
Paralysis or paresis
1 week after surgery
Pain on movement
Quadriplegia
Frail, needs assistance to transfer or ambulate
Severe pain
Unsteady gait
Activity medically restricted
In traction
Severe weakness
Patient is unable to safely leave home unattended

8. **Short-term goals**

RN	Pain relief
	Constipation resolving; plan for bowel management
	Medications regulated
HHA	Effective personal care
	ADL assistance
MSS	Problem identification
OT	Daily adherence to occupational therapy POC regimen
PT	Daily adherence to physical therapy POC regimen
	Safe mobility program implemented

9. **Long-term goals**

RN	Patient pain-free
	Safe with optimal mobility in own home
	Stable medication
	Understands self-care management program
HHA	Effective personal care
	ADL assistance
MSS	Community resources identified or problem resolution
OT	Independent ADLs
	Increased coordination, strength

| **PT** | Functional ambulation |
| | Return to mobility |

10. **Discharge plans for this patient**

Discharged when patient-centered goals achieved
No longer homebound, referred to outpatient services
Remains homebound, continues to need skilled, intermittent
    care
Discharged
Patient deterioration, admitted to inpatient facility
Return to self-care status, under MD supervision

11. **Patient, family, and caregiver educational needs**

Educational needs are the regimens that the patient or
caregiver will need to safely care for the patient between visits
or after discharge from home care. These include:

Safe and proper body mechanics to prevent further pain or
    injury
The importance of compliance to medical regimens
The home exercise program
Medications and their schedules, functions, possible side
    effects, and interactions with other medications
The importance of medical follow up
Other teaching specific to the patient's unique medical and
    other identified needs

12. **Specific tips for reimbursement**

In rehabilitative therapy, documentation should show that the
    services are restorative and directed toward safe mobility.
    Document the continued homebound status and specify why.

MYOCARDIAL INFARCTION

1. **General Considerations.** Home health care patients who have experienced a myocardial infarction have appropriate safety concerns. These patients need reassurance about the 24-hour on-call system and when emergency community personnel would be more appropriate to be contacted. These patients may also be appropriate for a personal emergency response system.

   Please refer to ''Cardiac Care'' or ''CABG Care'' should these be appropriate to your patient.

2. **Needs for initial visit**

   Specific initial physician orders
   Universal precautions supplies
   Other supplies or equipment, based on physician orders
   Vital signs equipment

3. **Some potential medical-surgical diagnoses and codes**

AMI	410.9
Anemia	285.9
Angina	411.1
Atrial fibrillation	427.31
Atrial flutter	427.32
Cardiomegaly	429.3
Cardiomyopathy	425.4
CHF	428.0
Chronic ischemic heart disease	414.9
COPD	496
Diabetes mellitus, with complications, adult	250.90
Diabetes mellitus, with complications, juv.	250.91
Digoxin toxicity	995.2 and E942.1
Electrolyte and fluid imbalance	276.9
HCVD	402.91
Heart block	426.9
Hypertension	401.9
Pacemaker, S/P	V45.0
Pericardial disease	423.9

Peripheral vascular disease	443.9
Pulmonary edema	518.4
Pulmonary edema with cardiac disease	428.1
Respiratory arrest, S/P	799.1
Venous thrombosis	453.8

4. **Associated nursing diagnoses**

Activity intolerance
Activity intolerance, high risk for
Anxiety
Body image disturbance
Breathing pattern, ineffective
Cardiac output, decreased
Caregiver role strain
Caregiver role strain, high risk for
Constipation
Coping, ineffective family: compromised
Decisional conflict (treatment)
Denial, ineffective
Diversional activity deficit
Family processes, altered
Fatigue
Fear
Fluid volume excess
Gas exchange, impaired
Grieving, anticipatory
Home maintenance management, impaired
Injury, high risk for
Knowledge deficit (disease process and management)
Mobility, impaired physical
Nutrition, altered: less than body requirements
Nutrition, altered: more than body requirements
Pain
Pain, chronic
Self-care deficit, bathing/hygiene
Self-care deficit, dressing/grooming
Self-care deficit, feeding
Self-care deficit, toileting
Skin integrity, impaired, high risk for
Sleep pattern disturbance
Spiritual distress (distress of the human spirit)
Tissue perfusion, altered (cardiopulmonary)

5. **Service skills identified**

Observation and complete systems assessment of the patient
S/P myocardial infarction
RN to teach care and safety regarding oxygen therapy at home
RN to instruct patient and caregiver regarding multiple
medications, including schedule, functions, routes,
knowledge, compliance, and possible side effects
RN to observe for signs of dig toxicity, including GI
symptoms such as vomiting or nausea and other possible
symptoms
RN to teach conservation of energy skills
RN to monitor for presence and amount of lower leg edema
Teach patient or caregiver record keeping for daily weights
and other aspects of self-observational care skills
RN to assess the patient's response to treatments and
interventions and report changes or unfavorable responses or
reactions to the physician
Management and evaluation of the patient POC
Measure vital signs, obtain baseline
Assess lungs, cardiovascular status, including peripheral pulses
Daily weights, patient or family to weigh patient
Venipuncture for prothrombin time, digoxin, electrolytes as
ordered q _____ (specify frequency ordered)
Assess for fluid retention, amount, site(s)
Assessment of any chest pain, including type, description,
frequency, duration, relief measures
Assess hydration, nutrition status
Teach regarding new medication regimen and side effects
Cardiac rehabilitation program per MD orders
Teach patient or family to take pulse
Assess for orthostatic hypotension
Implement bowel regimen
Teach low sodium, other diet as indicated
Teach patient signs and symptoms of pacemaker problems or
failure, including increased SOB, cough, pulse change,
increased edema, etc.
Teach patient ordered exercises, addressing issues of stair
climbing, lifting, and daily rest periods as indicated.

6. **Other services indicated**

HHA   Personal care duties
ADL assistance

MSS	Evaluation, indicated when the patient's social problems adversely impact the POC and impede the progress toward program goals
	Assess the patient's adjustment S/P AMI and associated problems
OT	Evaluation
	Teach energy conservation techniques
	ADL assessment
PT	Evaluation
	Strengthening exercises
	Gait training
	Endurance training

7. **Associated factors based on diagnosis justifying homebound status**

Bedridden
Chair dependence
Poor endurance S/P recent AMI
Cardiac restrictions on activity
Not to leave home for _____ weeks
Poor respiratory status, severe SOB
New pacemaker insertion after surgery
Frail, age _____, S/P AMI
Needs assistance of one or two persons to transfer or ambulate
Paralysis S/P CVA
Severe dizziness, weakness
Bathroom privileges only
Limited energy, endurance, and dyspnea on exertion
Angina with activity
Severe functional limitations
Lower extremity edema impairing ambulation
Patient cannot safely leave home unattended

8. **Short-term goals**

RN	Daily compliance with medication and POC
HHA	Effective personal hygiene
	ADL assistance
MSS	Problem identification
OT	Daily adherence to plan
	Patient uses conservation of energy techniques
PT	Daily adherence to PT program

9. **Long-term goals**

RN	Medications regulated
	Stable cardiovascular and respiratory status
	Vital signs and blood results in normal for patient range
HHA	Effective personal hygiene
	ADL assistance
OT	Patient independent in ADLs
	Effective integration of conservation of energy skills into daily living
PT	Functional independence in gait/ambulation

10. **Discharge plans for this patient**

Discharge when patient-centered goals achieved, self-care
No longer homebound, referred to outpatient services
Discharge home, self-care, under MD supervision

11. **Patient, family, and caregiver educational needs**

Educational needs are the regimens that the patient or caregiver will need to safely continue to care for the patient at home. These include:

The patient's medications and their relationship to each other
The importance of proper weight maintenance, rest, optimal nutrition, and the specified long-term exercise regimen
The importance of compliance to the regimen
The importance of medical follow up
Effective use of oxygen, including use, liter flow, and safety
The application of anti-embolic stockings as ordered
The symptoms that would appropriately necessitate calling emergency services (specify symptoms)
The need to quit or cut down on smoking
Other teaching specific to the patient and caregiver needs

12. **Specific tips for reimbursement**

Document the specific care provided including teaching instructions
Communicate any POC changes in your documentation
Document progress toward goals
Document any abnormal lab values in the clinical record
Document any medication changes in the clinical record

Document the specific teaching accomplished and the
behavioral outcomes of that teaching

Document any identified learning barriers

Document tachycardia, bradycardia, any pulse irregularity

Document any change in respiratory status, increased
respiratory rate, SOB, etc.

Document any episodes of chest pain and note the site,
severity, reaction, and notify physician

OSTEOMYELITIS

1. **General Considerations.** Home health care patients who have osteomyelitis usually have identified nursing needs of dressing changes, observation, and monitoring of antibiotic therapy.

   Please refer to ''IV Care,'' or ''Wound Care'' should those problems be appropriate for your patient.

2. **Needs for initial visit**

   Specific initial physician orders
   Universal precautions supplies
   Other supplies or equipment, based on physician orders
   Vital signs equipment

3. **Some potential medical-surgical diagnoses and codes**

Osteomyelitis (foot, ankle)	730.07
Osteomyelitis (lower leg, knee)	730.06
Osteomyelitis (pelvic region and thighs)	730.05
Osteomyelitis (site unspecified) acute	730.00

4. **Associated nursing diagnoses**

   Activity intolerance
   Anxiety
   Caregiver role strain
   Caregiver role strain, high risk for
   Fatigue
   Fear
   Home maintenance management, impaired
   Infection, high risk for
   Injury, high risk for
   Knowledge deficit (self-care regimen)
   Mobility, impaired physical
   Pain
   Pain, chronic
   Self-care deficit, bathing/hygiene
   Self-care deficit, dressing/grooming
   Self-care deficit, feeding
   Self-care deficit, toileting

Skin integrity impaired, high risk for
Sleep pattern disturbance

5. **Service skills identified**

Skilled observation and complete systems assessment of the
  patient with osteomyelitis of _____ (specify)
Dressing changes _____ site, per physician orders
Wash site gently and dry
Teach new antibiotic regimen
Measure temperature, redness of site, amount of swelling
Assess for signs of decreased circulation, report to physician
Evaluate healing process
Keep leg elevated at all times
Keep leg elevated when sitting
Wear Ace™ wrap or TED stocking whenever up
Observe for healing, infection
Culture open wound as ordered, send for C & S
Assess hydration and nutrition status
Instruct patient or caregiver on dressing change procedure
Assess peripheral circulation
Check pedal pulses
Assess amount, site(s) of edema
Assess amount, site(s) of pain
Medicate patient with pain medication prior to dressing change
Assess pain: site, frequency, duration, characteristics of pain
Teach new medication regimen
Measure vital signs
Teach signs and symptoms of further infection
Teach sterile or prescribed dressing techniques
Teach safe disposal of old soiled dressings
Management and evaluation of the POC

6. **Other services indicated**

HHA	Personal care
	ADL assistance
MSS	Evaluation
	Home safety assessment
	Financial counseling
	Problems impeding POC implementation
	Community resource referral(s)
PT	Evaluation
	Joint therapy

Active ROM
Resistive exercise program
Home exercise program
Gait training and progressive weight bearing
management (assistive devices as needed)

7. **Associated factors based on diagnosis justifying
homebound status**

Weakness
Limited activity resulting from leg wound
Medical restrictions, leg to be elevated, no weight
bearing
Heel wound, poor ambulation
Patient requires maximum assistance to ambulate
Unable to transfer without maximum assistance
Chairbound or bedbound
Open abdominal wound with large amount of bloody
drainage
Open, infected wound
Surgical restriction
Open, draining leg lesions
Severe arthritis
Morbid obesity (specify height, weight)
Multiple functional limitations including _____
Poor ambulation with frequent falls
Patient unable to safely leave home without assistance

8. **Short-term goals**

RN	Daily compliance with POC
	Pain control
HHA	Effective personal hygiene
	ADL assistance
MSS	Problem, resource identification
PT	Practices home exercise program

9. **Long-term goals**

RN	Wound site(s) healed, infection-free
	Patient compliance with regimen(s)
HHA	Effective personal hygiene
	ADL assistance
MSS	Community referral(s), as indicated
	Returned to self-care status

Able to implement POC effectively

PT   Increased joint function

Increased strength and mobility

10. Discharge plans for this patient

Discharge, self-care, when no longer homebound or in need of skilled services

Continue home health visits on patient who remains homebound and requires skilled care

Patient discharged self-care, under MD supervision

11. Patient, family, and caregiver educational needs

Educational needs are the regimens that the caregiver will be managing with the patient. These include:

Home safety assessment and counseling

The avoidance of injury or infection to compromised skin sites

The importance of medical follow up

Signs and symptoms that necessitate calling the MD

Support groups in the community that are available to patients and caregivers

Teach patient and caregiver all aspects of care related to wound, including effective handwashing, disposal of soiled dressings, and other infection control measures

The importance of nutrition in the healing process

Teach patient about all medications, including schedule, route, functions, and possible side effects

Other aspects of care that are based on your patient's unique medical condition and other needs

12. Specific tips for reimbursement

Document the wound, indicate stage, drainage, color, amount and the specific care provided

Communicate any POC changes in your documentation

Document communication with the MD in the clinical record

Document progress in wound healing or deterioration in wound status

Document your supplies needed on the form 485 and obtain a physician order for all supplies

If wound culture is obtained, document the results in the daily visit record

Document any other learning barriers

Document if patient or family member is unable to do dressing
    (retinopathy, severity of wound, or other reasons)

Document the specific teaching accomplished and the
    behavioral outcomes of that teaching

Document patient's level of independence in care

Document red, warm, or draining at wound site

Document any changes, including specific care provided

Document RN in contact with physician
    regarding _____ (specify)

Document the continued homebound status and specify why

Wound care is an area in which some managed-care companies and other payers are attempting to decrease allowed numbers of visits. It is the professional nurse's responsibility to remember that it is not just the dressing change that occurs. When a nurse makes the home visit, there is an assessment of the wound healing or deterioration, actual hands on wound care, and teaching that occurs. These skills usually require the skills of the nurse. All of these components contribute to effective and safe wound care.

Remember that for Medicare patients, daily is defined as 5, 6, or 7 days. If your patient needs daily or BID dressing changes, obtain an order from the physician with an estimate for the finite and predictable endpoint. This date needs to be a date, for example 10/10/9_, not "when the decubitus heals." Remember that a patient that needs daily home care for the rest of their lives, is probably not appropriate for Medicare. In addition, remember that daily insulin injections (and only in those cases where the patient is unable or unwilling) are the exception to daily. Please review the HIM-11 or information from your manager obtained from the home health intermediary for further information.

OSTEOPOROSIS

1. **General Considerations.** According to some research, osteoporosis is estimated to occur in 25% to 50% of women over 60 years of age. Furthermore, researchers have found that one out of every five women who reach the age of 90 will experience a hip fracture. Whether due to the trauma of falls or insidious pathologic fractures, this problem is emerging as a health problem for all women in the 1990s. Interestingly, a nasal spray of calcitonin is currently being tested.

   Please refer to ''Fracture Care,'' ''Care of the Bedbound Patient,'' and ''Care of the Patient with Pain'' should those problems be appropriate for your patient.

2. **Need for initial visit**

   Specific initial physician orders
   Universal precautions supplies
   Other supplies or equipment, based on physician orders
   Vital signs equipment

3. **Some potential medical-surgical diagnoses and codes**

Arthritis	716.90
Constipation	564.0
CVA	436
Degenerative joint disease (hip, thigh)	715.95
Degenerative joint disease (lower leg, knee)	715.96
Diabetes mellitus, with complications, adult	250.90
Diabetes mellitus, with complications, juv.	250.91
Dislocated hip	835.00
Dislocation right or left hip prosthesis	996.4
Fracture humerus	812.20
Fracture, pathological	733.1
Fracture right or left hip	820.8
Fracture tibula with fibula	823.82
Hip replacement, partial	81.52
Hip replacement, total	81.59
Hyperparathyroidism	252.0
Hyperthyroidism	242.9
Lumbar stenosis	724.02
Lymphoma	202.80
ORIF	79.35

Osteoarthritis	715.90
Osteomyelitis	730.05
Osteoporosis	733.00
Paget's disease	731.0
Rheumatoid arthritis	714.0
Spinal stenosis	724.0
Sprain (acute), lumbar	847.2
Sprain (acute), lumbosacral	846.0
Sprain (acute), sacral	847.3
Vertebral compression fracture	805.8

4. **Associated nursing diagnoses**

Activity intolerance
Activity intolerance, high risk for
Anxiety
Body image disturbance
Constipation
Fear
Home maintenance management, impaired
Injury, high risk for
Knowledge deficit (management of disease)
Mobility, impaired physical
Nutrition altered: less than body requirements
Pain
Pain, chronic
Peripheral neurovascular dysfunction, high risk for
Self-care deficit, bathing/hygiene
Self-care deficit, dressing/grooming
Self-care deficit, feeding
Self-care deficit, toileting
Trauma, potential for

5. **Service skills identified**

Skilled assessment of the patient with history of fracture due to osteoporosis
RN to assess home and health habits for safety risks of trauma or falls
RN to monitor hydration and nutrition status
RN to teach regarding calcitonin medication therapy, including administration and side effects
RN to obtain weights (specify frequency) per MD order
RN to administer injection of calcitonin (calcimar) (specify route dose and frequency)

RN to administer and to teach caregiver to apply warm, wet compresses for comfort and pain relief

RN to assess patient pain and implement pain relief program

RN to teach caregiver and patient about the importance of correct body mechanics, range of motion, and caution about lifting or pulling

RN to teach patient regarding importance of hormone replacement therapy and associated implications

Instruct patient in the importance of x-ray and/or bone density studies prior to calcitonin therapy

Assess bowel patterns and instruct patient in bowel management

RN to teach regarding the importance of vitamin D, need for sunshine, and calcium in diet

Home safety evaluation for patient at high risk for falls and fractures

RN to assess the patient's response to treatment or interventions and report changes or unfavorable responses or reactions to the physician

Management and evaluation of the patient's POC

6. **Other services indicated**

HHA	Personal care
	ADL assistance
	Assist with home exercise program
OT	Evaluation
	Teach conservation of energy techniques
	Evaluation of patient for assistive/adaptive equipment to maintain safety in home (i.e., meal preparation safety)
PT	Evaluation
	Strengthening and safe transfer program
	Teach ROM, correct body positioning, and safe body mechanics
	Teach caregiver and patient home exercise program

7. **Associated factors based on diagnosis justifying homebound status**

Patient has pain on movement

Recent pathologic fracture precludes patient from leaving home

Patient has bony pain from hip fracture

Patient cannot leave home without maximum assistance and walker

Patient has very poor vision and cannot leave home alone

8. **Short-term goals**

RN	Maintain patient's level of functioning while preventing falls
	Daily adherence to POC regarding daily injections
	Home safety being improved
HHA	Effective personal hygiene
	Safe ADL assistance
OT	Adherence to OT POC
	Safe use of assistive/adaptive devices
PT	Safe joint mobility and function

9. **Long-term goals**

RN	Fracture healed
	Decreased pain and pain controlled
	Patient or caregiver able to manage care needs
	Safety in home setting improved
	Effective pain and safety program established
	Patient able to remain safely in home with assistive devices and information learned integrated into daily activities
	Therapeutic levels of calcium achieved with injections
HHA	Effective personal hygiene
	ADL assistance
OT	Patient using OT techniques
	Patient using assistive/adaptive devices
PT	Increased strength and mobility
	Increased function
	Pain control program established
	Optimal nutrition with adequate calcium intake

10. **Discharge plans for this patient**

Patient discharge back to community in safe environment at home

Patient returned to self-care status under MD supervision

Caregiver taught injections and other management aspects of care

Patient to be admitted to skilled nursing facility for increased care needs and caregiver exhaustion

Patient in long-term calcium replacement therapy and remains homebound

11. **Patient, family, and caregiver educational needs**

Educational needs are the regimens that the caregiver or patient will be managing. These include:

The route, dose, frequency, and technique for safe injections

Importance of adequate hydration and nutrition, particularly calcium

Home safety concerns, issues, and teaching about identified hazards

Referral of patient to have a personal emergency response system at home should they fall and be alone

The importance of medical follow up, including prescribed bone scan, studies, or procedures

The importance of the exercise program

All aspects of prevention, safety, and maintenance related to osteoporosis

Other needed information based on the patient's unique medical and other needs

12. **Specific tips for reimbursement**

For Medicare patients, calcimar injections and the calcimar itself can be covered. This is true for postmenopausal women with a documented history of fracture due to osteoporosis. The actual RN and other home care visits are billed as usual to Part A. This is unusual because Medicare does not usually pay for drugs or biologicals. Remember to document that the patient is unable to administer the drug and the caregiver(s) is unable or unwilling. Remember to project an estimated endpoint to the daily visits for calcimar administration. This should be located in number 22 of the 485 form.

For these patients and others with osteoporosis, there are various skills utilized by the licensed nurse. They include observation and assessment (pain, med monitoring), injection administration, and management and evaluation of the patient POC.

Refer to the HIM-11, Section 460 for more information.

OSTOMY CARE

---

1. **General Considerations.**   The patient needing ostomy care
   in the home setting must learn to adapt to an altered body
   image, and the nurse assists in the integration of this process.
      Please refer to ''Wound Care,'' ''Decubitus Ulcer,'' or
   ''Cancer Care'' should these problems be appropriate for your
   patient.

2. **Needs for initial visit**

   Specific initial physician orders
   Universal precautions supplies, per agency protocol
   Other supplies or equipment, based on physician orders, per
      agency protocol
   Vital signs equipment
   Irrigation set(s); disposble enema container, tubing, clamp
   4×4s
   Stomahesive, paste, karaya seal
   Paper tape
   Skin prep
   Ostomy bags, belts
   Waterproof pad(s)
   Gloves

3. **Some potential medical-surgical diagnoses and codes**

Attention to colostomy	V55.3
Attention to cystostomy	V55.5
Attention to ileostomy	V55.2
Attention to other artificial opening of digestive tract	V55.4
Attention to other artificial opening of urinary tract	V55.6
Bladder, cancer	188.9
Bowel obstruction	560.9
Bowel perforation	569.83
Cancer of the colon	153.9
Cancer of the rectosigmoid	154.0
Cancer of the rectum	154.1
Colectomy, sigmoid	45.76
Colitis	558.9
Colostomy	46.10

Diverticulitis	562.11
Hemicolectomy with colostomy	45.75 and 46.10
Ileostomy or other intestinal appliance, fitting and adjustment	V53.5
Proctocolectomy	45.79
Radiation enteritis	558.1
Skin eruptions	782.1
Skin, excoriation of	919.8
Urinary devices, fitting and adjustment	V53.6
Wound evisceration	998.3

4. **Associated nursing diagnoses**

Anxiety
Body image disturbance
Bowel incontinence
Caregiver role strain
Caregiver role strain, high risk for
Constipation
Diarrhea
Fatigue
Fear
Fluid volume deficit, high risk for
Infection, high risk for
Injury, high risk for
Grieving, anticipatory
Knowledge deficit (self-management and disease process)
Management of therapeutic regimen (individuals), ineffective
Nutrition altered: less than body requirements
Pain
Pain, chronic
Self-care deficit, toileting
Sexuality patterns, altered
Skin integrity, impaired
Skin integrity, impaired, high risk for
Social interaction, impaired
Spiritual distress (distress of the human spirit)
Tissue integrity, impaired
Tissue perfusion, altered (gastrointestinal)
Urinary elimination, altered

5. **Service skills identified**

Assessment of wound status

Teach ostomy care

Teach regarding appropriate diet

Assess hydration and nutrition

Adjust size of karaya seal

Teach patient modification of appliance to preserve wound integrity

Closely assess stoma and wound progress

Instruct patient regarding skin care and air-dry procedures

Teach patient regarding avoidance of gas-producing foods such as cauliflower, cabbage, beans, cucumbers, onions, etc.

Document emotional or physical barriers to learning or coping (e.g., severe arthritis of hands)

Help patient find best ostomy equipment and supplies, based on patient needs and price

Teach regarding irrigation procedure(s)

Teach regarding skin care to protect from irritation and infection

Consult with enterostomal therapist for care planning as needed

Assess for allergy to sealant or appliances

Upon discharge, teach patient to be prepared for ''accidents,'' have cosmetic bag with supplies and one of each appliance or supply used and small plastic bag for disposal of soiled materials

Skilled observation and systems assessment of the patient with a _____ (specify) ostomy

RN to assess the patient's response to ordered interventions or treatments and report changes or unfavorable responses or reactions to the physician

Management and evaluation of the patient POC

6. **Other services indicated**

HHA	Effective personal hygiene
	ADL assistance
MSS	Assessment of social and emotional factors
	Counseling regarding body image changes that impede treatment plan implementation
	Financial assistance
	Nursing home placement
	Assess home situation
	Home evaluation

7. **Associated factors based on diagnosis justifying homebound status**

Weakness S/P major abdominal surgery
Medically restricted due to new colostomy
Pain S/P abdominal surgery
No driving, no lifting, homebound per physician orders
Severe weakness
Unsteady gait, continued weakness requiring assistive device
Patient unable to leave home without assistance

8. **Short-term goals**

RN	Daily adherence to nursing plan
HHA	Effective personal hygiene
	ADL assistance
MSS	Problem identification
	Counseling begun
	Patient able to implement care plan

9. **Long-term goals**

RN	Patient independent in colostomy care
	Normal vital signs
	Elimination regulated
	Returned to self-care status
	Infection-free
HHA	Effective personal hygiene
	ADL assistance
MSS	Community referral(s) initiated
	Returned to self-care status
	Patient adapting to altered body image

10. **Discharge plans for this patient**

Discharged, patient no longer homebound, referred to
   outpatient enterostomal therapist
Remains homebound, in need of skilled care
Nursing home placement
Returned to self-management, under MD supervision

11. **Patient, family, and caregiver educational needs**

Educational needs are the care regimens that the patient or
caregiver will be managing at home. These include:

Care of ostomy, including bag changes, skin care, and signs or
   symptoms to report

Teach patient self-observational skills regarding skin and other care regimens

Effective personal hygiene habits

The patient's medication and their relationship to each other

Temperature checking and reading

The importance of medical follow up

When to call the physician

Other instructions as needed, based on the patient's unique medical condition and other needs

For resources or support for patients there are two organizations that your patients can contact: The United Ostomy Association, 26 Executive Park, Suite 120, Irvine, CA 92714, (714) 660-8624, or The National Foundation for Ileitis and Colitis, 1-800-343-3637.

The American Cancer Society (ACS) has support groups such as ''I Can Cope'' and other programs. To locate the chapter nearest your patient, call 1-800-ACS-2345.

The ACS has a ''Look Good . . . Feel Better Program'' that offers support and makeover services by cosmetologists for women undergoing chemotherapy or radiation therapy. Call 1-800-395-LOOK for more information.

12. **Specific tips for reimbursement**

Document progress noted since admission and teaching started

Document up with assistance only

Document any changes, including specific care provided

Document physician changed medications to _____ (specify)

Document new onset (any problem)

Document pain not controlled

Document increased gas pain

Document inability of patient and caregiver to learn stoma or irrigation care procedures

Document all teaching done and outcomes of that teaching

Document all changes on the next form 486 and in the nursing notes

Document the specific type of ostomy, the type and size of the ordered appliances, and frequency of changes needed

Document the patient's skin condition, the specific skin care regimen ordered and provided

Document the patient's level of self-care and progress toward predetermined, patient-centered goals

There are usually many nursing needs of the patient with a new colostomy or the patient with a new caregiver who must be taught the established care regimens. These include:

Observation and assessment skills
Ostomy care including healing, complications, body
    image, etc.
Wound care (hands-on teaching and wound assessment/
    reassessment)
Teaching the safe care regimens to caregivers
Other skills, based on the patient's needs

PAIN (CARE OF THE PATIENT WITH)

1. **General Considerations.**   It has been said that the most frequently identified nursing diagnoses may be pain.

   It is important to remember that patients are the experts on their pain, their histories, and often even the relief measures they need. This information can be most easily elicited during the completion of the pain assessment tool. Once asked, patients will readily assess and discuss their pain perceptions. There are many options available to control patient's pain and other symptoms.

   Nurses are becoming the experts in this area as experienced hospice and specialized pain unit nurses develop accepted assessment tools, protocols for titration of medications, and overall management of pain. For effective pain management, efforts of the home care nurse and team need to be directed toward comfort and verbalization of relief, when possible.

2. **Needs for initial visit**

   Specific initial physician orders
   Universal precautions supplies
   Other supplies or equipment, based on physician orders
   Vital signs equipment

3. **Some potential medical-surgical diagnoses and codes**

   Pain can come from any cause, source, or diagnosis. Please refer to the other care guidelines for specific diagnoses codes such as arthritis, cancer, depression, hospice care, peripheral vascular disease, fracture care, or any other area that is appropriate for your patient's pain problems.

4. **Associated nursing diagnoses**

   Activity intolerance
   Activity intolerance, high risk for
   Anxiety
   Caregiver role strain
   Caregiver role strain, high risk for
   Constipation
   Coping, family: potential for growth
   Coping, ineffective family: disabling

Coping, ineffective individual: disabling
Fatigue
Fear
Home maintenance management, impaired
Hopelessness
Infection, high risk for
Injury, high risk for
Knowledge deficit (pain management)
Mobility, impaired physical
Pain
Pain, chronic
Powerlessness
Role performance, altered
Self-care deficit, bathing/hygiene
Self-care deficit, dressing/grooming
Self-care deficit, feeding
Self-care deficit, toileting
Self-esteem disturbance
Sensory/perceptual alterations (specify) (visual, auditory, kinesthetic, gustatory, tactile, olfactory)
Sleep pattern, disturbance
Spiritual distress (distress of the human spirit)

5. **Service skills identified**

Complete initial assessment of systems in patient with pain for baseline information

RN to assess patient's pain q visit to identify need for change, addition, or other plan or dose adjustment

RN to assess all aspects of pain (including site(s), character, description, relation to activity or position); type of pain (constant, spontaneous, episodic); or other factors patient identifies

RN to teach patient and caregivers about the importance of and rationale for round the clock schedule of analgesia for continuous pain

Assess relationship of pain to increase safety risks, such as falls, in the home; counsel regarding safety and precautions

RN to implement nonpharmacologic interventions with medication schedule, including therapeutic massage, imagery, progressive muscle relaxation, humor, music therapies, and biofeedback

RN to provide emotional support to patient and family

Evaluate pain in relation to other symptoms, including fatigue, confusion, constipation, depression, SOB, etc.

RN to evaluate need for noninvasive methods of pain control, including heat, cold applications, or a transcutaneous electrical nerve stimulation (TENS) unit

Administer antiemetic on round the clock basis to control nausea caused by narcotic analgesia ordered for continuous pain

RN to titrate the dose to achieve patient pain relief with minimal side effects (per the range noted in the physician orders)

RN to evaluate patient's bowel patterns, need for stool softeners, laxative, dietary changes, or increase in fluids

RN to develop bowel management plan

RN to evaluate for emotional and other factors having an impact on pain

RN to assess the patient's unique response to treatments and interventions for pain control, and report changes or unfavorable responses or reactions to the physician

Management and evaluation of the patient's POC

6. **Other services indicated**

HHA	Personal care
	ADL assistance
	Assist with nonpharmacologic pain relief measures under supervision of RN, PT, OT
MSS	Evaluation of psychosocial factors of the patient with pain, chronic illness, and poor prognosis
	Assessment of financial ability to comply with pain regimen
	Evaluate family and patient's coping skills regarding chronic pain and its management
	Emotional support to patient
	Financial resource information
	Referral to community programs
OT	Evaluation
	Teach conservation of energy techniques
	Home and patient safety evaluation for needs of assistive/adaptive devices or equipment
	Assessment of home and health factors having an impact on health and POC being successfully implemented
PT	Evaluation

Home safety assessment
Progressive muscle relaxation
Safety precautions counseling
Biofeedback
Heat/cold applications
Use and management of TENS
Joint safety management
Management and evaluation of the POC

7. **Associated factors based on diagnosis justifying homebound status**

Needs maximum assistance for all activities
Patient has extensive pain with movement
Homebound, safety of patient compromised due to medication therapy
Patient homebound due to pain relief measures and pathologic fracture
Patient has weakness due to (diagnosis), cannot leave home unattended
Patient on oxygen, needs assistive devices to leave home safely
Patient severely sight-impaired, cannot leave home unattended
Patient cannot leave home unattended due to weakness, pain
Limited activity due to pain, shortness of breath
Chairbound or bedridden
Unable to transfer without maximum assistance
Patient on PCA pump for pain relief

8. **Short-term goals**

RN	Daily control of pain and other symptoms
	Patient without symptoms that impact daily function and ability to interact with friends and family
HHA	Effective personal care
	Patient clean and comfortable
MSS	Problem identification
	Home care team and patient adhering to POC to safely achieve pain control, and other symptom relief
OT	Daily adherence to occupational therapy POC
	Patient practicing use of conservation of energy techniques

	Patient using assistive devices or equipment
	Home exercise program
PT	Daily adherence to ordered POC
	Pain relief/control

9. Long-term goals

RN	Effective pain control and other symptom relief
	Functional mobility
	Early detection of problems/effects of bedridden patient by caregivers
	Patient and caregivers knowledgeable about side effects (e.g., constipation)
	Optimal hydration/nutrition status
	Patient and caregiver knowledgeable about pain relief measures and care for optimal relief and control
	Safety measures taught and implemented
HHA	Safe, effective personal care provided
	Patient clean and hygiene maintained
	Patient comfortable
MSS	Problem identification and referral to appropriate resources
	Referral to community support group
OT	ADL level maintained at optimal for patient's level
	Increased functional mobility
	Safe, effective use of assistive/adaptive devices
PT	Effective pain control
	Function maintained

10. Discharge plans for this patient

Patient discharged from home care, able to self-manage pain control care, under MD supervision

Caregivers taught and demonstrate ability to manage pain and symptom regimens

Symptom controlled death at home with caregiver and family support

Discharge from home care when patient stabilized and able to go to outpatient clinic for follow up

11. Patient, family, and caregiver educational needs

Educational needs are the regimens that the caregiver will be managing with or for the patient. These include:

Importance of all aspects of the pain control regimen

Importance of adequate hydration, nutrition, and rest

The importance of medical follow up

Support groups in the community that are available to patients and caregivers

Other information based on the patient's unique medical and other needs

12. **Specific tips for reimbursement**

The nursing skills used primarily in the area of pain and other symptom management will be: (1) observation and assessment; (2) management and evaluation of the patient POC; (3) administration of IM, SQ, or, in some cases, depending on the patient's unique medical condition; and (4) teaching and training activities related to the medication regimen, side effects, and how to administer the medication safely and effectively.

Examples of teaching or training activities may be, for example, teaching the patient and family the use of the PCA pump, how to safely administer medication, or care of the bedbound patient.

Document all care provided, including that related to pain management and the patient response to those interventions. Document any changes to the POC, MD communications, and obtain orders for any changes. Document changes or alterations to the POC and the patient's response to the changed interventions.

PARKINSON'S DISEASE

1. **General Considerations.** In home health care, patients with Parkinson's disease are usually admitted after an acute exacerbation of debilitating symptoms or a new diagnosis of the disease.

   Please refer to "Care of the Bedbound Patient" if that problem is appropriate to your patient.

2. **Needs for initial visit**

   Specific initial physician orders
   Universal precautions supplies
   Other supplies or equipment, based on physician orders
   Vital signs equipment

3. **Some potential medical-surgical diagnoses and codes**

Parkinson's, idiopathic primary (paralysis agitans)	332.0
Parkinson's, secondary, due to drugs	332.1 and E947.9
Sciatica	724.3

4. **Associated nursing diagnoses**

   Activity intolerance
   Activity intolerance, high risk for
   Airway clearance, ineffective
   Anxiety
   Caregiver role strain
   Caregiver role strain, high risk for
   Communication, impaired verbal
   Constipation
   Coping, ineffective family: compromised
   Family processes, altered
   Fatigue
   Fear
   Home maintenance management, impaired
   Incontinence, functional
   Infection, high risk for
   Injury, high risk for
   Knowledge deficit (self-care)
   Mobility, impaired physical

Nutrition, altered: less than body requirements
Pain
Pain, chronic
Role performance, altered
Self-care deficit, bathing/hygiene
Self-care deficit, dressing/grooming
Self-care deficit, feeding
Self-care deficit, toileting
Sensory/perceptual alterations (specify) (visual, auditory, kinesthetic, gustatory, tactile, olfactory)
Sexuality patterns, altered
Skin integrity, impaired
Skin integrity, impaired, high risk for
Sleep pattern disturbance
Social interaction, impaired
Spiritual distress (distress of the human spirit)
Swallowing, impaired
Thought processes, altered
Trauma, high risk for
Urinary elimination, altered

5. **Service skills identified**

Skilled observation and complete systems assessment of the patient with Parkinson's disease
RN to provide support and instruct primary caregiver regarding multiple medications, including specific schedule, function, and possible side effects
RN to assess and provide home safety instruction
RN to observe patient q visit for increased tremor, decreased cognitive function, weight, or other changes
RN to assess the patient's response to treatments and interventions and report changes, unfavorable responses, or reactions to the physician
Management and evaluation of the patient's POC

6. **Other services indicated**

HHA	Effective personal hygiene
	ADL assistance
MSS	Evaluation counseling of problem(s) impeding POC implementation
	Financial resources assessment
	Nursing home placement

	Community resource referral(s)
OT	Evaluation of patient and home safety
	Increase upper or lower extremity strength
	Assistive device evaluation
	Increase coordination
	Instruction in therapeutic exercises
	ADL retraining
	Teach alternative ADL skills
PT	Evaluation of patient and home safety factors
	Balance coordination exercises
	Therapeutic strengthening exercises
	Gait training with assistive device
	Use of assistive device
	Gentle stretching and joint ROM management
	Home exercise program
	Stair climbing
	Active ROM
	Teach patient and caregiver safety program
	Gait safety assessment
	Transfer mobility
	Safety awareness
S-LP	Evaluation
	Swallowing testing and evaluation
	Food texture recommendations
	Speech dysphagia instruction program
	Lip, tongue, and facial exercises to improve swallowing and vocal skills
	Short-term memory skills
	Establish home maintenance program

7. **Associated factors based on diagnosis justifying homebound status**

Bedridden
Chairbound
Paralysis, paresis
Pain on movement
Frail, needs assistance to transfer, ambulate
Severe pain
Unsteady gait and dizziness
Activity medically restricted to home
Patient cannot safely leave home without assistance

8. **Short-term goals**

HHA	Effective personal hygiene
	ADL assistance
MSS	POC implemented
OT	Daily adherence to occupational therapy plan
PT	Daily adherence to physical therapy plan
S-LP	Safe swallowing
	Improved communication
	Improved breath control
	Increased volume control

9. **Long-term goals**

HHA	Effective personal care
	ADL assistance
MSS	Community resources identified or problem resolution
OT	ADL retraining provided using adaptive equipment
	Independent ADLs
	Increased coordination, strength, sensation
PT	Safe, functional ambulation
	Return to mobility
	Safe use of assistive devices
	Trained in maintenance program, including ROM, strength, coordination, and safety
S-LP	Patient communicates
	Swallows safely

10. **Discharge plans for this patient**

Discharged, maintained in community, under MD supervision
Discharged, goals achieved
No longer homebound, referred to outpatient services
Remains homebound, continues to need skilled care
Discharged or patient deterioration with admission to inpatient facility

11. **Patient, family, and caregiver educational needs**

Educational needs are the regimens that the patient or caregiver will need to safely care for the patient at home. These include:

The importance of compliance to the regimen and medical
follow up

The need for the patient to maintain optimal nutrition and
exercise

Information about support groups in the community

Facts about safety concerns in the home, particularly the
bathroom as it is the most dangerous room in the house, fire
plans, electrical safety issues, and other environmental
dangers

The symptoms or problems that necessitate calling the RN
or MD

Other teaching specific to the patient's and caregiver's needs

12. **Specific tips for reimbursement**

Document the continued homebound status and specify why.

Obtain MD orders for *any* changes to the POC

Document all specific teaching accomplished and the
behavioral outcomes of that teaching

Document any POC changes on the next form 486

Document any POC changes, including specific care provided.
Many of these patients are admitted to home care because
they have Foley catheters or tube feedings. For catheters,
document the type, the size, the ordered frequency of
changes (also get 2-3 prn visits), teaching that occurs, and
the patient's response to interventions. For tube feedings, the
orders and the documentation also needs to be specific;
include the type, size, site, skin condition, change (frequency
of orders to change), the feeding schedule, and the ordered
feeding.

Document communication with the MD related to the POC.

PERIPHERAL VASCULAR DISEASE

1. **General Considerations.** Peripheral vascular disease is often seen in home health care as the initial diagnosis or in conjunction with problems, such as S/P AMI, CHF, or cellulitis.

    Please refer to ''IV Care,'' ''Wound Care,'' or ''Decubitus Ulcer'' if those problems are appropriate for your patient.

2. **Needs for initial visit**

    Specific initial physician orders
    Universal precautions supplies
    Other supplies or equipment, based on physician orders
    Vital signs equipment
    Measuring tape

3. **Some potential medical-surgical diagnoses and codes**

AMI	410.9
Amputation, infected right or left BKA, AKA	997.62
Amputation, transmetatarsal (right or left)	84.12
Arterial graft, S/P	39.58
Arterial insufficiency	447.1
Arterial occlusive disease	447.1
Bullous pemphigoid	694.5
Cellulitis of the arm	682.3
Cellulitis of the trunk	682.2
Cellulitis RLE, LLE	682.6
Chronic, ischemic heart disease	414.9
Congestive heart failure (CHF)	428.0
Coronary artery disease	414.0
Debridement right or left BKA, AKA	86.22
Decubitus ulcer	707.0
Diabetes mellitus, with complications, adult	250.90
Diabetes mellitus, with complications, juv.	250.91
Diabetic neuropathy	250.60 and 357.2
Diabetic retinopathy	250.50 and 362.01

Excoriation of skin	919.8
Femoral-popliteal bypass (right or left)	39.29
Foot abscess	682.7
Gangrene, toe	785.4
Hypertension	401.9
I and D stitch abscess	86.04 and 998.5
Leg injury	959.7
Open wound lower leg (right or left)	891.1
Open wound upper leg (right or left)	890.1
Osteomyelitis, acute	730.00
Osteomyelitis lower leg, right or left	730.06
Osteomyelitis of foot	730.07
Peripheral vascular disease	443.9
Skin eruption	782.1
Skin, excoriation of	919.8
Skin graft	86.69
Staph infection	041.1
Stasis ulcer	454.2
Stitch abscess, excision	998.5 and 86.22
Thrombophlebitis	451.9
Ulcer, heel with cellulitis	682.7
Ulcer right or left heel	707.1
Varicose leg ulcer	454.2
Vascular insufficiency	459.9
Vascular shunt bypass	32.29
Venous insufficiency	459.81
Wound, open lower leg (right or left)	891.1
Wound, open upper leg (right or left)	890.1

4. **Associated nursing diagnoses**

Activity intolerance
Adjustment, impaired
Anxiety
Body image disturbance
Body temperature, altered, high risk for
Cardiac output, decreased
Caregiver role strain
Caregiver role strain, high risk for
Coping, ineffective individual
Denial, ineffective
Family processes, altered
Fatigue

Fear
Fluid volume deficit, high risk for
Fluid volume excess
Gas exchange, impaired
Grieving, anticipatory
Home maintenance management
Infection, high risk for
Injury, high risk for
Knowledge deficit (self-care management)
Mobility, impaired physical
Noncompliance (specify, for example, self-care regimen)
Pain
Pain, chronic
Self-care deficit, bathing/hygiene
Self-care deficit, dressing/grooming
Self-care deficit, feeding
Self-care deficit, toileting
Sensory/perceptual alterations (specify) (visual, auditory, kinesthetic, gustatory, tactile, olfactory)
Sexuality patterns, altered
Skin integrity, impaired, high risk for
Sleep pattern disturbance
Social interaction, impaired
Spiritual distress (distress of the human spirit)
Tissue integrity, impaired
Tissue perfusion, altered (specify type) (renal, cerebral, cardiopulmonary, gastrointestinal, peripheral)

5. **Service skills identified**

Skilled observation and complete systems assessment of the patient with PVD
Weigh patient q visit
Dressing change _____ site, per physician orders
Wash site gently and dry
Teach new antibiotic regimen
Assess temperature, redness of site, amount of swelling
Assess for signs of decreased circulation, report to physician
Evaluate healing process
Teach to keep leg elevated at all times
Teach to keep leg elevated when sitting
Teach to wear Ace™ wrap or TED hose whenever ''up''
Observe for healing, infection

Culture open wound as ordered, send for culture and
  sensitivity
Assess hydration and nutritional status
Instruct patient or caregiver on dressing change procedure
Assess peripheral circulation
Check pedal pulses for equality, rate, and strength
Assess amount, site(s) of edema
Teach about aspirin therapy and side effects
Pain management, relief interventions
Apply occlusive dressing to wound
Teach patient correct application of compression stockings
Medicate patient with pain medication before dressing change
Assess pain, site, frequency, duration
Teach new medication regimen
Measure vital signs
Teach effective personal hygiene and proper handwashing
  techniques
Teach signs and symptoms of (further) infection
Teach sterile or prescribed dressing techniques
Teach safe disposal of soiled dressings or other supplies
Management and evaluation of the patient POC

6. **Other services indicated**

HHA	Personal care
	ADL assistance
MSS	Evaluation
	Home safety assessment
	Financial counseling
	Problems impeding POC implementation
	Community resource referral

7. **Associated factors based on diagnosis justifying
   homebound status**

Weakness and decreased or no weight bearing
Limited activity because of leg wound
Medical restriction, leg to be elevated
Heel wound, poor ambulation
Patient requires assistance to ambulate
Unable to transfer without assistance
Chairbound or bedbound
Pain on movement
Open, infected wound

Surgical restriction S/P abdominal surgery
Open, draining leg lesions
Severe arthritis
Morbid obesity
Multiple functional limitations including _____
Poor ambulation

8. **Short-term goals**

RN	Daily compliance with regimen
	Pain control
HHA	Effective personal hygiene
	ADL assistance
MSS	Problem, resource identification

9. **Long-term goals**

RN	Wound site(s) healed
	Infection free
	Patient compliance with regimen(s)
	Optimal circulation for patient
HHA	Effective personal hygiene
	ADL assistance
MSS	Community referral(s), as indicated
	Returned to self-care status
	POC effectively implemented

10. **Discharge plans for this patient**

Referred to outpatient services
Discharged, self-care, when no longer homebound or in need
   of skilled services
Continue home health visits on patient who remains
   homebound and requires skilled care
Self-care in home under MD supervision
Discharged when patient-centered, realistic goals achieved

11. **Patient, family, and caregiver educational needs**

Educational needs are the care regimens that the
patient or caregiver will be managing at home. These
include:

Teach patient self-observational skills regarding skin or wound
   site changes

The importance of medical follow up

The care and long-term regimens for this chronic
  disease

Optimal nutrition and home exercise program

When to call the RN or the physician

Other instructions as needed, based on the patient's unique
  medical condition and other identified needs

12. **Specific tips for reimbursement**

Document the wound, indicate stage, drainage, color, amount,
  and the specific care provided

Communicate any POC changes in your documentation

Document progress in wound healing or deterioration in
  wound status and measure in progress notes at least one
  time a week, noting other pertinent diagnoses that impede
  progress

Document supplies needed on the form 485 and obtain
  physician orders for all new or changed supplies

Decrease visit frequency as appropriate

If wound culture is obtained, document the results

Document if patient or family member unable to do dressing
  (retinopathy, severity of wound, etc.)

Document any other learning barriers

Document the specific teaching accomplished and the
  behavioral outcomes of that teaching

Document patient's level of independence in care

Wound care is an area in which some managed-care
companies and other payers are attempting to decrease the
allowed numbers of visits. It is the professional nurse's
responsibility to remember that it is not just the dressing
change that occurs. When a nurse makes the home visit, there
is an assessment of the wound healing or deterioration and
teaching that occurs. These skills usually require the skills of a
nurse. All of these components contribute to safer, effective
wound care.

Remember that for Medicare patients, daily is defined as 5,
6, or 7 days. If your patient needs daily or BID dressing
changes, obtain an order from the physician with an estimate
for the finite and predictable endpoint. This date needs to be a
date, for example 10/10/9_, not ''when the decubitus heals.''
In addition, remember that daily insulin injections (and only in

those cases where the patient is unable or unwilling) is the exception to daily. Please review the HIM-11 or information from your manager obtained from the home health intermediary for further information.

PNEUMONIA

1. **General Considerations.**   Pneumonia, especially in the elderly, remains a major cause of death.

    Please refer to "IV Care," "Chronic Obstructive Pulmonary Disease," and "Care of the Bedbound Patient" should those problems be appropriate for your patient.

2. **Needs for initial visit**

    Specific initial physician orders
    Universal precautions supplies, including masks, per agency
       policy
    Other supplies or equipment, based on MD orders
    Vital signs equipment
    Physical assessment skills

3. **Some potential medical-surgical diagnoses and codes**

Asthma, acute exacerbation	493.90
Bronchitis	466.0
CHF	428.0
COPD	496
Cor pulmonale	415.0
Dehydration	276.5
Electrolyte and fluid imbalance	276.9
Emphysema	492.8
Hypertension	401.9
Lung biopsy	33.27
Lung cancer	162.9
Pleural effusion (left or right)	511.9
Pneumonia	486
Pneumonia, pneumocystic carinii	136.3
Pulmonary edema	518.4
Tuberculosis (pulmonary)	011.90

4. **Associated nursing diagnoses**

    Activity intolerance
    Activity intolerance, high risk for
    Airway clearance, ineffective
    Anxiety
    Aspiration, high risk for

Body temperature, altered, high risk for
Breathing pattern, ineffective
Communication, impaired verbal
Fatigue
Fear
Fluid volume deficit, high risk for
Gas exchange, impaired
Home maintenance management, impaired
Infection, high risk for
Injury, high risk for
Knowledge deficit (self-care management)
Mobility, impaired physical
Nutrition altered: less than body requirements
Oral mucous membrane, altered
Pain
Pain, chronic
Protection, altered

5. **Service skills identified**

Skilled observation and complete systems assessment of the patient with pneumonia
Assess respiratory status, respiratory rate, pattern
Teach, evaluate new antibiotic regimen
Venipuncture, for CBC as ordered q _____ (specify ordered frequency)
Teach patient, family, and caregiver safe, effective oxygen therapy at home
Teach other pulmonary treatment as indicated
Teach effective coughing and deep breathing exercises
Assess breath, lung sounds
Evaluate vital signs
Teach patient, family, and caregiver use of nebulizer therapy
Postural drainage as ordered
Pain management due to cough and chest pain
Assess for signs and symptoms of hypoxia
Evaluate hydration and nutrition status
Management and evaluation of the patient's POC

6. **Other services indicated**

HHA	Personal care
	ADL assistance
MSS	Psychosocial assessment

	Home evaluation
	Financial counseling
	Community resources
	NHP placement
OT	Evaluation
	Conservation of energy techniques
	Assistive devices and home safety evaluation
PT	Evaluation
	Therapeutic exercises
	Home exercise program
	Gait training

7. **Associated factors based on diagnosis justifying homebound status**

   Severe SOB
   Limited mobility
   Severe weakness, nausea
   Respiratory distress with any movement or talking
   Patient on oxygen
   Profound weakness
   Chairbound
   Bedbound
   Needs assistance to ambulate or transfer safely
   Unable to transfer independently
   Needs assistance for all ADLs
   Severe arthritis
   Mobility severely restricted because of _____ (specify)
   Dizziness or weakness
   Severe SOB on any activity
   Severe functional limitations, including age
   Oxygen dependence
   Patient unable to safely leave home without assistive device

8. **Short-term goals**

RN	Daily compliance with medications, diet, POC
	Improved air exchange
	Decreased SOB
	Temperature in normal for patient range
HHA	Effective personal hygiene
	ADL assistance
MSS	Patient able to follow POC

OT	Utilizing conservation of energy techniques in daily regimen
	Safe use of adaptive equipment
PT	Home exercise regimen
	Pulmonary program
	Increased mobility and strength
	Discharged ambulating

9. Long-term goals

RN	Patient returning to good health
	Patient's pneumonia resolved
	Caregiver able to effectively care for patient
	Clear lung sounds
	Stable respiratory status
	Vital signs normal for patient
	Optimal hydration and nutrition
HHA	Effective personal hygiene
	ADL assistance
MSS	Resolution of problems
	Referred to community resources
	Successful implementation of POC
OT	Patient integrates conservation of energy tecnniques into daily life
	Using adaptive equipment safely
PT	Maximum oxygen exchange
	Patient able to do pulmonary care
	Maximum mobility, strength, and endurance

10. Discharge plans for this patient

Discharged when goals achieved
No longer homebound, referred to outpatient services
Patient discharged to 24-hour care services
Patient remains homebound, needing skilled care
Discharged to self-care, under MD supervision

11. Patient, family, and caregiver educational needs

Educational needs are the care regimens that the patient or caregiver will need to safely provide care between visits or at discharge. These include:

Effective handwashing techniques and other aspects of infection control

The patient's medication and their relationship to each other

The importance of compliance to the regimen and medical follow up

The symptoms that would appropriately necessitate calling emergency services (specify symptoms)

The importance of optimal nutrition, hydration, and the home exercise regimen

Other teaching specific to the patient and caregiver based on their unique needs

12. **Specific tips for reimbursement**

Document all abnormal breath and lung sounds heard

Obtain a telephone order for any POC changes and document these changes

These patients are usually sick, so be objective and document what the patient looks like (frail, pale, poor intake, SOB, unable to do ADLs, etc.)

Document patient's continued poor activity level because of SOB

Document the ordered rate of oxygen flow, mode, and specific hours needed

Discuss patient at case conference with physical therapy, occupational therapy, home health aide, and other ordered services

Document any increased SOB

Document any change, including medications, on the POC

Document RN contacted physician regarding _____ (specify)

Document RN in frequent communications with physician regarding _____ (specify)

Document febrile at _____ or tachycardia at _____ irr. irr.

New onset (any symptom)

Document patient deteriorating or progressing well

Document dehydration, dehydrating

Document stable, unstable

Document pain uncontrolled, any other symptom not controlled

Document positive sputum culture; physician started patient on _____ (specify ordered medication)

Document medications being regulated

Document bony prominences, red or opening skin sites

Document unable to do ADLs, personal care (for HHA services)

Refer to HCFA HHA manual for specifics on physical therapy or occupational therapy indications

PROSTATE CANCER

1. **General Considerations.** For patients who have prostate cancer in home health care, the nursing focus is often catheter care and pain or other symptom control measures. The documentation must clearly show that the patient is homebound and requires skilled nursing care.

   Please refer to ''Cancer Care,'' and hospice or pain Clinical Guidelines if appropriate.

2. **Needs for initial visit**

   Specific initial physician orders
   Universal precautions supplies
   Other supplies or equipment, based on physician orders
   Vital signs equipment
   Urinary catheter(s)
   Catheterization sets
   Drainage bag(s)
   Irrigation set

3. **Some potential medical-surgical diagnoses and codes**

Bladder cancer	188.9
Bone metastasis	198.5
Cancer of the prostate	185
Prostatectomy (TURP)	60.2
Prostatitis	601.9
Urinary tract infection	599.0
Urine incontinence	788.3
Urine retention	788.2

4. **Associated nursing diagnoses**

   Activity intolerance
   Activity intolerance, high risk for
   Adjustment, impaired
   Airway clearance, ineffective
   Anxiety
   Aspiration, high risk for
   Body image disturbance
   Body temperature, altered, high risk for

Bowel incontinence
Breathing pattern, ineffective
Cardiac output, decreased
Caregiver role strain
Caregiver role strain, high risk for
Constipation
Coping, ineffective family: compromised
Decisional conflict (treatments)
Denial, ineffective
Diarrhea
Family processes, altered
Fatigue
Fear
Grieving, anticipatory
Home maintenance management, impaired
Incontinence, total
Infection, high risk for
Injury, high risk for
Knowledge deficit (disease and management)
Mobility, impaired physical
Nutrition, altered: less than body requirements
Oral mucous membrane, altered
Pain
Pain, chronic
Parenting, altered
Protection, altered
Role performance, altered
Self-care deficit, bathing/hygiene
Self-care deficit, dressing/grooming
Self-care deficit, feeding
Self-care deficit, toileting
Sensory/perceptual alterations (specify) (visual, auditory,
    kinesthetic, gustatory, tactile, olfactory)
Sexual dysfunction
Skin integrity, impaired
Skin integrity, impaired, high risk for
Sleep pattern disturbance
Social interaction, impaired
Spiritual distress (distress of the human spirit)
Thought processes, altered
Tissue integrity, impaired
Urinary elimination, altered
Urinary retention

5. **Service skills identified**

Skilled observation and systems assessment of the patient with
  prostate cancer
Teach family or caregiver care of the patient
Assess bowel regimen and implement program as needed
Assess pain, other symptoms
Teach care of the bedridden patient
Measure vital signs
Assess cardiovascular, pulmonary, and respiratory status
Assess nutrition and hydration status
Teach new pain or symptom control medication regimen
Diet counseling for patient with anorexia
Check for and remove impaction as needed
Condom catheter or indwelling catheter care as ordered
Teach feeding tube care to family
Teach caregivers symptom control and relief measures
Assess weight as ordered
Measure abdominal girth for ascites and edema; document
  sites, amount
Oxygen on at _____ liters per _____ (specify orders)
Assess mental status, sleep disturbance changes
Assess disease process progression
Obtain venipuncture as ordered q _____ and prn
Teach new medications and effects
Decubitus ulcer care as indicated
Assess for electrolyte imbalance
Teach catheter care to caregiver
Teach family or caregiver IM injection technique and assess
  for complications
Assess amount and frequency of urinary output
Teach patient or family regarding conservation of energy
  techniques
Teach family regarding home safety and fall precautions
Teach and observe regarding side effects of chemotherapy,
  including constipation, anemia, and fatigue
RN to provide and teach effective oral care and comfort
  measures
RN to teach family about patient's need for small, high-calorie
  meals of his or her choice
RN to assess patient's pain or other symptoms q visit, to
  identify need for change, addition, or other plan or dose
  adjustment
RN to provide emotional support to patient and family

RN to evaluate the patient's bowel patterns, need for stool softeners, laxatives, and dietary adjustments, and develop bowel management plan

Assess the patient's response to treatments and interventions and report changes or unfavorable responses to the physician

RN to teach patient and caregiver regarding disease process and management

Management and evaluation of the patient POC

6. Other services indicated

HHA	Personal care
	ADL assistance
MSS	Evaluation of patient with illness of a chronic or terminal nature
	Problems impeding POC implementation
	Financial counseling
	Community resource referral(s)
OT	Evaluation of patient and home setting safety assessment
	Assess need for adaptive assistive devices
	Energy conservation techniques
	Muscle reeducation

7. Associated factors based on diagnosis justifying homebound status

Chairbound
Bedridden
Needs maximum assistance to ambulate
Needs assistance for all activities
Lower extremity paresis, paralysis, or paraplegia
Severe pain lower back (or other site)
Impending death, dying
Mobility severely restricted due to _____ (specify)
Weakness, dizziness
Severe SOB on any activity with oxygen dependency
Severe functional limitations, including age
Indwelling catheter
Patient unable to leave home without assistive device

8. Short-term goals

RN	POC followed as instructed by RN
	Pain, other symptom control

	Patent catheter
	Infection-free
HHA	Effective personal hygiene
	ADL assistance
MSS	POC implementation
	Problems, resources identified
OT	Patient using adaptive devices
	Patient implementing conservation of energy program and muscle reeducation skills

9. **Long-term goals**

RN	Pain and symptom control
	Patient able to care for self
	Caregiver able to care for patient
	Patent catheter
HHA	Effective personal hygiene
	ADL assistance
MSS	Community resources identified
	Problem resolution or referrals initiated
OT	Quality of life improved through use of adaptive devices, other skills taught by occupational therapist

10. **Discharge plans for this patient**

Discharge when goals achieved
Patient death
No longer homebound, referred to outpatient services
Remains homebound, continues to need skilled care
Discharged, patient needs 24-hour skilled care
Patient discharged, self-care, under MD supervision

11. **Patient, family, and caregiver educational needs**

Educational needs are the regimens that the caregiver will be managing for or with the patient. These include:

The importance of handwashing and effective hygiene
The availability of adequate pain relief measures
The need for keeping records related to and assessing for constipation
The safe use of oxygen therapy at home
The therapeutic and palliative value of nonpharmacologic comfort measures such as positioning, massage, progressive muscle relaxation, and other interventions of patient choice

The patient's medications and their relationship to each other

The importance of round-the-clock analgesia

Teach patient management of hair loss

The importance of medical follow up

Care of the catheter, changing bags, signs of catheter problems

The availability of support and hospice programs, if appropriate

Teach regarding the avoidance of infection and the signs and symptoms of infection

Other teaching specific to the patient and caregiver needs

The American Cancer Society has support groups such as ''I Can Cope'' and other programs. To locate the chapter nearest your patient call 1-800-ACS-2345.

12. **Specific tips for reimbursement**

Document all patient changes in the clinical record

Document an exacerbation of symptoms

Document dehydration or dehydrating

Document unstable, not stable

Document urine culture obtained and the results

Document RN in communication with physician regarding _____ (specify)

Document any POC change in the documentation and obtain orders for all changes

RENAL FAILURE

1. **General Considerations.** Patients with varying degrees of renal failure, including patients receiving dialysis for chronic renal failure, are primarily cared for at home. This continuum is very broad. The home health nurse's efforts are often directed toward the other pathologies that are present. Common examples include DM, CVA, hypertension, and skin care problems. The skills frequently utilized by the home health nurse include venipuncture, observation and assessment, and wound care.

2. **Needs for initial visit**

   Specific initial physician orders
   Universal precautions supplies
   Other supplies or equipment, based on physician orders
   Vital signs equipment

3. **Some potential medical-surgical diagnoses and codes**

Acute myocardial infarction	410.92
Acute pyelonephritis	590.10
Acute renal failure	584.9
Anemia	285.9
Angina pectoris	413.9
Ascites	789.5
Benign prostatic hypertrophy	600
Bronchitis, acute	466.0
CAPD (continuous ambulatory peritoneal dialysis)	54.98
Chronic ischemic heart disease	414.9
Chronic renal failure	585
Cirrhosis of the liver	571.5
Congestive heart failure	428.0
Constipation	564.0
Convulsions	780.3
CVA	436
Debility	799.3
Decubitus ulcer	707.0
Dehydration	276.5
Diabetes Mellitus, with complications, adult	250.90

Diabetes Mellitus, with complications, juv.	250.91
Diabetic nephropathy	250.41 and 583.81
Emphysema	492.8
Gastritis	535.50
Glomerulonephritis	583.9
Heart disease, chronic ischemic	414.9
Heart failure	428.9
Heart failure left	428.1
Hemiplegia	342.9
Hepatitis	573.3
Hepatitis B	070.30
Hepatitis (viral)	070.9
Hypercalcemia	275.4
Hyperosmolality	276.0
Hypertension	403.91
Hypoglycemia	251.2
Hypopotassemia	276.8
Kidney transplant (S/P)	V43.0
Kidney transplant (surgical code)	55.69
Liver disorder	573.9
Lung disease	518.89
Malaise and fatigue	780.7
Myocardial infarction	410.92
Nephrosclerosis	403.91
Nephrotic syndrome	581.9
Pericardial effusion	423.9
Pericarditis	423.9
Peripheral neuropathy	356.9
Peripheral vascular disease	443.9
Peptic ulcer	533.90
Pneumonia	486
Postoperative infection	998.5
Postoperative wound disruption	998.5
Psychosis	298.9
Pyelonephritis	590.80
Renal failure	586
Renal polycystic disease	753.12
Septicemia	038.9
Shunt, arteriovenous	V45.1
Shunt, infected	996.62
Shunt, peritonvas	54.94
Skin eruptions, nonspecific	782.1

Stomach ulcer	531.90
Systemic lupus erythematosus	710.0
Tubular necrosis (acute)	584.5
Wound debridement	86.28

4. **Associated nursing diagnoses**

Activity intolerance
Anxiety
Body image disturbance
Bowel incontinence
Cardiac output, decreased
Caregiver role strain
Caregiver role strain, high risk for
Constipation
Coping, family: potential for growth
Coping, ineffective family: compromised
Coping, ineffective family: disabling
Coping, ineffective individual
Diarrhea
Family processes, altered
Fatigue
Fear
Fluid volume deficit, high risk for
Fluid volume excess
Gas exchange, impaired
Health maintenance, altered
Home maintenance management, impaired
Hopelessness
Infection, high risk for
Injury, high risk for
Knowledge deficit (related to renal disease and care)
Mobility, impaired physical
Management of therapeutic regimen (individuals) ineffective
Noncompliance (specify)
Nutrition, altered: less than body requirements
Nutrition, altered: more than body requirements
Oral mucous membrane, altered
Pain
Pain, chronic
Peripheral neurovascular dysfunction, high risk for
Powerlessness
Protection, altered
Self-care deficit, bathing/hygiene

Self-care deficit, dressing/grooming
Self-care deficit, feeding
Self-care deficit, toileting
Sensory/perceptual alterations (specify) (visual, auditory,
  kinesthetic, gustatory, tactile, olfactory)
Sexual dysfunction
Skin integrity, impaired
Skin integrity, impaired, high risk for
Sleep patterns, altered
Spiritual distress (distress of the human spirit)
Thought processes, altered
Tissue perfusion, altered (renal)
Urinary elimination, altered

5. **Service skills identified**

Assessment of cardiovascular and other systems in patient with
  impaired renal function
RN to draw blood for digoxin level or other reasons (specify
  frequency)
Wound care, teaching and observation and assessment of the
  wound site and healing process
RN to assess patient and home safety factors for patient to
  have CAPD
RN to change dressing site using aseptic technique
RN to instruct on all medications, including schedule,
  functions, and side effects
Observe and assess all symptoms and systems
Teach signs and symptoms of bleeding and precautions
Administer EPO sq _____ (specify dose and frequency) to
  patient on CAPD
RN to teach patient and caregiver self-observational and care
  skills (e.g., TPR, I and O, BP, weight and record keeping)
Report changes, including signs and symptoms to MD
Teach caregiver wound care regimen
Assessment/dressing/teaching to patient and caregiver about
  subclavian access
Teach regarding application of topical lotion to pruritic areas
Monitor for signs and symptoms of infection
Venipuncture to monitor patient's hematocrit related to anemia
  and epoetin therapy
Assessment of shunt, graft, or fistula sites
Monitor bowel patterns, including frequency and evaluate need
  for stool softeners, diet changes, or laxatives

Teach patient and caregiver regarding skin care, including the need for frequent position changes, pressure pads or mattresses, and prevention of breakdown

Monitor blood pressure and other vital signs

Teach regarding effective oral hygiene measures

Teach about the availability of and the importance of wearing a Medic Alert™ bracelet

Teach emergency measures related to shunt site

Teach regarding new medications and their effects

RN to assess for complications of new medication therapy

RN to teach patient and caregiver nutrition and hydration regimen

Observation and assessment of the patient with DM and RF

Instruct about diet (e.g., low protein with fluid or other specified dietary orders and restrictions)

Venipunctures for fasting blood sugars

Teach patient and family regarding use of home glucose monitoring

Teach insulin administration and other DM care regimens including foot care, skin care, and emergency measures for signs and symptoms of hyper/hypoglycemia

Provide emotional support to patient and family with chronic illness

Teach patient and family emergency measures related to DM and RF

Assess and monitor patient's weights and intake and output

Management and evaluation of the patient POC

6. Other services indicated

HHA	Personal care
	ADL assistance
	Home exercise program
MSS	Evaluation
	Patient assessment including adjustment to health problems and diagnosis with long-term implications. Determine factors having an impact on POC not being effectively implemented or followed.
	Identify eligibility for services or benefits
	Financial counseling
	Community resource referral
	Referral to support group(s)
OT	Evaluation

	Conservation of energy techniques
	Adaptive assistive devices
PT	Evaluation
	Strengthening program, transfer training, progressive gait training
	Instruct, supervise, and teach caregiver home exercise regimen
	Management and evaluation of the patient POC

7. **Associated factors based on diagnosis justifying homebound status**

Fatigue due to anemia
SOB during all activities
Bed rest
Needs maximum assistance to ambulate
Transfers with assistance only
Needs assistance for all activities
Mobility severely restricted due to _____ (specify)
Patient medically restricted to home because of the threat of additional infection
Patient has significant lower extremity edema
Limited mobility or pain
Unsteady ambulation

8. **Short-term goals**

RN	Daily compliance to medical regimens (medications, fluid/dietary restrictions, recording I and O, others)
	Patient able to exert some control over activities, whenever possible, with all safety measures met
	BP within normal range for patient
	Cardiovascular, other systems, and renal function maintained
	Patient infection-free
	Patient able to spend time with friends and family
	Patient experiences an improved quality of life due to care interventions
	No significant weight gain, absence of edema
	Skin integrity maintained or improved
	Wound site infection-free
	Effective oral hygiene maintained

	Patient wearing Medic Alert™ bracelet
	Patient cared for safely at home
HHA	Effective personal hygiene
	ADL assistance
	Mobility maintained
MSS	Problem identification
	Counseling initiated
	Patient able to implement POC
OT	Daily adherence to occupational therapy POC
PT	Daily adherence to physical therapy POC

9. Long-term goals

RN	Patient adheres to dialysis regimen
	Patient and family integrate information about the disease process and care into their daily activities
	Patient experiences an improved quality of life due to care interventions
	Patient and caregivers effective in care management and know when to call physician or other professionals for assistance
	Patient able to make long-term decisions about care. This can include renal transplantation, kind of dialysis, or the stopping of treatment, if and when appropriate.
	Maintenance of goal weight
	Stable CV/renal status as demonstrated by _____ (specify)
	Skin integrity maintained
	Wound site healed
	Support patient on CAPD
	Access sites are patent and infection-free
	Optimal nutrition/protein restriction diet maintained
HHA	Safe, effective personal care
	Patient clean and feels better
	ADL assistance
MSS	Community resources identified
	Problem resolution
	Team and patient able to implement and integrate POC
	Effective adjustment to diagnosis and implications

	Referral of patient and spouse for continued support through community support services
OT	Patient able to use conservation of energy techniques in daily life activities
	Patient using adaptive or assistive devices
PT	Caregiver taught safe home exercise regimen, including transfers
	Patient practices exercise regimen and maintains schedule
	Patient has increased mobility
	Patient experiences or verbalizes increased strength and endurance

10. **Discharge plans for this patient**

Wound healed, patient infection-free, discharged back to the dialysis center

Discharge when patient-centered goals achieved

Diabetes mellitus stabilized, discharged from HHA

Patient no longer homebound, referred back to physician for outpatient care

Patient death

Discharged from HHA, patient needs 24-hour and/or full-time care and has been admitted to a long-term care facility.

Patient will continue to need daily wound care by the RN. The projected finite and predictable endpoint is _____ (stated by a projected date) according to physician.

Discharged from home care, caregiver trained, and under MD supervision in the community

Patient will remain in home with spouse as primary caregiver, providing safe care and under the supervision of the MD

Patient requires continued injections

11. **Patient, family, and caregiver educational needs**

Educational needs are the regimens that the caregiver will be managing with the patient. These include:

Fluid/dietary restrictions and monitoring daily weights

Effective personal hygiene habits

Effective bowel management program

The avoidance of infections, including effective handwashing techniques

Safety factors related to shunt site and care

The patient's medications and their relationship to each other

The importance of medical follow up

Aspects of self-care observation, including Tenckhoff catheter or site care of arteriovenous fistula between dialysis or home health nurse visits for observation and assessment

Temperature checking and recording of fluid and intake and output monitoring

The availability of the National Kidney Foundation as a resource for information and support

Support groups in the community that are available to patients and caregivers

Any other care regimens that the patient will need to manage care needs successfully after discharge

12. **Specific tips for reimbursement**

For Medicare patients, know that when a patient has end stage renal disease (ESRD), that this is a special and separate Medicare benefit from home care. All dialysis-related care needs to be provided by the dialysis center. Therefore, the patients that are seen in home care, usually have another medical problem separate from the ESRD or renal dialysis problems. These can include hypertension and the monitoring and medication regulation that occurs, diabetes mellitus, CVA wound care, insulin or EPO administration, and other problems not **directly** related to the dialysis condition.

When completing form 485, ESRD is usually not the principle diagnosis; the principle diagnosis is the reason that skilled care is needed. For example, it would be the wound, DM, or the hypertension. The documentation should reflect the actual care provided for the wound (i.e., hands-on care, teaching or observation, and assessment) and your patient's response to those care interventions. Wound care of infected shunt sites are not usually covered under the home health benefit.

For epoetin therapy, nursing visits to administer epoetin are usually covered as long as the drug frequency and duration are reasonable and necessary, based on the patient's unique medical condition and whether all coverage criteria are met. Remember that the actual drug epoetin is not covered under Medicare homecare.

Document the coordination occurring based on the POC between team members. Have the multidisciplinary conference notes reflected in the clinical record.

If any service has to be put on hold because the patient is "too sick," this should be reflected in the record and an MD order for that period should be obtained. Otherwise, it appears that the PT is not making visits as ordered on the POC.

SCIATICA

1. **General Considerations.**   For patients in home health care who have sciatica, the nursing focus is pain control and the physical therapy emphasis is functional mobility.

2. **Needs for initial visit**

   Specific initial physician orders
   Universal precautions supplies
   Other supplies or equipment, based on physician orders
   Vital signs equipment

3. **Some potential medical-surgical diagnoses and codes**

Arthritis, spine	721.90
Back contusion	922.3
Cancer of the lumbar spine	170.2
Compression fracture, vertebrae	733.1
Laminectomy	03.09
Lumbar fracture	805.4
Lumbar stenosis	724.02
Osteoarthritis, spine	721.90
Quadriplegia	344.0
Rheumatoid arthritis, spine	20.0
Sciatica	724.3
Spinal cord compression	336.9
Spinal cord tumor	239.7
Spinal stenosis	724.00

4. **Associated nursing diagnoses**

   Activity, intolerance
   Anxiety
   Constipation
   Fatigue
   Fear
   Home maintenance management, impaired
   Injury, high risk for
   Knowledge deficit (self-care management)
   Mobility, impaired physical
   Pain
   Pain, chronic

Self-care deficit, bathing/hygiene
Self-care deficit, dressing/grooming
Self-care deficit, feeding
Self-care deficit, toileting
Sleep pattern disturbance

5. **Service skills identified**

Skilled observation and complete systems assessment of the
    patient with sciatica
RN to monitor patient's bowel habits and assess for bowel
    management program
Assessment of patient's pain and relief with analgesia or other
    pain relief measures
RN to instruct patient and caregiver regarding medications,
    including schedule, functions, and possible side effects
RN to assess the patient's response to treatments and
    interventions and report changes or unfavorable responses or
    reactions to the physician
Management and evaluation of the patient POC

6. **Other services indicated**

HHA	Personal care
	ADL assistance
MSS	Evaluation
	Counseling on problem(s) impeding POC implementation
	Financial resources assessment
	Nursing home placement
	Community resource referral(s)
OT	Evaluation
	Increased upper or lower extremity daily living skills
	Increased coordination
	Instruction in therapeutic tasks and exercises
	ADL retraining
	Assessment of need for adaptive and safety equipment
PT	Evaluation
	Therapeutic exercises
	Strengthening exercises
	Progressive gait training with assistive device
	Home exercise program

Stair climbing
Active ROM
Teach patient use and application of TENS unit
Ultrasound to _____
Transfer mobility
Moist heat pack
Therapeutic massage

7. Associated factors based on diagnosis justifying homebound status

Bedridden
Chair dependent
Bed rest
Paralysis or paresis
One week after surgery
Pain on movement
Quadriplegia
Frail, needs assistance to transfer or ambulate
Severe pain
Unsteady gait and dizziness S/P surgery
Activity medically restricted
In traction
Severe weakness
Patient cannot leave home without maximum assistance

8. Short-term goals

RN	Adherence to pain control regimen
HHA	Effective personal hygiene
	ADL assistance
MSS	POC successfully implemented
OT	Daily adherence to occupational therapy POC program
PT	Daily adherence to physical therapy POC program

9. Long-term goals

RN	Pain control
	Safe mobility
HHA	Effective personal care
	ADL assistance
MSS	Community resources identified or problem resolved
OT	Independent ADLs

	Increased coordination and strength
	Safe use assistive/adaptive equipment
PT	Functional ambulation
	Return to mobility
	Increased strength, endurance, and mobility

10. **Discharge plans for this patient**

Discharged when goals achieved
No longer homebound, referred to outpatient services
Remains homebound, continues to need skilled care
Discharged, patient deterioration, admitted to inpatient facility
Returned to self-care, under MD supervision

11. **Patient, family, and caregiver educational needs**

Educational needs are the regimens that the patient or caregiver will need to safely care for the patient between visits or after discharge from home care. These include:

Safe and proper body mechanics to prevent further pain or injury
The importance of compliance to medical regimens
The home exercise program
Safety education, including bathroom safety, electrical, fire, and any identified environmental hazards
The importance of medical follow up
Other teaching specific to the patient's unique medical and other identified needs

12. **Specific tips for reimbursement**

Document the homebound status throughout your clinical documentation
Document the coordination occurring between team members based on the POC. The multidisciplinary conference notes should be reflected in the nursing notes. Refer to these meetings in planning further care and care coordination.

If PT is put on hold because the patient is too sick or other medical reasons, this should be reflected in the clinical documentation. Obtain an MD order for this change, otherwise it appears that the PT is not making visits as ordered on the POC.

SEIZURE DISORDERS

1. **General Considerations.** The patients seen in home health care with seizures may have other diagnoses such as cerebral vascular accident or cancer with metastatic disease that causes the seizures.

    Please refer to those clinical guidelines, ''Cerebral Vascular Accident,'' ''Cancer Care,'' or ''Brain Tumor'' should those topics be appropriate for your patient.

2. **Needs for initial visit**

    Specific initial physician orders
    Universal precautions supplies
    Other supplies or equipment, based on physician orders
    Vital signs equipment
    Flashlight

3. **Some potential medical-surgical diagnoses and codes**

CVA	436
Hypertension	401.9
Seizure disorder	780.3
TIAs	435.9

4. **Associated nursing diagnoses**

    Airway clearance, ineffective
    Anxiety
    Aspiration, high risk for
    Body image disturbance
    Bowel incontinence
    Caregiver role strain
    Caregiver role strain, high risk for
    Coping, ineffective family: compromised
    Coping, ineffective individual
    Fatigue
    Fear
    Grieving, anticipatory
    Home maintenance management, impaired
    Incontinence, total
    Injury, high risk for
    Knowledge deficit (self-care management)

Mobility, impaired physical
Noncompliance (specify)
Oral mucous membrane, altered
Parenting, altered
Personal identity disturbance
Powerlessness
Sensory/perceptual alterations (specify) (visual, auditory, kinesthetic, gustatory, tactile, olfactory)
Skin integrity, impaired
Social isolation
Spiritual distress (distress of the human spirit)
Thought processes altered
Trauma, high risk for

5. **Service skills identified**

Skilled observation and complete systems assessment of the patient with seizures
Measure vital signs
Assess neurological status
Teach patient and family seizure precautions
Teach new medication regimen
Assess need for a personal emergency response system
Assess effectiveness and side effects of new medication regimen
Teach signs and symptoms of TIA or stroke
Teach safety factors related to seizure disorder
Venipuncture for blood levels as ordered q _____ (specify orders)
Teach family to record characteristics of seizures

6. **Other services indicated**

HHA	Personal care
	ADL assistance
MSS	Evaluation
	Evaluation of problems impeding POC implementation
	Financial counseling
	Community resource referral(s)
PT	Patient evaluation
	Strengthening exercises
	Establish home exercise program

Gait training with walker
Teach patient and family safety precautions

7. **Associated factors based on diagnosis justifying homebound status**

Impaired neurological status, cannot walk
Paralysis left side S/P CVA
Dependence for all care
Severe weakness
Unsteady ambulation
Frail, needs assistance to ambulate
Severe SOB
Bedridden
Wheelchair dependent
Patient cannot safely leave home without assistance

8. **Short-term goals**

RN	Injury protection, safe care at home
	Daily compliance to treatment plan
HHA	Effective personal hygiene
PT	Daily adherence to exercise regimen

9. **Long-term goals**

RN	Stable neurological status
	Patent airway
	Injury protection
	Control of seizures and medication regulation
HHA	Effective personal hygiene
	ADL assistance
PT	Functional ambulation
	Return to mobility
	Increased strength, function, and balance

10. **Discharge plans for this patient**

Discharge, self-care, no longer homebound or in need of skilled services, referred to outpatient services
Continue home health visits to patient who remains homebound and requires skilled care
Discharged, medications regulated, self-care, under MD supervision

11. **Patient, family, and caregiver educational needs**

   Educational needs are the regimens that the patient or caregiver will need to safely care for the patient between visits or after discharge from home care. These include:

The symptoms that necessitate calling community emergency services
The importance of compliance to medical regimens
Safety precautions in the home environment
Other teaching specific to the patient's unique medical or other identified needs

12. **Specific tips for reimbursement**

   Occasionally, physical therapy services are indicated for those patients whose seizures or CVA result in hemiplegia or paralysis. This physical therapy is usually restorative in nature.

Document any seizure activity
Document any medication-related side effects
Document any communication with physician concerning patient changes or problems
Document any change in the POC
Document specific teaching accomplished and the behavioral outcomes of that teaching

SICKLE-CELL ANEMIA

1. **General Considerations.** The care listed below may also be appropriate for patients with sickle-cell trait, sickle cell-hemoglobin C (HbSC), and thalassemia should the patient be symptomatic or in the posthospitalization period after a crisis.

   Please refer to "IV Care" or "Care of the Patient with Pain" should those topics be appropriate to your patient.

2. **Needs for initial visit**

   Specific initial physician orders
   Universal precautions supplies
   Other supplies or equipment, based on physician orders
   Vital signs equipment

3. **Some potential medical-surgical diagnoses and codes**

Aseptic necrosis	733.40
Cardiomegaly	429.3
Cerebral hemorrhage	431
Cerebral vascular accident	436
Cholelithiasis	574.20
Congestive heart failure	428.0
CVA with dysphagia	436 and 787.2
Dehydration	276.5
Depression	300.4
Hematuria	599.7
Hemiparesis (right or left)	436 and 342.9
Hemiplegia	436 and 342.9
Hypertension	401.9
Hypertensive nephrosclerosis	403.90
Nephropathy	282.60 and 583.81
Osteomyelitis	730.00
Pneumonia	486
Priapism	607.3
Renal failure	586
Sickle-cell anemia (disease)	282.60
Splenomegaly	789.2
Stasis ulcer	454.0
Thalassemia	282.4
Thrombosis, leg	453.8

4. **Associated nursing diagnoses**

Activity intolerance
Activity intolerance, high risk for
Anxiety
Body image disturbance
Caregiver role strain
Caregiver role strain, high risk for
Constipation
Diarrhea
Fatigue
Fear
Fluid volume deficit
Fluid volume deficit, high risk for
Growth and development, altered
Infection, high risk for
Injury, high risk for
Knowledge deficit (disease management)
Mobility, impaired physical
Noncompliance (specify)
Nutrition, altered: less than body requirements
Pain
Pain, chronic
Role performance, altered
Self-care deficit, bathing/hygiene
Self-care deficit, dressing/grooming
Self-care deficit, feeding
Self-care deficit, toileting
Sexual dysfunction
Skin integrity, impaired
Skin integrity, impaired, high risk for
Tissue perfusion, altered (specify type) (renal, cerebral,
    cardiopulmonary, gastrointestinal, peripheral)

5. **Service skills identified**

Observation and complete assessment of all body systems of
    patient with sickle-cell disease
RN to assess patient for signs and symptoms of infection, S/P
    multiple blood transfusions, evaluation for internal/external
    bleeding
RN to monitor amount and site of pain
RN to observe for chronic leg ulcers, other sites of thrombosis

RN to counsel patient on importance of adequate hydration, nutrition, rest, and infection resolution and control

RN to teach patient about safe, effective use of oxygen therapy

RN to observe and assess patient for signs of impending crisis

RN to monitor patient's respiratory, mental status, and other functions for evidence of change or impending crisis

RN to monitor vital signs

Venipuncture for CBC, sedimentation rate (specify frequency ordered)

RN to monitor patient's weight, record q visit, report weight loss to MD

RN to start and monitor IV of _____ for hydration (specify MD orders)

RN to assess IV's patency and site for redness, tenderness, swelling, or other signs of infection/infiltration

RN to monitor intake and output of patient recently discharged from the hospital S/P crisis

RN to assess for alterations in bowel elimination patterns and instruct in bowel management program

RN to dress leg wound sites with (specify per MD orders) q (specify frequency)

RN to monitor patient's pain control regimen, including teaching caregivers the importance of adherence to the ordered, fixed medication schedule

RN to teach patient relaxation techniques, imagery, and other nonpharmacologic interventions that may assist in relief of pain/discomfort

RN to provide emotional support to patient and family with chronic illness and associated implications

RN to care for and change Groshong catheter site dressing; assess for adverse effects of IV antibiotic therapy

RN to auscultate lung sounds for signs and symptoms of infection

RN to teach patient and caregiver regarding all aspects of sickle-cell disease self-management

RN to assess the patient's response to treatments or interventions and report changes, unfavorable responses, or reactions to the physician (including diet, rest, hydration, infection control, and other high-risk activities that may precipitate a crisis)

Management and evaluation of the patient POC

6. **Other services indicated**

HHA	Personal care
	ADL assistance
	Participation in home exercise regimen
MSS	Evaluation
	Psychosocial assessment of patient with chronic illness, prognosis, and implications for future care needs
	Financial resource information
	Referral to community programs
OT	Evaluation
	Conservation of energy techniques
	Home and patient safety evaluation of needs for assistive/adaptive devices
	Assessment of home and health factors having an impact on health and POC being successfully implemented
PT	Evaluation
	Home exercise program assures ADLs, safety in home
	Teach safe use of assistive or adaptive devices

7. **Associated factors based on diagnosis justifying homebound status**

Patient posthospitalization with SOB, weakness
Patient on oxygen, needs assistive devices to leave home safely
Patient cannot leave home unattended
Patient severely sight-impaired, cannot leave home alone
Patient with joint pain (or other pain) uses _____ (specify assistive device) to ambulate
Mobility severely restricted due to _____ (specify)

8. **Short-term goals**

RN	Daily adherence to POC
	Return to self-care status, under care of MD
	Pain, other symptoms controlled
	Patient afebrile, infection controlled
	Patient hydrated
	Patient learning needed information about self-care
	Compliance with medication regimen

HHA	Effective personal care
	Patient clean and comfortable
MSS	Problem identification
	Home care team and patient adhering to POC
	Evaluate need for genetic counseling and referral
OT	Daily adherence to occupational therapy POC
	Patient practicing conservation of energy techniques
PT	Daily adherence to home exercise program

9. Long-term goals

RN	Patient discharged with functional mobility, pain-free, afebrile, and able to manage care
	Patient knowledgeable about factors that can precipitate a crisis
	Patient returned to self-care under MD supervision
	Avoid exposure to infections
	Pain, other symptoms controlled
	Adequate hydration/nutrition status
	Leg ulcers healing, clean, infection-free; patient able to self-manage care
	Patient knowledgeable about factors that can precipitate a crisis
HHA	Safe, effective personal care provided
	Patient clean and comfortable
MSS	Problem identification and referral to appropriate resources
	Referral to community support group
OT	Patient able to use conservation of energy techniques taught
	Patient able to safely use assistive/adaptive device
	Increased functional mobility
	Independent ADLs
PT	Patient knows and practices home exercise regimen
	Patient mobility maintained or improved

10. Discharge plans for this patient

Patient discharged from home care, able to manage care under MD supervision

Caregivers taught and demonstrated ability to manage care of patient in home with medications

Discharged from home care, caregiver and patient able to care effectively for patient, under MD supervision

Patient readmitted to acute care setting in crisis with need for transfusions

11. **Patient, family, and caregiver educational needs**

Educational needs are the regimens that the caregiver will be managing with or for the patient. These include:

Importance of adequate rest, hydration, and nutrition

The avoidance of infections

Self-observational skills of leg infections or wounds

Availability of genetic counseling

Pain management program

The importance of medical follow up

Support groups in the community that are available to the patient and their caregivers

Other information based on the patient's unique and other identified needs

For you and your patient's information, the following resource is available: National Association for Sickle Cell Disease, Inc., 4221 Wilshire Boulevard, Suite 360, Los Angeles, California 90010.

12. **Specific tips for reimbursement**

Patients with sickle-cell disease have a long history of interactions with health care settings and professionals. The patients know their histories, what pain medications bring relief most effectively, and other important information that assists the home care nurse in meeting patient and home care goals.

The nursing skills needed include observation and assessment, wound care for chronic leg ulcers, and management and evaluation of the patient POC.

SUBDURAL HEMATOMA AND FALLS

1. **General Considerations.**   Trauma is the most frequent cause of subdural hematomas. Other factors can be anticoagulation therapy, dialysis, renal failure, alcohol, and other drug abuse. The elderly and frail are at risk, often with a slow onset of symptoms after a fall. These patients, who live alone or spend most of the day alone, are very appropriate referrals for a personal emergency response system.

   Please refer to the section entitled ''Cerebral Vascular Accident,'' and, specifically, the services of PT, OT, and S-LP if mobility, paralysis, or impaired physical functioning occurs.

2. **Needs for initial visit**

   Specific initial physician orders
   Universal precautions supplies
   Other supplies or equipment, based on physician orders
   Vital signs equipment
   Flashlight for neurological checks

3. **Some potential medical-surgical diagnoses and codes**

Craniotomy	01.24
Hypertension	401.9
Subdural hematoma evacuations	01.09
Subdural hematoma (nontraumatic)	432.1
Subdural hematoma (traumatic)	852.20

4. **Associated nursing diagnoses**

   Anxiety
   Coping, ineffective family: compromised
   Coping, ineffective individual
   Fatigue
   Fear
   Grieving, anticipatory
   Home maintenance management, impaired
   Injury, high risk for
   Knowledge deficit (self-care management)
   Mobility, impaired physical
   Personal identity disturbance
   Powerlessness

Sensory/perceptual alterations (specify) (visual, auditory, kinesthetic, gustatory, tactile, olfactory)
Skin integrity, impaired
Spiritual distress (distress of the human spirit)
Thought processes, altered
Trauma, high risk for

5. **Service skills identified**

Skilled observation and complete systems assessment of the patient with a subdural hematoma
Assess blood pressure, observe for symptoms
Assess neurological status, including unsteady gait
Assess incisional site, care of sutures or staples
Medications (new) regimen teaching and observations
Physician regulating steroid therapy dose regimen
Teach family members symptoms of increased intracranial pressure
Teach family about and assess home safety
Assess need for personal emergency response system
Management and evaluation of the patient POC

6. **Other services indicated**

HHA	Personal care
	ADL assistance
MSS	Psychosocial assessment
	Evaluation of problems impeding POC implementation

7. **Associated factors based on diagnosis justifying homebound status**

Severe weakness S/P neurologic surgery
Weakness unsteady gait S/P surgery
Patient needs assistive device or assistance to ambulate

8. **Short-term goals**

RN	Daily compliance with medication regimen
	Blood pressure in normal range for patient
	No withdrawal symptoms from steroids
HHA	Effective personal hygiene
	ADL assistance
MSS	Resources identified
	Return to self-care status

9. **Long-term goals**

RN	Patient able to remain in home safely
	Medications regulated
	Blood pressure in normal range
	Stable neurological status
HHA	Effective personal hygiene
	ADL assistance
MSS	POC implementation
	Community referral

10. **Discharge plans for this patient**

Discharged, self-care in the community when no longer homebound

Patient returned to self-care status, under MD supervision

Patient no longer homebound, refer to outpatient services

Remains homebound, continues to need skilled care, remains in home health care service

11. **Patient, family, and caregiver educational needs**

Educational needs are the regimens that the patient or caregiver will need to safely manage care for the patient between visits or after discharge from home care. These include:

The symptoms that necessitate calling community emergency services

The importance of compliance to medical regimens

Safety precautions in the home environment

Other teaching specific to the patient's unique medical or other identified needs

12. **Specific tips for reimbursement**

Communicate any POC changes

Document any abnormal blood pressure readings in the clinical documentation

Obtain a telephone order for any POC change or additonal visit frequency

Document the continuing need for patient personal care
   services of the home health aide

Document specific teaching accomplished and the behavioral
   outcomes of that teaching

Document the patient's safety status

SURGICAL CARE

1. **General Considerations.** The kinds of patients seen at home with postsurgical problems are many and varied. The nursing problems that need management are also challenging and wide ranging. There are four areas that need to be assessed in all patients at home postoperatively. Sometimes these are referred to as the four Ws. They are wind, water, wound, and walk, and they correspond to the areas that are most at risk after surgery. The wind is lung problems or pneumonia; the wound is the operative wound that can become a site of infection; walk refers to phlebitis or leg thrombophlebitis; and the water refers to urinary tract infections. Other areas needing nursing care can include other systems, activity levels, and psychosocial concerns in the postoperative patient.

   Please refer to other specific, more common surgical diagnoses seen in home care, such as amputation, cardiac surgery, cellulitis, mastectomy, ostomy, tracheostomy, and hip fracture care.

2. **Needs for initial visit**

   Specific initial physician orders
   Universal precautions supplies
   Other supplies or equipment, based on physician orders
   Vital signs equipment

3. **Some potential medical-surgical diagnoses and codes**

Abdominal aortic aneurysm	441.4
Appendectomy	47.0
Appendicitis (perforation with abscess)	540.9
Attention to surgical dressing and sutures	V58.3
Bowel impaction	560.30
Cellulitis, RLE, LLE	555.9
Cholecystectomy	51.22
Cholecystitis (acute)	575.0
Cholecystostomy	51.04
Colitis	558.9
Colostomy, attention to	V55.3
Constipation	564.0
Crohn's disease	555.9

Cystocele	300.4
Decubitus ulcer	707.0
Diabetes mellitus, with complications, adult	250.90
Diabetes mellitus, with complications, juv.	250.91
Dehydration	276.5
Diverticulitis	562.11
Diverticulosis	618.4
Gastrojujunstomy	V45.3
GI bleeding (rectal)	569.3
Hemicolectomy	45.75
Hickman catheter insertion	39.98
Hysterectomy (abdominal)	68.4
I and D of abscess	86.04
Ileus	560.1
Intestinal obstruction	560.9
Other aftercare following surgery	V58.4
Pancreatitis (Acute)	577.0
Peritonitis, postoperative infection	998.7
Pneumonia	486
Posthemorrhage anemia	285.1
Quadriplegia	344.0
Thrombophlebitis (leg)	451.2
Urinary incontinence	788.3
Urinary tract infection	599.0
Wound dehiscence	998.3
Wound infection	998.5

4. **Associated nursing diagnoses**

Activity intolerance
Activity intolerance, high risk for
Adjustment, impaired
Anxiety
Body image disturbance
Body temperature, altered, high risk for
Bowel incontinence
Caregiver role strain
Caregiver role strain, high risk for
Constipation
Coping, ineffective family: compromised
Coping, ineffective individual
Denial, ineffective
Diarrhea
Diversional activity deficit

Family processes, altered
Fatigue
Fear
Fluid volume deficit, high risk for
Grieving, anticipatory
Health maintenance, altered
Home maintenance management, impaired
Incontinence, functional
Infection, high risk for
Injury, high risk for
Knowledge deficit, specify
Mobility, impaired physical
Noncompliance
Nutrition, altered: less than body requirements
Oral mucous membrane, altered
Pain
Pain, chronic
Powerlessness
Role performance, altered
Self-care deficit, bathing/hygiene
Self-care deficit, dressing/grooming
Self-care deficit, feeding
Self-care deficit, toileting
Self-esteem disturbance
Sensory/perceptual alteration (specify) (visual, auditory,
    kinesthetic, gustatory, tactile, olfactory)
Sexual dysfunction
Sexuality patterns, altered
Skin integrity, impaired
Skin integrity, impaired, high risk for
Sleep pattern disturbance
Social interaction, impaired
Spiritual distress (distress of the human spirit)
Tissue integrity, impaired
Tissue perfusion, altered (specify type) (renal, cerebral,
    cardiopulmonary, gastrointestinal, peripheral)
Urinary elimination, altered
Urinary retention

5. **Service skills identified**

Assessment of wound and systems in patient discharged from
    the hospital post-op _____ (specify surgery or disease
    identified)

RN to wrap site in _____ (specify) as ordered

Teach patient about new antibiotic regimen

RN to provide aseptic wound care to site (specify supplies, frequency, other MD orders)

Observation and assessment of wound

RN to evaluate patient pain and implement pain control/relief regimen

Teach patient and caregiver care related to wound including infection control measures

RN to assess lower extremity for signs and symptoms of compromised circulation or decreased sensation

RN to instruct on all medications, including route, schedule, functions, and side effects

Evaluate medication effectiveness

RN to assess and monitor pain, patient's response to interventions and effective pain relief measures

Teach patient and caregiver safe use of PCA pump

Monitor postoperative patient's bowel patterns, including frequency and evaluation of need for stool softeners, laxatives, or dietary changes

Assessment of blood pressure and other vital signs

RN to teach patient and caregiver on importance of nutrition postoperatively and dietary regimen

Teach patient and family safety issues postoperatively, including no pushing, pulling, or lifting until physician approves

RN to observe patient for signs and symptoms of infections postoperatively

Patient observed for signs and symptoms of infection postoperatively, including urinary and lung infections

Patient and caregiver taught signs and symptoms of when to call RN or MD

RN to medicate patient with pain medication prior to dressing change

RN assessment and observation of nutrition/hydration status

RN to culture wound site for C and S and send to lab

Teach regarding application of support hose

Ordered venipunctures to be obtained (specify frequency and diagnosis as needed) (e.g., fasting blood sugar for DM)

RN to administer IM or SQ medication _____ (specify) as ordered

Assess the patient's response to treatments and interventions

and report changes, unfavorable responses, or reactions to
the physician

Management and evaluation of the patient's POC

6. **Other services indicated**

HHA	Personal care
	ADL assistance
	Ambulation or assistance with home exercise program
MSS	Evaluation
	Assessment of social and emotional factors having an impact on health and effective POC implementation
	Identification of factors impeding POC from being successfully implemented
	Identify eligibility for services or benefits
	Financial assistance
	Community resource referral
	Counseling
OT	Evaluation
	Teach conservation of energy techniques
	Adaptive or assistive devices evaluation
	Teach use of adaptive/assistive devices
PT	Evaluation
	Strengthening home exercise program
	Safe transfer training
	Progressive gait training
	Instruct, supervise, and teach caregiver home exercise regimen
	Management and evaluation of the patient POC
	Teach application of and rationale for TENS unit

7. **Associated factors based on diagnosis justifying homebound status**

Patient is S/P _____ surgery (specify) has weakness and pain on movement

Patient is medically restricted for 3 weeks not to leave home except for visits to the vascular surgeon

Patient has open wound site and is unable to leave home without assistance

Multiple functional limitations, including blindness

Patient needs assistance to ambulate safely

Limited ambulation due to postoperative pain
Surgically restricted after abdominal surgery
Patient can transfer only with assistance of others
Patient requires maximum assistance to transfer and ambulate
Unsafe, unsteady gait in new post-op patient
Bathroom privileges only
Patient has compromised immune status (due to medications or disease),
Patient requires oxygen therapy and cannot handle portable without assistance
No or very limited weight bearing due to cardiopulmonary insufficiency

8. **Short-term goals**

RN	Daily adherence to POC
	Optimal nutrition for healing
HHA	Effective personal care
	ADL assistance
MSS	Identification of problem interfering with patient's or caregiver's ability to follow POC
	Initial counseling begun
	Care team and patient adhering to POC
	Referral initiated to community resources
OT	Daily adherence to occupational therapy POC
PT	Daily adherence to physical therapy POC

9. **Long-term goals**

RN	Patient and family caregivers adhere to implemented, effective POC
	Patient and family integrate information about the disease process and care into their daily activities
	Patient experiences an improved quality of life due to care interventions
	Patient and caregivers effective in care management and know when to contact RN, MD, or other care professionals for assistance
	Skin integrity intact
	Wound site healed without evidence of infection
	Patient is discharged without postoperative complications
HHA	Safe, effective personal care

	Patient clean and comfortable
	ADL assistance
MSS	Community resources identified
	Problem resolution
	Care team and patient able to implement and integrate POC into daily life
	Financial assistance
	Effective adjustment to diagnosis and implications
	Referral of patient and spouse caregiver to community services for continued support
OT	Patient able to use conservation of energy techniques taught in daily activities
	Patient using adaptive or assistive devices
PT	Caregiver taught safe home exercise regimen, including transfer techniques
	Patient practices exercise regimen and maintains schedule
	Patient has increased mobility
	Patient experiences or verbalizes improved strength or endurance

10. **Discharge plans for this patient**

Discharge when wound is healed or patient no longer requires skilled care

Patient infection-free with healed wound and discharged from home care program under care of local MD

Discharge when patient-centered goals achieved

Patient no longer homebound, referred to MD for outpatient visits

Patient will continue to need daily wound care by the RN. Medicare defines daily as 5, 6, or 7. The projected finite and predictable endpoint is _____ (stated in a projected date), according to MD.

Discharge from home care when nursing home bed becomes available per caregiver

Patient will remain in community with caregiver trained in patient care and under MD supervision

Discharged from home care, returned to self-care status

Discharged when patient and family able to safely and effectively provide patient care

11. **Patient, family, and caregiver educational needs**

Educational needs are the regimens that the patient or

caregiver will be managing with or for the patient. These include:

A home safety assessment and counseling regarding safety
Effective personal hygiene habits
The avoidance of infections
The importance of optimal hydration and nutrition
The patient's medications and their relationship to each other
The importance of medical follow up, including prescribed labwork
Self-care observation aspects of care, particularly the wound site
Support groups in the community that are available to your patient and their caregivers
Other information based on the patient's unique needs

12. Specific tips for reimbursement

Wound care appears to be an area in which some managed-care programs continue to reduce the number of approved visits. It is important, as the clinician actually seeing the patient and wound, that your input be heard. There are generally three parts to any wound care visit. They are: (1) the actual hands-on wound care and dressing change, (2) the observation and assessment of the wound and surrounding skin in relationship to healing and the patient's general health (i.e., temperature, swelling, pain), and (3) instruction or teaching skills that the professional nurse uses when educating the patient or caregiver for ultimate self-care. It is important that some third-party payers understand the nursing role and the components that comprise safe, effective wound care. Remember that Medicare defines daily as 5, 6, or 7 days a week. The projected finite and predictable endpoint should be realistic and stated as an actual date.

The way to help third-party payers understand these components is to clearly record the care you provided on each skilled visit. The specifics related to the wound size, drainage, odor, involvement of tissues/structures, and your skilled assessment of the healing or potential for healing will be helpful to those having to make a payment decision about the services provided.

TRACHEOSTOMY

1. **General Considerations.** Patients with extensive lung or cardiac surgery, tumors, foreign bodies, or edema return to the home setting needing tracheostomy care, which may be temporary or permanent, based on the pathophysiology causing this procedure.

2. **Needs for initial visit**

   Specific initial physician orders
   Universal precautions supplies
   Other supplies or equipment, based on physician orders
   Vital signs equipment
   Tracheostomy care supplies
   Gloves
   Water
   Suction supplies

3. **Some potential medical-surgical diagnoses and codes**

Airway obstruction, chronic	496
Attention to tracheostomy	V55.1
Bronchitis, acute	466.0
Cancer of the esophagus	150.9
Cancer of the larynx	161.9
Cancer of the pharynx	149.0
Cancer of the tongue	141.9
Cancer of the trachea	162.0
Laryngectomy	30.4
Tracheitis, acute	464.10
Tracheostomy closure	31.72
Tracheostomy permanent	31.29

4. **Associated nursing diagnoses**

   Airway clearance, ineffective
   Anxiety
   Aspiration, potential for
   Body image disturbance
   Caregiver role strain
   Caregiver role strain, high risk for
   Communication, impaired verbal

Fear
Home maintenance management, impaired
Infection, high risk for
Injury, high risk for
Knowledge deficit (self-care management)
Nutrition, altered: less than body requirements
Oral mucous membrane, altered
Pain
Pain, chronic
Skin integrity, impaired
Swallowing, impaired
Tissue integrity, impaired

5. **Service skills indentified**

Skilled observation and complete systems assessment of the
  patient with a tracheostomy
Assess pulmonary status
Assessment of respiratory status, draining amount, character of
  secretions
Assess vital signs
Suction per orders
Teach patient and caregiver infection control measures
  regarding cleaning cannula, etc.
Measure weight
Teach patient, family, and caregiver suction procedure(s)
Assess nutrition and hydration status
Provide and teach daily tracheostomy care
Teach patient, family, and caregiver regimen for inner cannula
  care
Teach patient, family, or caregiver environmental safety
  concerns regarding airway aspiration
Implement and teach respiratory therapy program
Teach care of tracheostomy
Teach signs and symptoms of respiratory infections
Teach CPR with tracheostomy
Management and evaluation of the patient POC

6. **Other services indicated**

HHA	Personal care
	ADL assistance
PT	Evaluation
	General conditioning exercises

	Gait training
	Safety assessment and teaching
	Home maintenance exercise program
S-LP	Comprehensive evaluation
	Teach and develop a communication system
	Care of voice prosthesis, including removal, cleaning, and safe site maintenance
	Articulation teaching

7. **Associated factors based on diagnosis justifying homebound status**

No driving, lifting, pushing, or pulling medical restrictions per physician orders
Limited mobility or pain
Copious secretions and SOB
Severe SOB
Braces on hips, very unsteady on walking
90° heat and humidity outside and patient has new surgery
Severe weakness after surgery
Pain or weakness
Weakness after multiple surgeries
Medically restricted because of risk of infection after surgery
Dyspnea on exertion requiring oxygen continuously
Patient needs maximum assistance to safely ambulate

8. **Short-term goals**

RN	Daily adherence to care regimen
	Patent airway
HHA	Effective personal hygiene
	ADL assistance
PT	Functional gait
	Functional home exercise program
S-LP	Patient able to communicate
	Safe swallowing

9. **Long-term goals**

RN	Patent airway with stable respiratory status
	Able to perform daily tracheostomy care
	Self-care regarding medical regimens
	No dyspnea
	Infection-free
	Optimal gas exchange

HHA	Effective personal hygiene
	ADL assistance
PT	Functional home exercise program
	Safe gait
S-LP	Patient able to communicate
	Functional communication
	Effective safe swallowing

10. **Discharge plans for this patient**

Discharged, goals achieved

Discharged, patient no longer homebound

Remains on service, in need of skilled care and remains homebound

Discharged, needs 24-hour acute care setting

Discharged, nursing home placement

Patient returned to self-care

11. **Patient, family, and caregiver educational needs**

Educational needs are the regimens that the caregiver will be managing with or for the patient. These include:

Importance of adequate hydration, optimal nutrition, and rest for healing and recovery

Effective handwashing techniques, the avoidance of infections, and particularly respiratory irritants such as smoking

All aspects of stoma site care include self-observational skills, cleansing routines, need for humidity, hygiene measures, and safety care related to stoma

Self-management aspects of care including daily trach care

Referral to a local support group for patients who have tracheostomies

The importance of continuing S-LP services on an outpatient basis when the patient is no longer homebound

Other information based on the patient's unique medical history and other identified needs

The American Cancer Society (ACS) has support groups such as "I Can Cope" and other programs. To locate the chapter nearest your patient, call 1-800-ACS-2345.

The ACS has a "Look Good . . . Feel Better Program" that offers support and makeover services by cosmetologists for women undergoing chemotherapy or radiation therapy. Call 1-800-395-LOOK for more information.

12. Specific tips for reimbursement

Document all care provided
Document the outcome of that care
Document any change in POC
Document amount and character of secretions
Document any respiratory changes
Document any increased temperature or other vital signs
    change
Document any change noted on the next form 486
Document the continuing homebound status
Document the teaching and training activities
Document suctioning
Document observation and assessment of _____ (specify)

WOUND CARE

1. **General Considerations.** Wound care is a common problem necessitating referrals to home health care. These patients utilize the nurse's ongoing assessment, teaching, and hands-on wound care skills through discharge.

2. **Needs for initial visit**

   Specific initial physician orders
   Universal precautions supplies
   Other supplies or equipment, based on physician orders
   Vital signs equipment
   Supplies (sterile or clean)
   Tape
   Wound culture if ordered

3. **Some potential medical-surgical diagnoses and codes**

Amputation, infected right or left BKA, AKA	997.62
Amputation, transmetatarsal (right or left)	84.12
Anal rectal abscess	566
Arterial graft, S/P	39.58
Arterial insufficiency	447.1
Arterial occlusive disease	447.1
Bullous pemphigoid	694.5
Cellulitis of the arm	682.3
Cellulitis of the trunk	682.2
Cellulitis RLE, LLE	682.6
Chronic ischemic heart disease	414.9
Congestive heart failure (CHF)	428.0
Coronary artery disease	414.0
Debridement	86.22
Decubitus ulcer	707.0
Diabetes mellitus, with complications, adult	250.90
Diabetes mellitus, with complications, juv.	250.91
Diabetic neuropathy	250.60 and 357.2
Diabetic retinopathy	250.50 and 362.01
Excoriation of skin	919.8

Femoral-popliteal bypass (right or left)	39.29
Foot abscess	682.7
Foot wound, open	892.2
Gangrene, toe	785.4
Heel ulcer, decubitus, right or left	707.1
Hypertension	401.9
I and D stitch abscess	86.04 and 998.5
Infection, postoperative	998.5
Leg injury	959.7
Open wound, lower leg (right or left)	891.1
Open wound, upper leg (right or left)	890.1
Osteomyelitis, acute	730.00
Osteomyelitis, foot	730.07
Osteomyelitis, lower leg (right or left)	730.06
Peripheral vascular disease	443.9
Peritonitis	567.2
Quadriplegia	344.0
Skin eruption	782.1
Skin, excoriation of	919.8
Skin graft	86.69
Staph infection	041.1
Stasis ulcer	454.2
Stitch abscess, excision	998.5 and 86.22
Surgical wound, open	998.3
Thrombophlebitis	451.9
Ulcer, heel with cellulitis	682.7
Ulcer, right or left heel	707.1
Urinary incontinence	788.3
Vascular insufficiency	459.9
Vascular shunt bypass	32.29
Varicose leg ulcer	454.2
Venous insufficiency	459.81
Wound evisceration	998.3
Wound, open lower leg (right or left)	891.1

4. **Associated nursing diagnoses**

Activity intolerance
Anxiety
Body image disturbance
Body temperature, altered, high risk for
Caregiver role strain

Caregiver role strain, high risk for
Coping, ineffective individual
Denial, ineffective
Family processes, altered
Fatigue
Fear
Fluid volume deficit, high risk for
Fluid volume excess
Home maintenance management
Infection, high risk for
Injury, high risk for
Knowledge deficit (self care management)
Management of therapeutic regimen (individuals), ineffective
Mobility, impaired physical
Noncompliance (self-care regimen)
Nutrition, altered: less than body requirements
Pain
Pain, chronic
Self-care deficit, bathing/hygiene
Self-care deficit, dressing/grooming
Self-care deficit, feeding
Self-care deficit, toileting
Sensory/perceptual alterations (specify) (visual, auditory, kinesthetic, gustatory, tactile, olfactory)
Sexuality patterns, altered
Skin integrity, impaired
Sleep pattern disturbance
Social interaction, impaired
Spiritual distress (distress of the human spirit)
Tissue integrity, impaired
Tissue perfusion, altered (specify type) (renal, cerebral, cardiopulmonary, gastrointestinal, peripheral)

5. **Service skills identified**

Skilled observation and systems assessment of the patient with a _____ (specify site or type) wound
Assessment of healing process and site for sign of infection
Pack wound with betadine-soaked 2×2, cover with kerlix and Ace™ wrap
Culture wound prn
Teach patient or caregiver wound packing and irrigation techniques
Soak foot in Domeboro's solution

Venipuncture to check blood sugar once a week while wound is healing

Cleanse wound with dry sterile Q-tip™

Cover wound with _____ (specify orders)

Apply Xerofoam gauze

Wrap site

Assess wound on left extremity for signs and symptoms of infection

Measure vital signs q SNV

Teach regarding new antibiotic regimen

Assess hydration and nutrition status

RN to contact enterostomal therapist for assessment of wound and recommend plan

RN to provide aseptic wound care to site (specify supplies, frequency, and specific wound orders)

Skilled observation and assessment of wound q visit

RN to evaluate patient pain and implement pain control/relief program

Teach patient and caregiver regarding wound infection control measures

Assess the patient's response to treatments and interventions and report unfavorable changes or reactions to the physician

Management and evaluation of the patient POC

6. **Other services indicated**

HHA	Personal care
	ADL assistance
MSS	Home safety evaluation
	Assessment of social and emotional factors
	Counseling
	Financial assistance
	Evaluation of problems impeding POC implementation and goal achievement
PT	Assessment
	Whirlpool baths
	High voltage galvanic stimulation (HVGs)

7. **Associated factors based on diagnosis justifying homebound status**

Medical restrictions due to open wound

Open lesions, decreased mobility

Bedbound or chairbound
Surgically restricted after abdominal surgery
Requires maximum assistance to ambulate or transfer
Open infected wound with weakness
Continual oozing liquid drainage from site
Unsteady gait
No weight bearing
Multiple functional limitations due to severe pain (sx, burns on thigh)
Poor ambulation with history of falls
Bathroom privileges only
Leg lucer

8. **Short-term goals**

RN	Daily compliance to medical regimen
	Healing wound
HHA	Effective personal hygiene
	ADL assistance
MSS	Problems identified
	POC implemented
PT	Adherence to physical therapy POC

9. **Long-term goals**

RN	Wound healed
	Vital signs in normal for patient range
	Site infection-free
	Compliance with care regimens
HHA	Effective personal hygiene
	ADL assistance
MSS	Community resources identified, referral(s) as appropriate
PT	Increased wound healing
	Function maintained
	Wound clean, infection-free

10. **Discharge plans for this patient**

Discharge when patient-centered goals achieved
No longer homebound, refer for outpatient follow up
Remains homebound, in need of skilled care
Nursing home placement
Self-care at home, under MD supervision

11. **Patient, family, and caregiver educational needs**

Educational needs are the regimens that the caregiver will be managing with the patient. These include:

Signs and symptoms that necessitate calling the RN or MD
All aspects of the specific care related to wound care, including effective handwashing techniques, safe disposal of soiled dressings, and other infection control measures
Home safety assessment and counseling
The importance of compliance to the care regimens and medical follow up
The importance of optimal nutrition and when possible, exercise to speed the healing process
Medication instruction, including schedule, route, functions, and possible side effects
Other aspects of care, based on patient's unique medical condition and needs

12. **Specific tips for reimbursement**

Document progress toward wound healing
Document patient or wound deterioration
Document any change that impacts the provision of safe care
Document wound draining, amount and site
Document any medication change(s)
Document progress or deterioration in wound healing, take measurements at least once a week
If wound culture is obtained, document the results in the clinical record
Specify and document the specific teaching accomplished and the behavioral outcomes of that teaching
Document the patient's level of independence in care

Sometimes portable whirlpool therapy is used at home by the physical therapist. There are also patients who receive high voltage galvanic stimulation (HVGs) therapy by PTs. These are sometimes used on patients wtih wounds that do not respond to whirlpool or usual nursing management, particularly diabetic wounds. Again, services need to be based on your patient's unique medical history and condition and in collaboration with the patient's physician.

Wound care is an area in which some managed-care companies and other payors are attempting to reduce the number of visits. It is the professional nurse's responsibility to remember that it is not just the dressing change that occurs. When a nurse makes the home visit, there is (1) observation and assessment of the wound, (2) teaching and training activities related to the wound and associated care, and (3) the actual hand-on care provided. The observation and assessment should occur every visit and the documentation should be focused on the healing or deterioration of the wound. All three of these parts of wound care usually require the skills of a nurse and all of these components contribute to safe, effective wound care. In your documentation, clearly stress these three skills.

For wound care and all care regimens in which supplies or equipment are needed, a physician order must be obtained and filed on the clinical record. If a patient uses opsite, 4×4s, adaptic gauze, kerlix, Dakin's solution, montgomery straps, or duoderm, an order is needed for all these supplies. These are only examples and the supplies are as variable as the patient's needs; but remember, all the care provided is under the physician POC, the 485 form and, as such, all need orders.

Wound dressing or care orders should always include the specific orders such as aseptic or clean technique, wound location, frequency of change, and any special supplies needed to safely and effectively follow the POC.

Remember that for Medicare patients, daily is defined as 5, 6, or 7 days. If your patient needs daily or BID dressing changes, obtain an order from the physician with an estimate for the ''finite and predictable endpoint.'' This needs to be a date, for example 10/10/9_, not ''when the decubitus heals.'' In addition, remember that daily insulin injections (and only in those cases where the patient is unable or unwilling) is the exception to daily. Please review the HIM-11 or information from your manager obtained from the home health intermediary for further information.

PART FIVE

HOSPICE CARE

HOSPICE CARE

1. **General Considerations.** Hospice care is sometimes appropriate for patients with an illness of a terminal nature who have a limited life expectancy. The hospice focus is on quality of life, while supporting the patient and family in making every remaining day the best it can be. Hospice care can be given in many settings, including home, an inpatient hospice unit, or an extended-care facility. Palliative care, emotional support, pain control, and other symptom control are some of the specialty areas of the interdisciplinary hospice team. At team meetings, the medical director, the primary nurse, the spiritual counselor, the volunteer, the social worker, and any other identified services, including the physician, assist the patient and family in meeting their unique needs. After death, bereavement support provided to the family is a key component of continued hospice care.

   Please refer to ''Cancer Care,'' ''Acquired Immune Deficiency Syndrome,'' ''Care of the Patient with Pain,'' or ''Care of the Bedbound Patient'' if those needs are appropriate for your patient.

2. **Needs for initial visit**

   Physician order for hospice care, specific to the hospice
     program's admission criteria and policies
   Universal precautions supplies
   Other supplies or equipment, based on physician orders
   Vital signs equipment for baseline assessment

3. **Some potential medical-surgical diagnoses and codes**

   Any disease process that has a limited life expectancy may be appropriate for hospice care.

Acute myocardial infarction	410.9
Adrenal cancer	194.0
AIDS	042.9
Ascites, malignant	197.6
Bladder cancer	188.9
Bone metastases	198.5
Brain, cancer of	191.9
Breast cancer	174.9

Cancer of the head or neck	195.0
Cardiomyopathy	425.4
Cervix, cancer of the	180.9
CHF	428.0
Colon, cancer	153.9
Colon lymphoma	202.83
Colostomy, attention to	V55.3
COPD	496
CVA	436
Decubitus ulcer	707.0
Esophagus, cancer of the	150.9
Fracture, pathological	733.1
Gastric cancer, metastatic	51.9 and 199.1
Gastrostomy, attention to	V55.1
Heart failure	428.9
Ileostomy, attention to	V55.2
Kaposi's sarcoma	173.8
Kaposi's sarcoma with AIDS	042.2
Kidney, cancer of the (renal)	189.0
Laryngectomy	30.4
Larynx, cancer of the	161.9
Leukemia, acute	208.0
Leukopenia	288.0
Liver, metastatic cancer of	197.7
Lung cancer, squamous cell	162.9
Mastectomy, radical	85.46
Mastectomy, simple	85.42
Metastases, general	199.1
Multiple myeloma	203.0
Nasopharyngeal cancer	147.9
Ovarian cancer	183.0
Pancreas, cancer of the	157.9
Pharynx, cancer of the	149.0
Pleural effusion	197.2
Pneumocystic carinii	136.3
Pneumonia	486
Pneumonia, aspiration	507.0
Prostate, cancer of	185
Pulmonary edema with cardiac disease	428.1
Radiation enteritis	558.1
Radiation myelitis	990 and 323.8
Rectosigmoid, cancer of	154.0

Rectum, cancer of the	154.1
Renal cell cancer, metastatic	189.0 and 199.1
Renal failure, chronic	585
Respiratory failure	518.81
Spinal cord tumor	239.7
Stomach, cancer of the	151.9
Tongue, cancer of the	141.9
Trachea, cancer of	162.0
Tracheostomy, attention to	V55.0
Uterine sarcoma, metastatic	179 and 198.82
Uterus, cancer of the	179.0

4. **Associated nursing diagnoses**

Aspiration, high risk for
Body image disturbance
Body temperature, altered, high risk for
Bowel incontinence
Breathing pattern, ineffective
Cardiac output, decreased
Caregiver role strain
Caregiver role strain, high risk for
Communication, impaired verbal
Constipation
Coping, ineffective family: compromised
Coping, ineffective family: disabling
Coping, ineffective individual
Diarrhea
Disuse syndrome, high risk for
Family processes, altered
Fatigue
Fear
Fluid volume deficit, high risk for
Fluid volume excess
Gas exchange, impaired
Grieving, anticipatory
Growth and development, altered
Home maintenance management, impaired
Hyperthermia
Hypothermia
Incontinence, total
Infection, high risk for
Injury, high risk for
Knowledge deficit (specify)

Mobility, impaired physical
Noncompliance (specify)
Nutrition, altered: less than body requirements
Oral mucous membrane, altered
Pain
Pain, chronic
Parenting, altered
Protection, altered
Role performance, altered
Self-care deficit, bathing/hygiene
Self-care deficit, dressing/grooming
Self-care deficit, feeding
Self-care deficit, toileting
Sensory/perceptual alterations (specify) (visual, auditory, kinesthetic, gustatory, tactile, olfactory)
Sexual dysfunction
Sexuality patterns, altered
Skin integrity, impaired
Skin integrity, impaired, high risk for
Sleep pattern disturbance
Social interaction, impaired
Spiritual distress (distress of the human spirit)
Swallowing, impaired
Thought processes, altered
Tissue integrity, impaired
Tissue perfusion, altered (specify type) (renal, cerebral, cardiopulmonary, gastrointestinal, peripheral)
Trauma, potential for
Urinary elimination, altered
Urinary retention

5. **Service skills identified**

Presentation of hospice philosophy and services
Assess patient, family, and caregiver wishes and expectations regarding care
Assess patient, family, and caregiver resources available for care
Psychosocial assessment of patient and family regarding disease and prognosis
Teach family or caregiver care of the patient
Assess bowel regimen and implement program as needed
Assess pain and other symptoms, including site, duration, characteristics, and relief measures

Teach care of the bedridden patient

Measure vital signs

Assess cardiovascular, pulmonary, and respiratory status

Assess nutrition and hydration status

Teach new pain and symptom control medication regimen

Diet counseling for patient with anorexia

Check for and remove impaction as needed

Condom catheter or indwelling catheter as indicated

Teach feeding-tube care to family

Teach caregivers symptom control and relief measures

Assess weight as ordered

Measure abdominal girth for ascites and edema, document sites, amount

Oxygen on at _____ liters per _____ (specific MD orders)

Assess mental status, sleep disturbance changes

Assess disease process progression

Obtain venipuncture as ordered q _____ (ordered frequency)

Teach new medications and effects

Decubitus ulcer care as indicated

Assess for electrolyte imbalance

Identify and monitor pain, symptoms, and relief measures

Teach catheter care to caregiver

Teach patient and caregiver use of PCA pump

Assess amount and frequency of urinary output

Teach family regarding safety of patient in home

Teach patient and family regarding conservation of energy techniques

Assess skin integrity

Teach caregiver or family care of weak, terminally ill patient

Observation and evaluation of wound and surrounding skin

Evaluate patient's need for equipment, supplies to decrease pressure, alternating pressure mattress, gel foam seat cushion, heel, elbow protectors, etc.

Teach family to perform dressings between RN visits

RN to instruct in pain control measures and medications

Teach patient family or caregiver about proper body alignment and positioning in bed to prevent skin tears from shearing skin

Observation and skilled assessment of areas for possible breakdown including heels, hips, elbows, and ankles

Nonpharmacologic interventions of progressive muscle relaxation imagery, positive visualization, music, and humor therapy of patient's choice implemented

Teach caregiver regarding skin care needs, including the need for frequent position changes, pressure pads and mattresses available, and the prevention of breakdown

Nutrition/hydration to be maintained by offering patient high-protein diet and foods of choice as tolerated

RN to teach caregiver catheter daily care

RN to assess patient's pain or other symptoms q visit to identify need for change, addition, or other plan or dose adjustment

RN to provide emotional support to patient and family

RN to evaluate the patient's bowel patterns, need for stool softeners, laxatives, dietary adjustments, and develop bowel management plan

Comfort measures of back rub, hand, other therapeutic massage

Teach and observe regarding side effects of palliative chemotherapy, including constipation, anemia, and fatigue

Venipuncture q _____ (specify ordered frequency) for monitoring platelet count

RN to teach patient regarding care of irradiated skin sites

RN to provide and teach effective oral care and comfort measures

Observation and complete systems assessment of the patient with an indwelling catheter

RN to change catheter every 4 weeks and 3 prn visits for catheter problems, including patient complaints, signs and symptoms of infection, and other factors necessitating evaluation and possible catheter change

RN to assess the patient's response to treatments and interventions and report changes, unfavorable responses, or reactions to the physician

6. **Other services indicated**

HHA	Personal care
	ADL assistance, support
	Other duties
MSS	Psychosocial assessment of patient and family, including adjustment to illness and its implications
	Emotional support
	Facilitate communication among patient, family, and staff

	Referrals to resources as indicated
	Grief counseling
OT	Evaluation
	Adaptive/assistive devices
	Energy conservation techniques
	Muscle reeducation
	ADL assistance
PT	Evaluation
	Strengthening exercise program
	Safe transfer and gait training home program
	Bed mobility exercises, as tolerated
	Instruct and supervise caregiver and volunteers on home exercise regimen
	Teach safe use of assistive devices as indicated
	Assess gait safety
S-LP	Swallowing and speech evaluation
	Alaryngeal speech
	Swallowing disorders, aphasia, and so on
	Alternative functional communication

Dietary and nutritional counseling

Assessment of nutrition and hydration needs and status

Encourage small, frequent meals

Encourage fluids

Encourage nutritional supplements and snacks to increase protein and caloric intake

Counsel family that patient will have a decreased appetite and usually at some point may not eat

Food, dietary recommendations

Spiritual counseling

Provide emotional and spiritual support, identified by patient and family needs

Volunteer support

The central core service unique to hospice care

As indicated, based on patient and family, nursing and volunteer coordinator assessment

Duties may include personal care, companionship, running errands, and other needs identified by patient and family

7. **Associated factors based on diagnosis justifying homebound status**

Weakness or severe DOE because of lung cancer

Severe weakness resulting from terminal illness
Medical restriction to home because of risk of additional
 infection
Stage II sacral decubitus
Open wound site
Vomiting, dizziness, pain
Febrile at _____
Pain in neck and shoulder area
Continuous oxygen therapy
Severe lower extremity or sacral edema
Chairbound
Bedridden
Needs maximum assistance to ambulate
Needs assistance for all activities
Lower extremity paresis, paralysis, or paraplegia
Severe arthritis
Impending death, dying
Mobility severely restricted
Dizziness
Severe SOB on any activity with oxygen dependency
Severe functional limitations, including age

NOTE: The homebound factor is not a criteria in the Medicare
 hospice benefit. (See HCFA hospice manual for details on
 this program.)

8. Short-term goals

RN	Support to family and patient
	Pain and other symptom control
	Disease management at home
	Patient comfort
	Infection-free
HHA	Effective personal hygiene
	ADL assistance
MSS	POC implementation
	Problems and resources identified
	Psychosocial support and counseling initiated
OT	Patient using adaptive devices
	Patient implementing conservation of energy program or muscle reeducation skills
PT	Maintenance of function, prevention of complications, safe transfers
S-LP	Able to communicate, safe swallowing

Dietary and nutritional counseling

Optimal nutrition and hydration, based on
patient's condition

Spiritual counseling

Patient and family are provided with emotional
and spiritual support

Volunteer support

Patient or caregiver support

Activities as identified

9. **Long-term goals**

RN	Support, increased comfort
	Pain and other symptom control
	Caregiver able to care for patient at home
	Patient comfortable at home through death
	Patient and caregiver effective in care management and know when to call RN or MD for assistance
	Comfort maintained through death with dignity
HHA	Personal care
	ADL assistance
MSS	Psychosocial support
	Community resources identified
	Problem resolution
OT	Quality of life improved through use of adaptive devices and conservation of energy techniques
PT	Maintain function
	Prevent complication
	Safety in home transfers
S-LP	Patient able to communicate, swallow safely

Dietary and nutritional counseling

Optimal nutrition and hydration for patient

Spiritual counseling

Spiritual support provided to patient, family, and
caregivers

Volunteer support

Patient and caregiver support

10. **Discharge plans for this patient**

Symptom controlled death at home

Admission to inpatient hospice facility for 24-hour care needs

Remains homebound, continues to need skilled care

Dignified death at home (or other setting of patient's choice)

11. Patient, family, and caregiver educational needs

Educational needs are the care regimens that contribute to safe and effective care at home between the hospice team's visits. These include:

The basic tenets of hospice and the availability of support 24 hours a day, 7 days a week

Home safety assessment and counseling

The patient's medication regimen

Safe and proper body mechanics to promote patient comfort and avoid caregiver safety problems

Other teaching specific to the patient and family's unique needs

Support groups available to your patients family, such as the hospice program's "Caregiver Support Group" meetings for family members and friends of the patient

For more information about hospice, contact the National Hospice Organization (NHO), 1901 North Moore Street, Suite 901, Arlington, Virginia 22209, 1-800-658-8898. For more information about the Medicare hospice benefit, "The Medicare Handbook" is available free by calling 1-800-638-6833.

The ACS has a "Look Good . . . Feel Better Program" that offers support and makeover services by cosmetologists for women undergoing chemotherapy or radiation therapy. Call 1-800-395-LOOK for more information.

12. Specific tips for reimbursement

There are many models of hospice programs. Those that are home health agency-based must work within the framework of the Medicare home care program. For example, sometimes a hospice patient reaches a stable period in the illness and there are no further skilled needs or the patient is no longer homebound per Medicare home health care criteria. When this occurs, one option is to discharge the patient from Medicare home health agency reimbursement and maintain the patient on grant funds or other available resources. If the patient's status deteriorates and again meets the Medicare criteria, a new start of care is initiated on the form 485. Usually hospices continue volunteer support, nursing, and other services indicated during these periods of no reimbursement.

The Medicare hospice benefit does not require that the patient be homebound or have identified skilled needs. Though it is a needed and viable program, the Medicare hospice benefit may not be indicated for all Medicare eligible beneficiaries. For further information on this benefit, please refer to HCFA Hospice Manual 13.

Should the patient status deteriorate and increased personal care be needed, obtain a telephone order for the increased service noting frequency and estimating the duration.

Obtain a telephone order for all medication and treatment changes of the medical regimen and document these in the clinical record.

Unless the patient is in a hospice insurance program, some insurers will not pay for a skilled nurse visit that is made at death if the patient is dead upon the nurse's arrival to the home.

Document patient deterioration

Document dehydration, dehydrating

Document patient change or instability

Document pain, other symptoms not controlled

Document status after acute episode of _____ (specify)

Document positive urine, sputum, etc. culture; patient started on _____ (specify ordered antibiotic therapy)

Document patient impacted; impaction removed manually

Document RN in frequent communication with physician regarding _____ (specify)

Document febrile at _____, pulse change at _____, irr., irr.

Document change noted in _____

Document bony prominences red, opening

Document RN contacted physician regarding _____ (specify)

Document marked SOB

Document alteration in mental status

Document medications being adjusted, regulated, or monitored

Document unable to ADLs, personal care

Document all interdisciplinary team meetings and communications in the POC and in the progress notes of the clinical record

All disciplinaries involved should have input into the POC and document their interventions and goals

PART SIX

MATERNAL/CHILD CARE

ACQUIRED IMMUNE DEFICIENCY SYNDROME (AIDS) (CARE OF THE CHILD WITH)

1. **General Considerations.** There are three general groups of the pediatric population who have AIDS. There are (1) infants who were exposed in utero or in the birth process; (2) children and adolescents who received blood or blood products before the blood supply was adequately tested (e.g., hemophiliacs, etc.); and (3) adolescents who acquired the disease primarily through sexual contact or injection drug use, including steroids. All efforts in the care of these children are ultimately directed toward supportive care, infection control, and disease prevention.

   Please refer to "Acquired Immune Deficiency Syndrome" or "Care of the Child with Cancer" should those be appropriate for your patient.

2. **Needs for initial visit**

   Specific initial physician orders
   Universal precautions supplies, per agency protocol
   Other supplies or equipment, based on physician orders
   Vital signs equipment

3. **Some potential medical-surgical diagnoses and codes**

AIDS (general)	042.9
Anemia	285.9
Bacterial infections, recurrent	041.9 and 042.9
Candidias	112.9
Candidias, esophageal	112.84 and 042.9
Candidias, oral	112.0 and 042.9
Candidias, vaginal	112.1 and 042.9
Cervical cancer	180.9 and 042.9
Chorioretinitis	363.20 and 042.9
Cytomegalovirus	078.5 and 042.9
Cytomegalovirus retinitis	363.20 and 87.85
Developmental delays, neurologic	315.9 and 042.9
Diarrhea	558.9 and 042.9
Encephalitis	328.8
Encephalopathy, AIDS	348.3 and 042.9

Endocarditis	424.90 and 042.9
Esophagitis	530.1 and 042.9
Failure to thrive	783.4 and 042.9
Herpes simplex	054
Herpes zoster	053
Histoplasmosis	115.9
HTLV III	044.9
Kaposi's sarcoma	173.8 and 042.2
Lymphocytic interstitial pneumonia	516.8 and 042
Meningitis	047.9 and 042.9
Mycobacterium avium intracellulare	031.0 and 042.9
Neurologic developmental delays	315.9 and 042.9
Neuropathy, peripheral	357.4 and 042.9
Neutropenia	288.0 and 042.9
Peripheral neuropathy	357.4 and 042.9
Pneumocystic carinii pneumonia	136.3 and 042.0
Pneumonia (bacterial)	482.9 and 042.9
Pneumonia (NOS)	486 and 042.1
Pneumonia (viral)	480.8 and 042.1
Polymyositis	710.1
Polyradiculopathy	729.2
Quadriplegia	344.0
Retinal detachment	361.9
Retinal hemorrhage	362.81
Seizures	780.3
Sepsis	038.9 and 042.9
Shigella	004.9 and 042.9
Shigella, dysentery	004.0 and 042.9
Thrombocytopenia	287.5 and 042.9
Toxoplasmosis	130.9 and 042.9
Tuberculosis (pulmonary)	011.9 and 042.9
Wasting syndrome	799.4 and 042.9

4. **Associated nursing diagnoses**

Activity intolerance
Activity intolerance, high risk for
Airway clearance, ineffective
Anxiety
Body image disturbance
Body temperature, altered, high risk for
Bowel incontinence
Cardiac output, decreased
Caregiver role strain

Caregiver role strain, high risk for

Coping, ineffective family: compromised

Coping, ineffective family: disabling

Coping, ineffective individual

Family processes, altered

Fatigue

Fear

Fluid volume deficit, high risk for

Gas exchange impaired

Grieving, anticipatory

Growth and development, altered

Infection, high risk for

Injury, high risk for

Knowledge deficit, (related to managing disease)

Nutrition, altered: less than body requirements

Oral mucous membrane, altered

Pain

Pain, chronic

Powerlessness

Protection, altered

Self-care deficit, bathing/hygiene

Self-care deficit, dressing/grooming

Self-care deficit, feeding

Self-care deficit, toileting

Sensory/perceptual alterations (specify) (visual, auditory,
   kinesthetic, gustatory, tactile, olfactory)

Sexual dysfunction

Sexuality patterns, altered

Skin integrity, impaired

Skin integrity, impaired, high risk for

Social interaction, impaired

Social isolation

Spiritual distress (distress of the human spirit)

Swallowing, impaired

Thought processes, altered

Tissue integrity, impaired

Tissue perfusion, altered (specify type) (renal, cerebral,
   cardiopulmonary, gastrointestinal, peripheral)

Urinary elimination, altered

5. **Service skills identified**

Complete initial assessment of all systems in the child with
   compromised immune system and admitted to home care
   due to _____ (specify pathology necessitating care)

RN to instruct parents and caregivers regarding safety and universal precautions in the home

RN assessment of pulmonary status, including dyspnea, changed or abnormal breath sounds, retractions, respiratory rate, flaring, and other symptoms of respiratory compromise

RN to observe and assess all systems and symptoms every visit

RN to report changes or new symptoms to MD

RN to teach parents and caregivers all aspects of wound care, including safe disposal of dressing supplies

Instruct on pet care, avoidance of cross contamination, check with MD on certain types of pets

RN to weigh patient q visit and review food intake diary

RN to instruct parents or caregivers regarding prescribed diet

RN to assess and monitor child's use of and response to aerosol therapy medication

RN to assess child for candidal diaper rash or oral thrush

RN to teach child and parents safe use of oxygen therapy

RN to monitor for adverse effects of medication, particularly steroids

RN to evaluate caregiving ability, particularly if parents or other caregivers are HIV+

RN to monitor child's blood pressure and other vital signs

RN to teach parents and caregivers about new medications

RN to teach parents and caregivers about the importance of optimal hydration and nutrition

Instruct child, parents, and caregivers in all aspects of effective handwashing techniques and proper care of bodily fluids and excretions

RN to provide emotional support to child and caregivers with chronic/terminal illness and associated implications, especially if a parent is HIV+

RN to closely monitor parenteral feeding catheter site for infection and other problems

RN to instruct parents and caregivers to call MD for symptoms of fever, increased irritability, vomiting, diarrhea, suspected ear or other infection, decreased appetite, new cough, or any new symptom or complaint

RN to instruct parents regarding the need to isolate HIV+ child from anyone with known infections, such as other children at school who have chicken pox, measles, or other communicable infections that are life threatening for the child with AIDS

RN to teach parents and caregivers regarding all aspects of child's needed care for safe and effective management at home

RN to instruct parents or caregivers on all aspects of medications, including schedule, functions, and side effects

RN to instruct parents or caregivers regarding signs and symptoms that necessitate calling RN or MD

Observation and assessment of the child with an impaired immune response and multiple system infections

RN to provide support to child with new tumor, necessitating surgery, chemotherapy, or radiation

RN to address sexuality concerns with young adolescent with AIDS and the importance of safe sexual expression, including the use of condoms, abstinence, or other techniques

RN to assess the child's unique response to treatments and interventions and to report changes, unfavorable responses, or reactions to the physician

Assess grief, denial, and guilt of parents and caregivers

6. **Other services indicated**

HHA	Personal care
	Respite care for relief of family and caregivers
	Homemaker services to assist caregiver
	ADL assistance
MSS	Evaluation of psychosocial factors of the child and family with a chronic and terminal illness
	Financial assessment and counseling
	Emotional support to child, family, and caregivers
	Referral to community resources, (e.g., entitlement, nutrition assistance, early intervention/school)
OT	Evaluation
	Conservation of energy techniques
	Adaptive or assistive devices/supplies as indicated to meet child's needs
	ADL training program
PT	Evaluation
	Home exercise regimen

7. **Associated factors based on diagnosis justifying homebound status**

The homebound factor may or may not be a criterion for admission, based on the managed-care program or the third-party payer involved. However, the following are reasons the child would be homebound:

Oxygen therapy
Fatigue
Dyspnea
Infection control, protecting child from further infection
Pain or other symptoms necessitating care at home
Medically weak and fragile
Severe immune suppression
Weakness

8. **Short-term goals**

RN	Daily adherence to POC with optimal function maintained
	Prevention of further infection
	Symptom management stabilized and maintained
	Growth and developmental needs being met
	Child able to play and be symptom-free, when possible
	Child and family educational needs met
HHA	Effective personal care and hygiene
	ADL assistance
	Caregiver assistance and relief
MSS	Problems being identified
	Referral to community resources initiated
OT	Child practicing conservation of energy techniques
	Adaptive/assistive devices identified and ordered
PT	Child and caregiver practicing home exercise regimen
	Increased endurance

9. **Long-term goals**

RN	Patient maintained in safety, infections, and symptoms controlled
	Child is afebrile, and systems are stable in immunosuppressed child
	Child and caregivers demonstrate acceptable handwashing and other infection protection standards taught by RN to assure prevention of virus to caregivers and others and to help assure protection from new infections to child
	Palliative, curative, and symptomatic interventions to assure optimal level of functioning in child

	Child and caregiver integrating information about illness with life-threatening implications and the associated grieving process
	Support growth and developmental tasks of childhood
	Patient and family have adequate coping skills
HHA	Safe, effective personal care provided
	Patient clean and hygiene maintained
	Patient comfortable
	Family and caregiver receive appropriate respite
MSS	Problem identification and referrals made to appropriate resources
	Referral to community support group for family/caregiver
	Entitlement, food assistance, and financial counseling obtained
	Spiritual support and professional counseling referrals
	Educational level maintained
OT	Patient taught and practicing conservation of energy techniques
	Optimal function maintained
	Quality of life improved through use of techniques
	Family and child able to use skills and assistive devices
PT	Increased function and mobility
	Prevention of complications
	Family able to perform exercise program safely

10. Discharge plans for this patient

Patient maintained in comfort and safety of home with adequate hydration, nutrition, hygiene, and other needs met by family and caregiver

Discharge with caregivers taught and able to manage patient safely in home under MD supervision

11. Patient, family, and caregiver educational needs

Educational needs are the regimens that the parents or caregiver will be managing with or for the child. These include:

Symptom management

Importance of adequate hydration and nutrition

Universal precaution protocols

Home safety concerns, issues, and teaching

The avoidance of infection, when possible

The importance of medical follow up

Support groups and resources in the community available to the patient and family

Other identified information needed, based on the patient and family's unique medical and other needs

Resources include:

The Center for Disease Control and Prevention (CDC)

National AIDS Hotline: 1-800-342-2437 or 1-800-342-AIDS

The National AIDS Information Clearinghouse: 1-800-458-5231

The AIDS Pediatric Clinical Trials Information Service: 1-800-TRIALS-A (1-800-874-2572)

The National Hemophiliac Foundation: (212) 431-8541

12. **Specific tips for reimbursement**

AIDS is usually not what the home care nurse is specifically addressing. The care provided is directed toward symptom and infection control and treatment. These children and adolescents are usually so ill that there are many skills the professional nurse provides.

Document the coordination occurring, based on the POC among team members. The interdisciplinary conference notes should be reflected in the clinical record. Refer to these meetings or communications on any form used by third-party payers (e.g., your program's update form).

In addition:

Write the specific care and teaching instructions provided

Document your progress toward goals

Document any exacerbation of symptoms that necessitated another visit and be sure there is an MD order for that visit

Document all POC changes

Document all interactions/communications with the physician

Document the skills used in the provision of professional nursing care practice when caring for the child (e.g., teaching, training, observation, assessment, catheters, IV site care, venipuncture, etc.)

ANTEPARTAL CARE

1. **General Considerations.**   The antepartal patient referred to home health care usually has an associated medical problem, such as hypertension, that necessitates the initial referral for follow up.

2. **Needs for initial visit**

   Specific initial physician orders
   Universal precautions supplies
   Other supplies or equipment, based on physician orders
   Vital signs equipment

3. **Some potential medical-surgical diagnoses and codes**

Hypertension	642.92
Pregnancy	V23.4
Pregnancy, high risk	V23.8

4. **Associated nursing diagnoses**

   Activity intolerance
   Activity intolerance, high risk for
   Anxiety
   Body image disturbance
   Cardiac output, decreased
   Constipation
   Diversional activity deficit
   Family processes, altered
   Fatigue
   Fear
   Fluid volume excess
   Grieving, anticipatory
   Growth and development, altered
   Infection, high risk for
   Injury, high risk for
   Knowledge deficit (specify)
   Mobility, impaired physical
   Noncompliance (specify) (e.g., diet)
   Nutrition, altered: high risk for more than body requirements
   Nutrition, altered: less than body requirements
   Nutrition, altered: more than body requirements

Pain
Parental role conflict
Parenting, altered
Parenting, altered, high risk for
Role performance, altered
Sexual dysfunction
Sexuality patterns, altered
Skin integrity, impaired, high risk for
Sleep pattern disturbance
Spiritual distress (distress of the human spirit)

5. **Service skills identified**

Skilled assessment of patient with _____ (specify)
Assess medication response
Evaluate blood pressure
Teach patient and family regarding ordered diet
    therapy
Teach patient and family regarding decreased sodium
    diet
Teach patient safe, correct use of home uterine
    monitor
Teach patient and family regarding vitamin therapy
Teach patient and family regarding exercise and rest period
    needs
Teach patient and family regarding expected physiological
    changes
Teach patient and family regarding symptoms that need
    immediate physician notification
Monitor amount and site(s) of edema
Weigh daily and record
Dipstick urine for protein
Emotional support to patient and family
Teach patient self-observational skills (weights, results of urine
    dipsticks, edema, etc.)

6. **Other services indicated**

HHA	Personal care
	ADL assistance
MSS	Psychosocial assessment
	Problem identifications
	Financial counseling assistance, referral(s) to
	community resources as indicated

7. **Associated factors based on diagnosis justifying homebound status**

Bed rest with bathroom privileges only
Weakness, legs to be elevated
Decreased activity
Home confinement because of medical problems
Receiving IV care for hyperemesis

8. **Short-term goals**

RN	Patient understands POC and knows when to call MD
	Blood pressure stable
HHA	Effective personal hygiene
MSS	Problem identification

9. **Long-term goals**

RN	Healthy infant
	Mother self-care
	Blood pressure in normal for patient range
	Mother carries pregnancy to term
HHA	Effective personal hygiene
MSS	Community referrals

10. **Discharge plans for this patient**

Delivery of healthy infant
Self-care in community, under MD supervision

11. **Patient, family, and caregiver educational needs**

Educational needs are the aspects of care that the patient must understand to safely self-manage at home. These include:

The importance of compliance to the medical regimens and keeping scheduled OB appointments
The signs of preterm labor and other symptoms or changes that necessitate notifying the MD and being seen immediately (bleeding, premature rupture of membranes, etc.)
The need for optimal nutrition and frequent rest periods
The rationale and need for bed rest

Other care regimens as identified based on the patient's unique
needs

12. **Specific tips for reimbursement**

Document any abnormal blood pressure findings, protein in
urine or blood results
Document communications with physician in clinical record
Document the care given and the actions of that care
Document the specific teaching accomplished and the
behavioral outcomes of that teaching

CANCER (CARE OF THE CHILD WITH)

1. **General Considerations.**   It is said that cancer is the leading cause of death from disease in children who are 3 to 15 years old and the second cause of death from all causes, surpassed only by death from injuries.

   Cancer care in children utilizes all facets of nursing skills. Death at any age is sad, but the suffering and death of children magnifies the emotional turmoil. Parents know their child best and in this role they are the teachers for care providers. Parental control should be maintained as much as possible.

   Please refer to ''Cancer Care,'' ''Brain Tumor,'' or Part Five, ''Hospice Care,'' should those problems be appropriate for your patient.

2. **Needs for initial visit**

   Specific initial physician orders
   Universal precautions supplies
   Other supplies or equipment, based on physician orders
   Vital signs equipment

3. **Some potential medical-surgical diagnoses and codes**

Acute lymphocytic leukemia	204.0
Acute myelogenous leukemia	205.0
Aplastic anemia	284.9
Astrocytoma	191.9
Chronic leukemia	204.1
Chronic myelogenous leukemia	205.1
Leukopenia	288.0
Wilm's tumor	189.0

4. **Associated nursing diagnoses**

   Activity intolerance
   Activity intolerance, high risk for
   Adjustment, impaired
   Anxiety
   Aspiration, high risk for
   Body image disturbance
   Body temperature, altered, high risk for
   Breathing pattern, ineffective

Cardiac output, decreased
Caregiver role strain
Caregiver role strain, high risk for
Constipation
Coping, family: potential for growth
Coping, ineffective family: compromised
Coping, ineffective family: disabling
Decisional conflict (specify) (e.g., treatment regimen options)
Denial, ineffective
Diarrhea
Family processes, altered
Fatigue
Fear
Fluid volume deficit, high risk for
Grieving, anticipatory
Growth and development, altered
Infection, high risk for
Injury, high risk for
Knowledge deficit (diagnoses and treatment)
Mobility, impaired physical
Nutrition, altered: less than body requirements
Oral mucous membrane, altered
Pain
Pain, chronic
Parental role conflict
Parenting, altered
Protection, altered
Role performance, altered
Self-care deficit, bathing/hygiene
Self-care deficit, dressing/grooming
Self-care deficit, feeding
Self-care deficit, toileting
Sensory/perceptual alterations (specify) (visual, auditory, kinesthetic, gustatory, tactile, olfactory)
Sexuality patterns, altered
Skin integrity, impaired, high risk for
Sleep pattern disturbance
Social interaction, impaired
Spiritual distress (distress of the human spirit)
Swallowing, impaired
Tissue integrity, impaired

Tissue perfusion, altered (specify type) (renal, cerebral, cardiopulmonary, gastrointestinal, peripheral)

Urinary elimination, altered

5. **Service skills identified**

Skilled assessment of the child with _____ (specify)

Teach family and caregiver patient POC

Assess bowel regimen and implement program as needed

Assess pain and other symptoms

Teach care of the patient

Measure vital signs

Assess cardiovascular, pulmonary, and respiratory status

Assess nutrition and hydration status

Teach new pain and symptom control medication

Diet counseling for patient with anorexia

Check for and remove impaction as needed

Indwelling catheter as indicated

Teach feeding tube care to family and caregiver

Teach caregivers symptom and relief measures

Assess weight as ordered

Measure abdominal girth for ascites and edema, document sites and amount

Oxygen on at _____ liter per _____

Assess mental status, sleep disturbance changes

Obtain venipuncture as ordered q _____

Teach new medications and effects

Decubitus ulcer care as indicated

Assess for electrolyte imbalance

Teach catheter care to caregiver

Assess amount and frequency of urinary output

Teach family regarding safety

Teach patient and family regarding conservation of energy techniques

Provide emotional support to patient and family

Anticipate and encourage patient and family input into care regimen(s)

Assess patient and family coping skills

Symptom control for side effects of radiation or chemotherapy

Teach the importance of optimal nutrition and hydration

Teach caregivers observational aspects of care, including fever, bleeding, bruising, and other signs unique to the disease or treatment

RN to monitor for seizure activity and perform neurologic checks q visit

Teach the importance of effective handwashing and other infection control measures, including the avoidance of infection when possible

RN to provide emotional support to child and family with chronic or terminal illness and associated implications

RN to instruct caregiver to call MD for symptoms of fever, irritability, vomiting, diarrhea, suspected ear or other infection, decreased appetite, cough, or other complaint

RN to assess the child's unique response to treatments and interventions and to report changes or unfavorable responses or reactions to physician

6. **Other services indicated**

HHA	Effective personal care
	ADL activities
MSS	Psychosocial assessment of family with child who has cancer
	Problem evaluation
	Financial assistance counseling
	Support to patient and family
	Community resource referral(s) (American Cancer Society, Ronald McDonald™ House, etc.)

7. **Associated factors based on diagnosis justifying homebound status**

The homebound factor is not usually a criterion for this patient population; however, the following are the most common reasons:

Infection protection
Pain
Severe fatigue
SOB during any activity
Medical restrictions to home due to low blood count
NOTE: If the child is in an insurance hospice program, this requirement is usually waived

8. **Short-term goals**

| **RN** | POC implemented |

	Pain and symptom control
	Support to patient and family
HHA	Effective personal hygiene
	ADL assistance
	Respite care provided
MSS	Support to patient and family
	Plan of care implemented
	Problem identification

9. **Long-term goals**

RN	Child and parents are active participants in care planning and delivery
	Pain and symptom control
	Family able to care for patient
	Symptom control through cure, remission, or death
HHA	Effective personal hygiene
	ADL assistance
MSS	Parents and child will have effective support
	Community resources referral(s)
	Support to patient and family
	Grief counseling if appropriate

10. **Discharge plans for this patient**

Status stable
Discharged when goals achieved
Patient death with dignity maintained and family present
Admitted to acute care facility for 24-hour care
Patient discharged, family able to manage care, under MD supervision

11. **Patient, family, and caregiver educational needs**

Educational needs are the aspects of care that the parents or other caregivers need to safely care for the child between visits. These include:

The medication regimen, including schedule, route, functions, and side effects
Signs and symptoms that necessitate calling the MD or RN
The importance of round-the-clock medications for pain control
Pain and other symptom control measures

Information about the disease process

Based on the patient's prognosis and the family's preference, the availability of hospice and other support services for the patient, parents, and caregivers

The American Cancer Society has local support groups and can be reached at 1-800-ACS-2345.

For specific information on home care and children, contact the National Association for Home Care. For specific information on dying children, contact Children's Hospice International or The National Hospice Organization.

Radiotherapy Days, a 20-page, four-color paperback for children ages 8 to 12, is useful to caregivers who need to explain radiotherapy to children. To order, send $5.00 per copy to Mount Sinai Medical Center, Radiotherapy Days, Department of Pediatric Hematology/Oncology, Box 1208, One Gustave L. Levy Place, New York, NY 10029. Make check payable to MSMC.

The Make-A-Wish Foundation fulfills special wishes for children with a life-threatening illness and their families. 1-800-722-WISH (9474)

12. **Specific tips for reimbursement**

Document all care rendered and the outcomes of that care

Document any patient changes and communications with the physician

Document home care in lieu of hospitalization, when applicable

CESAREAN SECTION POSTCARE

1. **General Considerations.**   The nursing care of the new mother following cesarean section (C/S) surgery is usually directed toward wound care, catheter care, or other complications that necessitated the need for skilled services. Goals are directed to facilitate resolution of the medical problems to support bonding with the infant during this important perinatal period.

2. **Needs for initial visit**

   Specific initial physician orders
   Universal precautions supplies
   Other supplies or equipment, based on physician orders
   Vital signs equipment

3. **Some potential medical-surgical diagnoses and codes**

Anemia	285.9
Cesarean section (status post)	74.99
Constipation	564.0
Diabetes mellitus, with complications, adult	250.90
Diabetes mellitus, with complications, juvenile	250.91
Hemorrhoids, external	455.3
Hemorrhoids, internal	455.0
Hemorrhoids, postpartum	671.82
Urinary infection	599.0
Urinary retention	788.2
Wound dehiscence	674.1
Wound infection	674.3

4. **Associated nursing diagnoses**

   Activity intolerance
   Anxiety
   Body image disturbance
   Breast-feeding, effective
   Breast-feeding, ineffective
   Breast-feeding, interrupted
   Caregiver role strain
   Caregiver role strain, high risk for
   Constipation

Coping family: potential for growth
Family processes, altered
Fatigue
Fear
Fluid volume deficit, high risk for
Growth and development, altered
Home maintenance management, impaired
Infection, high risk for
Injury, high risk for
Knowledge deficit (regarding self-care, S/P C/S, infant care)
Mobility, impaired physical
Nutrition, altered: less than body requirements
Pain
Parenting, altered
Parenting, altered, high risk for
Role performance, altered
Self-esteem, situational low
Sexual dysfunction
Sexuality patterns, altered
Skin integrity, impaired
Sleep pattern disturbance
Spiritual distress (distress of the human spirit)
Urinary elimination, altered

5. **Service skills identified**

Skilled initial nursing assessment of the patient post-C/S
with _____ (specify problems necessitating skilled nursing
care)
RN to provide aseptic care to open wound site (specify
supplies, frequency, other MD orders)
Observation and assessment of wound site and surrounding
skin
RN to assess patient's pain on an ongoing basis to identify
need for change, alteration, addition, or other plan for pain
management
RN to provide emotional support to patient and family
RN to assess amount and character of lochia
RN to evaluate patient's bowel patterns, need for stool
softeners, laxatives, dietary changes, or increase in fluid
Evaluate pain in relation to other symptoms, including fatigue,
constipation, depression, or others
Assessment of breasts and nipples, engorgement, soreness,
cracking, or blisters

RN to obtain urine for culture and sensitivity

RN to instruct new mother regarding breast care comfort techniques

Assess patient and family stress/coping skills

RN to implement nonpharmacologic interventions with medication schedule, including massage, imagery, progressive relaxation exercises, humor, and music therapies

RN to teach new parents regarding infant safety measures, parenting skills, bathing, cord care, circumcision care, and well-child care, including need for immunizations at specified time intervals in the future

Assess nutrition and hydration status

Venipuncture for CBC (specify per MD orders)

RN to teach patient about wound care and infection control measures

RN to assess the patient's unique response to ordered interventions and treatments and report changes, unfavorable responses, or reactions to the physician

RN to teach regarding sexuality and family planning concerns

Management and evaluation of the patient POC

6. **Other services indicated**

HHA	Personal care
	ADL assistance
	Meal preparation
	Infant care

7. **Associated factors based on diagnosis justifying homebound status**

Though this is not usually an admission criteria, some managed-care programs will need rationale for why the patient cannot get to the MD's office. The following are some of the reasons:

Pain
Severe fatigue
SOB on any activity
Infection protection
Open wound site

8. **Short-term goals**

| **RN** | POC implementation |

Pain and symptom control through compliance to
medication regimen

Support to new mother and infant

Daily wound care (or specify) provided per MD
orders

Patient verbalizes signs and symptoms of
infection

HHA   Effective personal hygiene

ADL assistance

Safe, effective infant care

9. Long-term goals

RN   Wound healed, patient returned to self-care status

Patent catheter or catheter removed; without
evidence of UTI, catheter discontinued per MD
orders

Maternal-infant or parental bonding occurring

Positive, loving relationship with infant

Mother self-care and able to care for self and
infant

Patient pain- and infection-free

Adequate hydration and nutrition for mother and
baby

HHA   Effective personal hygiene

ADL assistance

Safe, effective infant care

10. Discharge plans for this patient

Discharge to care of new parents, with MD follow up for
well-child care, including planned immunization schedule

11. Patient, family, and caregiver educational needs

Educational needs are the regimens that the patient and
caregiver will be managing with the patient. These include:

Self-care of the mother

Wound care

Care of the infant

Home safety assessment (e.g., car seats, crib rails, playpens,
etc.)

Signs and symptoms that necessitate contacting MD

Effective personal hygiene habits

Handwashing and infection control with infant

The importance of medical follow up

Self-care observational aspects of care, particularly the wound and the infant

The importance of immunizations for the infant/child

Other information based on the patient's unique needs

12. **Specific tips for reimbursement**

Some third-party payers will want reasons for continued visits to see the patient when the wound is not infected, although still open. The professional nurse skills, however, are more than the actual hands-on packing of the wound and applying Montgomery straps or whatever the specific orders entail. It is the teaching and observation and assessment that usually justify the nurse not leaving before wound healing, closure, or the patient is able to go back to the MD for further care.

Document the specific care and teaching instructions provided

Document your progress toward patient-centered, realistic goals

Document all POC changes and obtain orders for any POC changes

CYSTIC FIBROSIS (CARE OF THE CHILD WITH)

1. **General Considerations.** With current treatments, the life expectancy of patients with cystic fibrosis has increased, and some patients are now in their 30s and 40s. In addition, there are some studies indicating that home therapy for CF with pulmonary exacerbations may be as effective for some patients as inpatient therapy.

    Please refer to "IV Therapy and Other Line Care," should your patient with CF be on IV antibiotic therapy at home.

2. **Needs for initial visit**

    Specific initial physician orders
    Universal precautions supplies
    Other supplies or equipment, based on physician orders
    Vital signs equipment

3. **Some potential medical-surgical diagnoses and codes**

Anemia	285.9
Bronchitis	490
Bronchopneumonia	485
Cholecystitis	575.1
Chronic obstructive pulmonary disease	496
Cirrhosis, biliary	571.6
Congestive heart failure	428.0
Constipation	564.0
Cor pulmonale	416.9
Cystic fibrosis	277.00
Dehydration	276.5
Diabetes mellitus, with complications, adult	250.90
Diabetes mellitus, with complications, juvenile	250.91
Emphysema	492.8
Failure to thrive	783.4
Heart-lung transplant (surgical code)	33.6
S/P heart-lung transplant care	V42.1 and V42.6

Hemoptysis	786.3
Ileus	560.1
Pancreatic insufficiency	577.8
Peptic ulcer	553.90
Pneumonia	486
Sinusitis	473.9
Rectum, prolapse of	569.1

4. **Associated nursing diagnoses**

Activity intolerance
Activity intolerance, high risk for
Airway clearance, ineffective
Anxiety
Body image disturbance
Breathing pattern, ineffective
Cardiac output, decreased
Caregiver role strain
Caregiver role strain, high risk for
Constipation
Coping, ineffective individual
Coping, family: potential for growth
Family processes, altered
Fatigue
Fear
Fluid volume deficit
Fluid volume excess
Gas exchange, impaired
Grieving, anticipatory
Growth and development, altered
Infection, high risk for
Injury, high risk for
Knowledge deficit (care management)
Nutrition, altered: less than body requirements
Pain
Pain, chronic
Sexuality patterns, altered
Skin integrity, impaired, high risk for
Social interaction, impaired
Spiritual distress (distress of the human spirit)
Suffocation, high risk for
Tissue perfusion, altered (specify type) (renal, cerebral,
    cardiopulmonary, gastrointestinal, peripheral)

5. **Service skills identified**

Skilled initial assessment of respiratory and other systems in child with cystic fibrosis

RN to teach parent and caregiver daily care chest physiotherapy regimen to maintain and help assure aeration and decrease secretions

RN to teach the need for the pancreatic enzyme replacements administered with each meal and snack

RN to instruct patient and caregiver on all aspects related to insulin-dependent diabetes

RN to teach caregiver signs and symptoms of the CF child that necessitate calling the MD

RN to instruct about the need for a well-balanced, high-calorie diet to help assure growth

RN to teach chest percussion and postural drainage on child

Instruct regarding infection control measures, including effective handwashing techniques and avoiding people with upper respiratory or other infections

Teach caregiver observational skills of weight loss or gain and to weigh and record daily weights

RN to evaluate home setting and caregiver for safe administration of IV antibiotic therapy with central venous access device

RN to teach child and caregiver effective conservation of energy techniques

RN to teach child and caregiver effective coughing techniques

RN to teach and monitor administration of aerosol bronchodilator medication to assist in expectoration

RN to assess patient's respiratory status and lung sounds, before and after CPT, consisting of clapping, drainage, and aerosol treatment and instructing caregiver about these skills

Observation and assessment of the amount and frequency of stools, abdominal distension, and other GI symptoms or complaints

RN to teach caregiver to watch for symptoms of infection, including change in child's behavior, increased irritability, fever, decreased appetite, or other signs

RN to assess the child's unique response to treatments and interventions and report changes or unfavorable responses or reactions to the physician

6. **Other services indicated**

HHA	Personal care
	ADL assistance
	Participation in home exercise program
MSS	Evaluation of psychosocial factors which have an impact on the family and child with a chronic illness, which impact POC implementation
	Counseling regarding financial and food assistance programs
	Emotional support to child, family, and caregivers
	Referral to community programs
PT	Evaluation of patient and learning needs of child, family, and caregiver
	Chest physical therapy
	Instruct regarding performance of chest PT, postural drainage, deep breathing exercises, and administration of treatments
	Home exercise regimen

7. **Associated factors based on diagnosis justifying homebound status**

Though homebound may or may not be an admission criterion, the following are some of the reasons that the child would be cared for at home:

Child with CF and chest process, MD wants cared for at home for infection control and to protect child from other sick children

SOB on any activity

Child with CF on home antibiotic regimen or TPN

8. **Short-term goals**

RN	Daily intake of adequate hydration and nutrition
	Daily adherence to medication regimen and POC
	Daily control of pulmonary infection, secretions
	Maintain bowel function or normal habits for patient
	Effective breathing and aeration with airway clear of mucous
	Beginning to integrate learned information into behavior
	Prevention of further infection

HHA	Effective personal care and hygiene
	ADL assistance
MSS	Problems being identified
	Referral to identified community resources
PT	Adherence to daily POC
	Pulmonary status stable
	Practicing exercise regimen

9. Long-term goals

RN	Patient maintains or increases weight
	Optimal growth and development in child with CF
	Patient afebrile and infection-free
	Child, family, and caregivers integrating information about illness with life shortening and chronic implications; grieving process initiated, family adapting through verbalization
	Functional and optimal bowel elimination
	Child's pulmonary status stable
	Family able to provide treatments effectively
HHA	Safe, effective personal care provided
	Patient clean and hygiene maintained
MSS	Problem identification and referrals made to appropriate resource
	Referral to community support group for caregiver
	Food assistance obtained
	Financial counseling accomplished
	Provide support to patient and family
	Support optimal participation of family members in aspects of care
PT	Effective chest physiotherapy regimen demonstrated by caregiver
	Home exercise regimen taught and patient able to practice

10. Discharge plans for this patient

Discontinued course of antibiotics

Discharged from home care, under MD supervision

Caregiver demonstrated knowledge of daily care, discharged from home care

Patient readmitted to hospital with acute exacerbation respiratory problems, discharged from home care

11. **Patient, family, and caregiver educational needs**

Educational needs are the regimens that the parents or caregiver will be managing with or for the child. These include:

The importance of adequate hydration, nutrition, and rest
The importance of medical follow up
Support groups in the community that are available to the child and caregivers
The importance of the correct administration of medications
Other information based on the patient's and family's unique medical and other needs

The Cystic Fibrosis Foundation is available to provide information and educational support to health care professionals and patients with CF, their families, and caregivers. They are located at: 6931 Arlington Road, Bethesda, Maryland 20814, 1-800-FIGHT CF.

12. **Specific tips for reimbursement**

Document the coordination occurring among team members based on the POC. The interdisciplinary conference notes should be reflected in the clinical record.
In addition:

Write the specific care and teaching instructions provided
Document progress toward patient-centered, realistic goals
Document the nursing actions and responses to the care interventions
Document the specific teaching accomplished and the behavioral outcomes of that teaching
Document the amount and character of secretions
Document any changes in the POC
Document any exacerbation of symptoms that necessitated another visit and be sure that there is an MD order for that visit in the Clinical record
Document the skills used in the provision of professional nursing care practice when caring for the child (e.g., teaching, training, observation, assessment, etc.)

DIABETES MELLITUS (CARE OF THE CHILD WITH)

1. **General Considerations.** Children with juvenile diabetes mellitus (DM) are often referred to home health care after a hospitalization or to prevent hospitalization. These children and their families have multiple defined teaching needs.

2. **Needs for initial visit**

   Specific initial physician orders
   Universal precautions supplies
   Other supplies or equipment, based on physician orders
   Vital signs equipment
   Venipuncture supplies
   Alcohol swabs
   Teaching skills
   Urine dipstick supplies
   Blood glucose monitoring machine

3. **Some potential medical-surgical diagnoses and codes**

Dehydration	250.81 and 276.5
Diabetes mellitus, insulin dependent	250.01
Diabetic retinopathy	250.51 and 362.01
Hyperglycemia	250.01
Hypoglycemia	251.2
Ketoacidosis	250.11

4. **Associated nursing diagnoses**

   Adjustment, impaired
   Anxiety
   Body image disturbance
   Body temperature, altered, high risk for
   Breathing pattern, ineffective
   Caregiver role strain
   Caregiver role strain, high risk for
   Denial, ineffective
   Family processes, altered
   Fatigue
   Fear
   Fluid volume deficit, high risk for

Gas exchange, impaired
Growth and development, altered
Infection, high risk for
Injury, high risk for
Knowledge deficit (specify) (e.g., care of the child with DM)
Management of therapeutic regimen (individuals), ineffective
Noncompliance (specify) (e.g., diet)
Nutrition, altered: high risk for more than body requirements
Nutrition, altered: less than body requirements
Nutrition, altered: more than body requirements
Pain
Pain, chronic
Parental role conflict
Parenting, altered
Parenting, altered, high risk for
Sexuality patterns, altered
Skin integrity, impaired
Social interaction, impaired
Spiritual distress (distress of the human spirit)
Thought processes, altered
Urinary elimination, altered

5. **Service skills identified**

Skilled assessment of child with DM
Administer _____ insulin q _____ am
Administer additional _____ insulin before meals
Teach parents and patient to draw up and give insulin
Teach diabetes management regimen(s)
Emotional support to child and parents with newly
   diagnosed DM
Teach regarding diet and importance of eating at regular,
   consistent times
Perform blood glucose monitor checks q _____, call physician
   if over _____ or less than _____
Teach patient and parents to mix insulins
Teach patient and parents blood glucose monitoring process
Teach signs and symptoms of hyperglycemia and
   hypoglycemia, teach emergency measures to patient and
   parents
Venipuncture for FBS as indicated
Teach patient and parents urine check procedures
Teach regarding new insulin and medication regimen
Teach disease process

Teach action of ordered insulin(s)

Assess long-term ability of patient and parents to comply with regimen

Teach patient and parents regarding site rotation and importance of site rotation

Teach patient and parents regarding dietary management and restrictions

Teach patient and parents regarding stressors that can increase the amount of insulin needed (e.g., infection)

Assess family and patient coping, refer as needed to support group

6. **Other services indicated**

MSS	Psychosocial assessment of patient and family with new illness of a chronic nature
	Problem identification
	Referral to community resource(s)
	Financial counseling and assistance

7. **Associated factors based on diagnosis justifying homebound status**

The homebound factor is usually not a criterion for this patient population, although the following are the most common:

Fatigue
Infection protection
Safety concerns while insulin is being regulated

8. **Short-term goals**

RN	Daily compliance to insulin and other regimens
MSS	Patient caregiver able to follow POC

9. **Long-term goals**

RN	Compliance with regimens related to DM
	Return to school
	Growth and development within normal range for patient
	Stable medical status and blood sugars
	Self-care of DM (age-related)
	Avoidance of complications of DM
MSS	Resources identified

Patient and family utilizing community resources
Effective POC implementation

10. Discharge plans for this patient

Discharged to self-care (age dependent), under MD supervision
Discharged, parent and family able to care for patient, with no
follow up
Goals achieved, return to self-care status

11. Patient, family, and caregiver educational needs

Educational needs are the aspects of care that the patient,
parent, and caregiver must know to safely manage at home.
These include:

Instructions in home blood glucose monitoring program
The importance of compliance with all the regimens related to
care
Instructions regarding "sick day" rules and care
Self-observational care recording, including blood sugars,
weights, etc.
The signs and symptoms of hyper/hypoglycemia and the
actions to take
Other care regimens and information based on the patient and
caregiver's unique needs

For resources, contact the American Diabetes Association,
1-800-ADA-DISC.

12. Specific tips for reimbursement

Document the actions of your care
Document the specific areas of education and care needed
Obtain a telephone order for any POC change
Document specific teaching accomplished and the behavioral
outcomes of that teaching

DIABETES MELLITUS IN PREGNANCY

1. **General Considerations.** Diabetes mellitus (DM) may be a complication of antepartum care characterized by an intolerance to glucose during pregnancy that usually reverts to normal glucose tolerance after delivery.

2. **Needs for initial visit**

   Specific initial physician orders
   Universal precautions supplies
   Other supplies or equipment, based on physician orders
   Vital signs equipment

3. **Some potential medical-surgical diagnoses and codes**

Dehydration	276.5
Diabetes mellitus, insulin dependent	648.03
Gestational diabetes mellitus, noninsulin dependent	648.03
Hyperglycemia	648.83
Hypoglycemia	251.2
Pregnancy, high-risk	V23.8

4. **Associated nursing diagnoses**

   Activity intolerance
   Activity intolerance, high risk for
   Adjustment, impaired
   Anxiety
   Body image disturbance
   Body temperature, altered, high risk for
   Cardiac output, decreased
   Caregiver role strain
   Caregiver role strain, high risk for
   Constipation
   Coping, family: potential for growth
   Coping, ineffective family: compromised
   Coping, ineffective family: disabling
   Denial, ineffective
   Diversional activity deficit
   Family processes, altered
   Fatigue

Fear

Fluid volume deficit, high risk for

Fluid volume excess

Gas exchange, impaired

Grieving, anticipatory

Growth and development, altered

Infection, high risk for

Injury, high risk for

Knowledge deficit (specify)

Mobility, impaired physical

Noncompliance (specify) (e.g., diet)

Nutrition, altered: high risk for more than body requirements

Nutrition, altered: less than body requirements

Nutrition, altered: more than body requirements

Pain

Pain, chronic

Parental role conflict

Parenting, altered

Parenting, altered, high risk for

Role performance, altered

Sexual dysfunction

Sexuality patterns, altered

Skin integrity, impaired, high risk for

Sleep pattern disturbance

Spiritual distress (distress of the human spirit)

Thought processes, altered

Urinary elimination, altered

5. **Service skills identified**

Skilled assessment of the patient with _____ (specify)

Teach insulin administration

Assess patient for asymptomatic urinary tract infections, obtain urine specimen and send for U/A, C and S

Teach patient or family member to correctly draw up and administer insulin

Teach diabetes management regimen(s)

Teach regarding diet and importance of eating at regular, consistent times

Teach regarding changing need of insulin amount as pregnancy advances

Perform blood glucose checks q _____, call physician if over _____ or less than _____

Teach patient and family to mix insulins

Teach patient and family member blood glucose monitoring process

Teach signs and symptoms of hyperglycemia and hypoglycemia

Teach emergency measures to patient and family

Teach regarding importance of reporting the following symptoms immediately to physician: nausea, vomiting, and infection

Venipuncture for FBS as ordered

Teach patient and family urine check procedures

Teach regarding new insulin, diet, and medication regimen

Teach action of different ordered insulins

Reassurance and support to pregnant patient regarding disease and appropriate concerns

6. **Other services indicated**

   MSS   Psychosocial evaluation
   Financial counseling assistance
   Referral(s) to community resources
   Support to high-risk patient

7. **Associated factors based on diagnosis justifying homebound status**

   Confined to home because of instability of DM
   Weakness, SOB
   Medically restricted because of high-risk pregnancy
   Activity restriction per obstetrician
   Patient on bed rest

8. **Short-term goals**

   RN   Daily compliance with new medication and diet regimens
   Prevention of infections
   No further complications to infant or mother
   MSS   Effective POC implementation
   Referral(s) to community resources

9. **Long-term goals**

   RN   Patient delivers a healthy, full-term infant
   Patient and family self-care regarding DM
   Prevention of infections
   Blood sugar in normal for patient range

Stable medical status
No adverse complications to mother or infant
from DM
MSS Resources identified
Patient utilizing community resources
Effective POC implementation

10. Discharge plans for this patient

Return to self-care status, under MD supervision
Continuing need for home health care because patient remains
medically confined to home and needs nursing care to
prevent hospitalization
Delivery of infant

11. Patient, family, and caregiver educational needs

Educational needs are the aspects of care that the patient and
caregiver must understand to safely self-manage at home.
These include:

The importance of compliance to the DM care regimens and
keeping scheduled OB appointments
The signs of labor and other symptoms or changes that
necessitate notifying the MD and being seen immediately
(e.g., bleeding, premature rupture of membranes, etc.)
The need for optimal nutrition and frequent rest periods
Self-observational skills including home blood glucose
monitoring findings, daily weights, etc.
Other care regimens as identified based on the patient's unique
needs

12. Specific tips for reimbursement

Document your care and the actions of your care
Document any abnormal findings in the clinical record and the
notification of the MD
Document initial knowledge level and progress achieved
through the teaching process
Document specific teaching accomplished and the behavioral
outcomes of that teaching

NEWBORN CARE

1. **General Considerations.**   Many commercial insurers encourage mothers and newborns to receive care at home after shortened inpatient stays (12 to 24 hours). At home, the infant is assessed, protected against infection, provided with adequate nutrition, and has more opportunity for infant-parent attachment.

2. **Needs for initial visit**

   Specific initial physician orders
   Universal precautions supplies
   Other supplies, or equipment, based on physician orders
   Vital signs equipment
   Infant scale with liner
   For state required tests (e.g., PKU), consent form, lancet,
      alcohol sponge, collection form, and bandages

3. **Some potential medical-surgical diagnoses and codes**

C-section with complications	674.14
Delayed development, newborn	764.90
Failure to thrive	783.4
Jaundice, fetal/neonatal	774.6
Newborn apnea, apnea/brady monitors	770.8
Vaginal delivery, single liveborn	V30.0
Vaginal delivery, twin-mate liveborn	V31.0

4. **Associated nursing diagnoses**

   Airway clearance, ineffective
   Anxiety
   Breast-feeding, effective
   Breast-feeding, ineffective
   Breast-feeding, interrupted
   Caregiver role strain
   Caregiver role strain, high risk for
   Family processes, altered
   Fear
   Infection, high risk for
   Injury, high risk for
   Knowledge deficit (care of newborn)

Nutrition, altered: less than body requirements
Nutrition, altered: more than body requirements
Parenting, altered
Thermoregulation, ineffective

5. **Service skills identified**

Assessment of all systems of newborn infant
Observation of mother, family, and infant bonding and
interactions
Assess apical pulse, respiration, rectal temperature
Teach regarding importance of effective handwashing to
mother and family
Assess for jaundice and instruct regarding care of same
Weigh infant q visit, lining, and balancing scale
Observe and record infant stool pattern
Record infant voiding pattern, noting frequency, color,
volume
Measure head circumference q visit
Heel stick to obtain blood per state regulations (e.g., PKU)
Assess head, thorax, skin, and genitals
Evaluate reflexes
Care of circumcision site per specific physician orders
Care of cord per specific physician orders
Evaluate baby's total nursing and feeding time(s)
Teach mother and family regarding bathing of infant
Teach mother and family regarding circumcision care
Teach mother and family regarding care of infant skin
Teach mother and family regarding cord care
Teach mother and family regarding well-child care
Teach mother and family regarding infant safety instructions
(e.g., car seat, playpen, crib rails)
Teach mother and family regarding clothing and other
identified areas needing information
Teach mother regarding sitz bath and indications
Assess skin/sclera coloring for jaundice

6. **Other services indicated**

HHA	Personal care
	ADL assistance, including bathing and dressing the infant, meal preparation for the family, and assisting with other siblings as indicated
MSS	Psychosocial assessment

Referral to community resources
Financial assistance counseling

7. **Associated factors based on diagnosis justifying homebound status**

   Usually not a requirement for early discharge maternity program, but the mothers and infants are confined to home for infection control, feeding reasons for the infant, and the increased rest needs of the new postpartal mother

8. **Short-term goals**

RN	Optimal nutrition for growth and development of the infant
	Daily, safe care provided by new parents and family
HHA	Effective personal care
	ADL assistance
MSS	Problem, resource identification

9. **Long-term goals**

RN	Cord site clean, drying, infection-free
	Positive relationship demonstrated between infant, parent, and family
	Parent and family comfortable with and able to provide care to infant
	Optimal nutrition for growth and development of the infant
	Stable, healthy newborn
HHA	Personal care
	ADL assistance
MSS	Referral(s) to needed community resources
	Effective POC implementation

10. **Discharge plans for this patient**

    Discharged to care of parents and family, under MD care

11. **Patient, family, and caregiver educational needs**

    Educational needs are the aspects of care that the mother and other caregivers need to safely care for the infant. These include:

The importance of medical follow up and keeping pediatrician appointments

Safety aspects of newborn care, including the projected immunization/well-child schedule

Care related to feeding and breast-feeding

Cord care, bathing, clothing, sleeping, and other infant habits

Other care regimens as identified based on the patient's and family's unique needs

The La Leche League International is available for local resources on breast-feeding. In addition, many hospitals have nurse consultants whose expertise is breast-feeding should your client need this service or support.

12. **Specific tips for reimbursement**

Document all nursing care and the actions of that care

Usually there is one clinical record for both mother and infant

Document feeding schedule in progress notes

Two to three visits is usually the number of nursing visits covered by insurance, depending on specific policies

Home health aides are usually involved and can stay as long as up to 8 hours daily in some insurance benefit programs

POSTPARTAL CARE

1. **General Considerations.** Because many female consumers of health care are opting for early maternity discharge programs, postpartal and newborn care are increasingly being provided by HHAs. Usually, the mothers and infants go home within 24 hours after birth and the home health nurse evaluates the mother and baby the next day.

2. **Needs for initial visit**

   Specific initial physician orders
   Universal precautions supplies
   Other supplies or equipment, based on physician orders
   Vital signs equipment

3. **Some potential medical-surgical diagnoses and codes**

C/S with complications	674.14
Forceps delivery, uncomplicated	72.9
Postpartum care, uncomplicated delivery	V24.0
Spontaneous vaginal delivery, uncomplicated	73.59

4. **Associated nursing diagnoses**

   Activity intolerance
   Anxiety
   Body image disturbance
   Breast-feeding, effective
   Breast-feeding, ineffective
   Breast-feeding, interrupted
   Caregiver role strain
   Caregiver role strain, high risk for
   Constipation
   Coping family: potential for growth
   Family processes, altered
   Fatigue
   Fear
   Fluid volume deficit, high risk for
   Growth and development, altered
   Home maintenance management, impaired
   Infection, high risk for
   Injury, high risk for

Knowledge deficit (regarding self-care S/P C/S and infant care)
Mobility, impaired physical
Nutrition, altered: less than body requirements
Pain
Parenting, altered
Role performance, altered
Self-esteem, situational low
Sexual dysfunction
Sexuality patterns, altered
Skin integrity, impaired
Sleep pattern disturbance
Spiritual distress (distress of the human spirit)
Urinary elimination, altered

5. **Service skills identified**

Skilled assessment of postpartal patient
Evaluation of patient
Assessment of breast and nipples, engorgement, soreness, cracking blisters
Assessment of Homan's sign
RN to assess patient's pain on an ongoing basis to identify need for change, alteration addition, or other plan for pain management
RN to teach new parents regarding infant safety measures, parenting skills, bathing, cord care, circumcision care, and well-child care
RN to obtain urine for culture and sensitivity
Assessment of amount, character of lochia
Assessment of episiotomy site
Assessment of episiotomy pain
Check fundus
Teach regarding parenting
Teach regarding breast-care regimen(s)
Teach regarding infant safety
Teach regarding activity level
Teach regarding exercise level
Teach regarding family planning
Teach regarding sexuality questions

6. **Other services indiated**

HHA   Personal care

	ADL assistance, may assist mother with meal preparation, light housekeeping, assisting with other siblings as indicated
MSS	Psychosocial evaluation
	Referral to community resources
	Financial assistance counseling
	Home safety assessment and counseling

7. **Associated factors based on diagnosis justifying homebound status**

   Usually not a requirement for early discharge maternity program, but the mothers and infants are confined to home for infection control, feeding reasons for the infant, and the increased rest needs of the new postpartal mother

8. **Short-term goals**

   Optimal nutrition and fluids
   Optimal nutrition and fluids to nourish infant if breast-feeding
   Daily care of peritoneal site
   Satisfaction for mother to enhance bonding
   Able to care for infant

9. **Long-term goals**

   Pain-free, comfortable patient
   Positive relationship with infant
   Mother self-care and able to care for infant
   Optimal nutrition and fluids for mother and infant
   Satisfaction for mother to enhance bonding
   Healing episiotomy or laceration
   Patient infection-free

10. **Discharge plans for this patient**

    Return mother to self-care status in community, effectively caring for infant, under MD supervision

11. **Patient, family, and caregiver educational needs**

    Educational needs are the regimens that the new mother and caregiver will need to safely care for herself and the infant between visits and after discharge. These include:

    Infant care, including well-child care and the need for immunizations in the future

The importance of optimal hydration, nutrition, and rest for
   healing and breast-feeding

Signs and symptoms of episiotomy infection

Management of pain, including hemorrhoid discomfort

Infection control, including effective handwashing

The importance of medical follow up

Other aspects of care related to the patient's unique needs

12. **Specific tips for reimbursement**

Document all nursing care and the actions of that care

Usually, there is one clinical record for both mother and infant

Two to three visits is usually the number of nursing visits
   covered by insurance, depending on specific policies

Home health aides are usually involved and can stay up to 8
   hours daily in some insurance benefit programs

SICKLE CELL ANEMIA (CARE OF THE CHILD WITH)

1. **General Considerations.** Children and adolescents with sickle cell anemia are occasionally referred to home health agencies for follow up after hospitalization. The emphasis at home utilizes nursing teaching skills.

2. **Needs for initial visit**

   Specific initial physician orders
   Universal precautions supplies
   Other supplies or equipment, based on physician orders
   Vital signs equipment

3. **Some potential medical-surgical diagnoses and codes**

Dehydration	276.5
Sickle cell anemia	282.60
Sickle cell crisis	282.62

4. **Associated nursing diagnoses**

   Activity intolerance
   Activity intolerance, high risk for
   Anxiety
   Body image disturbance
   Caregiver role strain
   Caregiver role strain, high risk for
   Family processes, altered
   Fatigue
   Fear
   Fluid volume deficit
   Fluid volume deficit, high risk for
   Growth and development, altered
   Infection, high risk for
   Injury, high risk for
   Knowledge deficit (disease management)
   Mobility, impaired physical
   Noncompliance (specify)
   Nutrition, altered: less than body requirements
   Pain
   Pain, chronic

Sexual dysfunction

Skin integrity, impaired

Skin integrity, impaired, high risk for

Tissue perfusion, altered (specify type) (renal, cerebral, cardiopulmonary, gastrointestinal, peripheral)

5. **Service skills identified**

Observation and complete systems assessment of the child with SC anemia

Assess pain, site, frequency, and character

Provide emotional support to patient and family

Assess pain medication regimen and response to therapy

Assess respiratory status

Assist with management of sickle cell crisis

Encourage nutritional supplements as ordered

Teach regarding importance of nutrition and hydration

Assess amount and site of any swelling

Teach regarding importance of contacting RN and MD regarding fever, SOB, or crisis onset

Teach patient to avoid factors that may predispose to crisis episode

RN to assess patient for signs and symptoms infection, S/P multiple blood transfusions

RN to monitor amount and site of pain

RN to observe for chronic leg ulcers and other sites of thrombosis

RN to counsel patient on importance of adequate hydration, nutrition, rest, and infection resolution and control

RN to teach patient about safe, effective use of oxygen therapy

RN to observe and assess patient for signs of impending crisis

RN to monitor patient's respiratory, mental status, and other functions for evidence of change or impending crisis

RN to monitor vital signs

Venipuncture of CBC, sedimentation rate (specify frequency ordered)

RN to monitor patient's weight

RN to start and monitor IV of _____ for hydration (per specific MD orders)

RN to assess IV's patency and site for redness, tenderness, swelling, or other signs of infection/infiltration

RN to monitor intake and output of patient recently discharged from the hospital S/P crisis

RN to dress leg wound sites with (specify per MD orders) q (specify frequency)

RN to monitor patient's pain control regimen, including teaching caregivers the importance of adherence to the ordered and fixed medication schedule

RN to teach patient relaxation techniques, imagery, and other nonpharmacologic interventions that may assist relief

6. Other services indicated

HHA	Personal care
	ADL assistance
MSS	Psychosocial assessment
	Problem identification
	Financial assistance counseling
	Referral(s) to community resources
	Home safety assessment
OT	Evaluation
	Conservation of energy techniques
	Adaptive/assistive devices as indicated

7. Associated factors based on diagnosis justifying homebound status

Pain, weakness
Decreased activity, bed rest to decrease oxygen

8. Short-term goals

RN	Daily pain relief
	Increase in appetite, nutrition, and hydration
HHA	Effective personal care
	ADL assistance
MSS	Problem identification
	POC implementation
OT	Daily adherence to OT regimen

9. Long-term goals

RN	Infection-free
	Management of pain
	Parents able to care for patient
	Optimal hydration and nutrition
	Decreased hospitalizations
	Pain, symptom contol at home

HHA	Effective personal hygiene
MSS	Referral to community resource(s)
	Problem resolution
	Counseling related to chronic illness
	Effective POC implementation
OT	Conservation of energy techniques utilized
	Adaptive/assistive devices used, safely and effectively

10. Discharge plans for this patient

Discharged, family able to provide care, under MD supervision

Discharged to 24-hour acute facility for pain-control management

11. Patient, family, and caregiver educational needs

Educational needs are the regimens that the caregiver will be managing with or for the patient. These include:

Importance of optimal rest, hydration, and nutrition
The avoidance of infections
Availability of genetic counseling
The importance of medical follow up
Support groups in the community that are available to the patient and their caregivers
Other aspects of care, based on your patient's unique needs

For you and your patient's information, the following resource is available: National Association for Sickle Cell Disease, Inc., 4221 Wilshire Boulevard, Suite 360, Los Angeles, CA 90010.

12. Specific tips for reimbursement

Document hematocrit and hemoglobin values
Ultimately, any organs can be affected and have clinical involvement, document these changes
Document the nursing care provided and the outcomes of that care
Document the specific teaching accomplished and the behavioral outcomes of that teaching

Patients with sickle cell disease have a long history of interactions with health care settings and professionals. The patients know their histories, what pain medications bring relief most effectively, and other important information that assists the home care nurse in meeting patient and home care goals.

SURGICAL (POSTOPERATIVE) CARE OF THE CHILD

1. **General Considerations.** Accidents continue to be the leading cause of death in children younger than 18 years of age. The care of the child at home after hospitalization and surgery is often due to trauma, particularly car accidents. Depending on the circumstances, care will usually be directed toward wound healing, restorative nursing, and rehabilitation goals.

2. **Needs for initial visit**

   Specific initial physician orders
   Universal precautions supplies
   Other supplies or equipment, based on physician orders
   Vital signs equipment

3. **Some potential medical-surgical diagnoses and codes**

Amputation, infected right or left BKA	997.62
Appendectomy	47.0
Appendicitis (perforation with abscess)	540.1
Attention to other artificial opening of urinary tract	V55.6
Attention to surgical dressing and sutures	V58.3
Bowel impaction	560.30
Cellulitis, RLE, LLE	682.6
Colitis	558.9
Colostomy, attention to	V55.3
Constipation	564.0
Crohn's disease	555.9
Cystocele	618.0
Dehydration	276.5
Depression, reactive	300.4
Diabetes mellitus, with complications, juvenile	250.91
Fitting and adjustment of urinary devices	V53.6
Hemiplegia	342.9
Hernia repair, inguinal	53.00
Hernia repair, umbilical	53.49
Hickman catheter insertion	86.07
Hypertension	401.9

I and D of abscess	86.04
Ileal conduit, post-op, infected	997.5
Ileus	560.1
Incontinence of urine	788.30
Osteomyelitis, lower leg	730.26
Other aftercare following surgery	V58.4
Paraplegia	344.1
Peritonitis	567.9
Peritonitis, postoperative infection	998.7
Pneumonia	486
Quadriplegia	344.0
Spinal cord injury, traumatic	952.9
Wound dehiscence	998.3
Wound infection	998.5
Urinary incontinence	788.3
Urinary tract infection	599.0

4. **Associated nursing diagnoses**

Activity intolerance
Activity intolerance, high risk for
Adjustment, impaired
Anxiety
Body image disturbance
Body temperature, altered, high risk for
Bowel incontinence
Caregiver role strain
Caregiver role strain, high risk for
Constipation
Coping, ineffective family: compromised
Coping, ineffective individual
Denial, ineffective
Diarrhea
Diversional activity deficit
Family processes, altered
Fatigue
Fear
Fluid volume deficit, high risk for
Grieving, anticipatory
Growth and development, altered
Hopelessness
Incontinence, functional
Infection, high risk for
Injury, high risk for

Knowledge deficit (care management)
Mobility, impaired physical
Noncompliance (specify)
Nutrition, altered: less than body requirements
Pain
Pain, chronic
Parenting, altered
Parenting, altered, high risk for
Self-care deficit, bathing/hygiene
Self-care deficit, dressing/grooming
Self-care deficit, feeding
Self-care deficit, toileting
Sexual dysfunction
Sexuality patterns, altered
Skin integrity, impaired
Sleep pattern disturbance
Social interaction, impaired
Social isolation
Spiritual distress (distress of the human spirit)
Tissue integrity, impaired
Tissue perfusion, altered (specify type) (renal, cerebral, cardiopulmonary, gastrointestinal, peripheral)
Urinary elimination, altered

5. **Service skills identified**

Skilled nursing assessment of wound and systems in child/adolescent with _____ (specify)

RN to care for wound site q (specify ordered frequency and dressing orders)

RN to teach child and caregiver about all medications, including schedule, functions, and side effects

RN to assess lower extremities for signs and symptoms of compromised circulation or decreased sensation

Skilled observation and assessment of wound and other (specify)

RN to evaluate patient pain and implement pain control/relief regimen per MD orders

RN to teach parent and caregiver safe use and care of PCA pump

Observation and assessment of postoperative patient's bowel patterns, including frequency and evaluation of need for stool softener, laxatives, or dietary changes

Assessment of blood pressure and other vital signs

RN to teach caregiver importance of nutrition and dietary regimen and requirements postsurgery

RN to teach child and caregiver about safe postoperative care; no pushing, pulling, lifting, roughhousing, or horseplay with siblings

Patient observed for signs and symptoms of recurrent infection

Caregiver instructed by RN on what signs and symptoms to watch for that would necessitate calling RN or MD

RN to consult with nurse enterostomal therapist about wounds with surrounding skin involvement

RN to teach family how to safely care for patient in traction or with pins

RN to assess and monitor pain, patient's response to interventions, and effective pain relief measures

RN to medicate patient with (specify MD order) for pain relief prior to extensive dressing change

RN to teach caregivers care of the adolescent in *halo* brace traction

RN to assess hydration and nutrition through review of food diary, intake and output records, and ordered weights

Assess the child's unique response to treatments and interventions and report changes, unfavorable responses, or reactions to the physician

Instruct on signs and symptoms, infection control, and the avoidance of those with upper respiratory or other infections

Teach child and caregivers effective handwashing techniques and other infection control measures

6. Other services indicated

HHA	Personal care
	ADL assistance
	Meal preparation
	Home exercise program
MSS	Evaluation
	Assessment of the social and emotional factors impacting effective POC implementation
	Determination of factors impeding POC from being successful
	Psychosocial assessment of the child and family with multiple social problems
	Financial counseling
	Community resources referral
	Facilitation of school reconnection or

	identification for tutoring needed for missed school work
OT	Evaluation
	Conservation of energy techniques
	ADL assistance and retraining
	Assessment of patient and home for assistive/ adaptive devices or equipment
PT	Evaluation
	Home exercise strengthening program
	Safe transfer training
	Instruct, supervise, and teach caregiver home exercise regimen
	Evaluate patient for overbed trapeze to facilitate bed mobility
	Gait training

7. **Associated factors based on diagnosis justifying homebound status**

Patient is status post_____ surgery (specify) and has weakness and pain

Patient is medically restricted for 4 weeks; not to leave home except for scheduled visits with vascular surgeon for flap assessment

Patient has open wound site and is unable to leave home without assistance

Patient is only partial or nonweight bearing

8. **Short-term goals**

RN	Patient comfort
	Daily compliance to wound care and other medical regimens
	Healing wound without infection
HHA	Effective personal hygiene
	ADL assistance
MSS	Problems identified
	POC being successfully implemented
OT	Daily adherence to OT POC
	Patient using assistive devices
PT	Daily adherence to PT POC
	Patient integrating bed mobility exercise regimen into daily plan
	Overbed trapeze

9. **Long-term goals**

RN	Wound healed
	POC successfully implemented
	Child becomes independent with self-care when possible
HHA	Safe, effective personal hygiene
	Patient clean and feels better
MSS	Community resource identified
	Problem resolution
	Care team able to implement POC
	Appropriate adjustment occurring to diagnoses and problems
	Referral of patient and caregivers to community services for continued support
OT	Patient using conservation of energy techniques taught in daily activities
	Patient using assistive/adaptive devices
PT	Caregiver taught safe home exercise program, including transfer techniques
	Patient practices bed mobility exercises and maintains schedule
	Patient experiences or verbalizes improved strength or endurance

10. **Discharge plans for this patient**

Patient-centered, realistic goals achieved, discharge from home care, self-care under MD supervision

Can get to outpatient clinic for care and will have peer-support groups available, discharge per MD order

Patient to be admitted to rehabilitation hospital when bed available

11. **Patient, family, and caregiver educational needs**

Educational needs are the regimens that the parent and caregiver will be managing for or with the child. These include:

Home safety assessment and teaching
Effective personal hygiene habits
The avoidance of infections
The patient's medications and their relationship to each other

The importance of medical follow up

Self-care observational aspects of care, particularly for the wound or other (specify) site

Support groups in the community that are available to your patient and their caregivers

Specific care of the wound and other precautions postsurgery

Assisting the child to continue growth and development phases, including seeing peers, stimulation, and maintaining or completing schoolwork

Other information based on the child's and family's unique needs

12. **Specific tips for reimbursement**

Document progress toward wound healing or other specified, patient-centered goals

Document patient or wound deterioration or problems

Document the specific nursing care and teaching instructions provided

Document the patient and caregivers response to care interventions

Document any exacerbation of symptoms or problems that necessitated additional visits and be sure that there are orders for all visits

Document all POC changes

Document all the skills used in the provision of professional nursing care practice when caring for the child (e.g., teaching, training, observation and assessment, catheters, IV site care, venipuncture, etc.)

Document the coordination occurring, based on the POC, among team members. The interdisciplinary conference notes should be reflected in the clinical record. Refer to these meetings or communications on the forms used by the insurer as an update on the patient's status.

PART SEVEN

MEDICARE GUIDELINES

COVERAGE OF SERVICES
(REVISION 222)

Covered and Noncovered Home Health Services

203.   CONDITIONS TO BE MET FOR COVERAGE OF HOME HEALTH SERVICES

Home health agency services are covered by Medicare when the following criteria
are met:

○   The person to whom the services are provided is an eligible Medicare beneficiary.

○   The home health agency which is providing the services to the beneficiary
has in effect a valid agreement to participate in the Medicare program.

○   The beneficiary qualifies for coverage of home health services as described
in §204.

○   The services for which payment is claimed are covered as described in §§205
and 206.

○   Medicare is the appropriate payer.

○   The services for which payment is claimed are not otherwise excluded from
payment.

203.1   Reasonable and Necessary Services

A.   Background.—In enacting the Medicare program, Congress recognized that the
physician would play an important role in determining utilization of services. The law requires
that payment can be made only if a physician certifies the need for services and establishes
a plan of care. The Secretary is responsible for ensuring that the claimed services are
covered by Medicare, including determining whether they are "reasonable and necessary."

B.   Determination of Coverage.—The beneficiary's health status and medical need
as reflected in the home health plan of care and medical record provide the basis for
determinations as to whether services provided are reasonable and necessary. A finding
that services are reasonable and necessary must be based on information available in
these documents, although clear inferences may be drawn from information provided in
the plan of care (form HCFA 485) or in supplementary forms (forms HCFA 486, 487, 488).

A finding that care is not reasonable and necessary must be based on information provided
on the forms and in the medical record with respect to the unique medical condition of the
individual beneficiary. That is, a coverage denial may not be made based solely on the
reviewer's general inferences about patients with similar diagnoses or on data related to
utilization generally, but must be based upon objective clinical evidence regarding the
patient's individual need for care.

392

203.1 (Cont.) COVERAGE OF SERVICES 04-89

Both payment and denial decisions may be based on summary information contained in the relevant HCFA data forms; however, additional information from the medical records (either via Form 488 or a copy of the medical record) must be requested when medical information needed to support a decision is not clearly present. The following examples illustrate this statement.

Examples of cases in which development of the case is needed:

EXAMPLE 1: A plan of care provides for daily skilled nursing visits for care of a pressure sore, but the description of the pressure sore and the dressing which is contained on the form causes the reviewer to question why daily skilled care is needed. The intermediary would not reduce the number of visits but would either request additional information to support the need for daily care or would request the nursing notes to determine if the beneficiary required daily skilled care.

EXAMPLE 2: A beneficiary with a diagnosis of congestive heart failure (CHF) has been hospitalized for 5 days. Posthospital skilled nursing care is ordered 3 × wk × 60 days for skilled observation, teaching of diet medication compliance and signs and symptoms of the disease. The documentation on the HCFA 485-486 shows that the patient has had CHF for 10 years with an exacerbation requiring recent hospitalization. The medications are not shown as changed or new. The clinical findings are contradictory. There is a possibility that this beneficiary requires skilled observation and teaching although the documentation does not give a clear picture of the beneficiary's needs. Therefore, the case would be developed further to determine if the criteria for coverage were met.

Examples of cases which would be denied without further development:

EXAMPLE 3: A plan of care calls for vitamin B12 injections 1 × mo × 60 days for a beneficiary who has been discharged from the hospital following a recent hip fracture. The beneficiary has generalized weakness but there is no diagnosis or clinical symptoms shown which support that the Medicare requirements governing coverage of skilled nursing care for B12 injections are met. The claim would be denied without development for further information since there is no support for coverage of the skilled nursing care for the B12 injections.

EXAMPLE 4: A beneficiary has a primary diagnosis of back sprain for which he was hospitalized for 7 days. The beneficiary also has a secondary diagnosis of emphysema with an onset 2 years prior to the start of care. Following the hospitalization, the physician ordered skilled nursing 2 × wk × 4 weeks for skilled observation of vital signs and response to medication and aide services 2 × wk × 4 weeks for personal care. The documentation on the HCFA 485-486 shows that the beneficiary is up as tolerated, is able to walk

10 feet without resting and is alert. Cliniclal facts show normal vital signs, and no reference to emphysema. The beneficiary is on phenobarbital PO 30 mg TID. The documentation clearly does not support the medical necessity for skilled nursing care and the claim for the services would be denied without development.

Examples of cases in which payment may be made without further development:

EXAMPLE 5:   A beneficiary with a diagnosis of CHF has been hospitalized for five days. Post-hospital skilled nursing care is ordered 3 × wk × 60 days for skilled observation, teaching of a new diet regimen, compliance with multiple new medications, and signs and symptoms of the disease state. The documentation on the HCFA 485-486 shows the beneficiary had had an acute exacerbation of a pre-existing CHF condition which required the recent acute hospitalization. The beneficiary is discharged from the hospital with a medication regimen changed from previous medications. The HCFA forms documenting the clinical evidence of the recent acute exacerbation of the beneficiary's cardiac condition combined with changed medications support the physician's order for care. Payment may be made without further development.

EXAMPLE 6:   A plan of care provides for physical therapy treatments 3 × wk × 45 days for a beneficiary who has been discharged from the hospital following a recent hip fracture. The beneficiary was discharged using a walker 7 days before the start of home care. The HCFA form 485 and supplementary form HCFA 486 shows that the beneficiary was discharged from the hospital with restricted mobility in ambulation, transfers, and climbing of stairs. The beneficiary had an unsafe gait which indicated a need for gait training and the beneficiary had not been instructed in stair climbing and a home exercise program. The goal of the physical therapy was to increase strength, range of motion and to progress from walker to cane with safe gait. Information on the relevant HCFA forms also indicates that the beneficiary had a previous functional capacity of full ambulation, mobility, and self care. The claim may be paid without further development, since there are no objective clinical factors in the medical evidence to contradict the order of the beneficiary's treating physician.

203.2   Impact of Other Available Caregivers and Other Available Coverage on Medicare Coverage of Home Health Services.—Where the Medicare criteria for coverage of home health services are met, beneficiaries are entitled by law to coverage of reasonable and necessary home health services.

Therefore, a beneficiary is entitled to have the costs of reasonable and necessary services reimbursed by Medicare without regard to whether there is someone available in the home to furnish them. However, where a family member or other caring person is or will be providing services that adequately meet the patient's needs, it would not be reasonable and necessary for home health agency personnel to furnish such services. Ordinarily it can be presumed that there is no able and willing person in the home to provide the services being rendered by the home health agency unless the beneficiary or family indicates otherwise, and objects to the provision of the services by the home health agency, or unless the home health agency has first hand knowledge to the contrary.

394

203.2 (Cont.) COVERAGE OF SERVICES 04-89

EXAMPLE: A beneficiary, who lives with an adult daughter and who otherwise qualifies for Medicare coverage of home health services, requires the assistance of a home health aide for bathing and assistance with an exercise program to improve endurance. The daughter is unwilling to bathe her elderly father and assist him with the exercise program. Home health aide services to provide these services would be reasonable and necessary.

Similarly, a beneficiary is entitled to have the costs of reasonable and necessary home health services reimbursed by Medicare even if the beneficiary would qualify for institutional care (e.g., hospital care or skilled nursing facility care).

EXAMPLE: A beneficiary who is being discharged from a hospital with a diagnosis of osteomyelitis and who requires continuation of the IV antibiotic therapy that was begun in the hospital was found to meet the criteria for Medicare coverage of skilled nursing facility services. If the beneficiary also meets the qualifying criteria for coverage of home health services, payment may be made for the reasonable and necessary home health services the beneficiary needs, notwithstanding the availability of coverage in a skilled nursing facility.

Medicare payment should be made for reasonable and necessary home health services where the beneficiary is also receiving supplemental services that do not meet Medicare's definition of skilled nursing care or home health aid services.

EXAMPLE: A patient who needs skilled nursing care on an intermittent basis also hires an licensed practical nurse (LPN) to provide nighttime assistance while family members sleep. The care provided by the LPN, as respite to the family members, does not require the skills of a licensed nurse (as defined in §205.1) and therefore has no impact on the beneficiary's eligibility for Medicare payment of home health services even though another third party insurer may pay for that nursing care.

203.3   Use of Utilization Screens and "Rules of Thumb".—Medicare recognizes that determinations of whether home health services are reasonable and necessary must be based on an assessment of each beneficiary's individual care needs. Therefore, denial of services based on numerical utilization screens, diagnostic screens, diagnosis or specific treatment norms is not appropriate.

204.   CONDITIONS THE BENEFICIARY MUST MEET TO QUALIFY FOR COVERAGE OF HOME HEALTH SERVICES

To qualify for Medicare coverage of any home health services, the beneficiary must meet each of the criteria specified in this section. Beneficiaries who meet each of these criteria are eligible to have payment made on their behalf for services which are discussed in §205 and §206.

204.1 Confined to the Home.—

A. Patient Confined to His Home.—In order for a beneficiary to be eligible to receive covered home health services under both Part A and Part B, the law requires that a physician certify in all cases that the beneficiary is confined to his home. (See §240.1.) An individual does not have to be bedridden to be considered as confined to his home. However, the condition of these patients should be such that there exists a normal inability to leave home and, consequently, leaving their homes would require a considerable and taxing effort. If the patient does in fact leave the home, the patient may nevertheless be considered homebound if the absences from the home are infrequent or for periods of relatively short duration, or are attributable to the need to receive medical treatment. Absences attributable to the need to receive medical treatment include attendance at adult day centers to receive medical care, ongoing receipt of outpatient kidney dialysis, and the receipt of outpatient chemotherapy or radiation therapy. It is expected that in most instances absences from the home which occur will be for the purpose of receiving medical treatment. However, occasional absences from the home for nonmedical purposes, e.g., an occasional trip to the barber, a walk around the block or a drive, would not necessitate a finding that the individual is not homebound so long as the absences are undertaken on an infrequent basis or are of relatively short duration and do not indicate that the patient has the capacity to obtain the health care provided outside rather than in the home.

Generally speaking, a beneficiary will be considered to be homebound if he has a condition due to an illness or injury which restricts his ability to leave his place of residence except with the aid of supportive devices such as crutches, canes, wheelchairs, and walkers, the use of special transportation, or the assistance of another person or if he has a condition which is such that leaving his home is medically contraindicated. Some examples of homebound patients which are illustrative of the factors to be taken into account in determining whether a homebound condition exists would be: (1) a beneficiary paralyzed from a stroke who is confined to a wheelchair or who requires the aid of crutches in order to walk; (2) a beneficiary who is blind or senile and requires the assistance of another person in leaving his place of residence; (3) a beneficiary who has lost the use of his upper extremities and, therefore, is unable to open doors, use handrails on stairways, etc., and therefore, requires the assistance of another individual in leaving his place of residence; (4) a patient who has just returned from a hospital stay involving surgery who may be suffering from resultant weakness and pain and, therefore, his actions may be restricted by his physician to certain specified and limited activities such as getting out of bed only for a specified period of time, walking stairs only once a day, etc.; and (5) a patient with arteriosclerotic heart disease of such severity that he must avoid all stress and physical activity, and (6) a patient with a psychiatric problem if his illness is manifested in part by a refusal to leave his home environment or is of such a nature that it would not be considered safe for him to leave his home unattended, even if he has no physical limitations.

396

The aged person who does not often travel from his home because of feebleness and insecurity brought on by advanced age would not be considered confined to his home for purposes of receiving home health services unless he meets one of the above conditions. A patient who requires speech therapy but does not require physical therapy or nursing services must also meet one of the above conditions in order to be considered as confined to his home.

Although a patient must be confined to his home to be eligible for covered home health services, some services cannot be provided at the patient's residence because equipment is required which cannot be made available there. If the services required by an individual involve the use of such equipment, the home health agency may make arrangements with a hospital, SNF, or a rehabilitation center to provide these services on an outpatient basis. (See §§200.2 and 206.5.) However, even in these situations, for the services to be covered as home health services the patient must be considered as confined to his home; and to receive such outpatient services it may be expected that a homebound patient will generally require the use of supportive devices, special transportation, or the assistance of another person to travel to the appropriate facility.

If for any reason a question is raised as to whether an individual is confined to his home, the agency will be requested to furnish the intermediary with the information necessary to establish that the beneficiary is homebound as defined above.

     B.   _Patient's Place of Residence._—A patient's residence is wherever he makes his home. This may be his own dwelling, an apartment, a relative's home, a home for the aged, or some other type of institution. However, an institution may not be considered a patient's residence if it:

     1.   Meets at least the basic requirement in the definition of a hospital, i.e., it is primarily engaged in providing by or under the supervision of physicians, to inpatients, diagnostic and therapeutic services for medical diagnosis, treatment, and care of disabled, or sick persons, or rehabilitation services for the rehabilitation of injured, disabled, or sick persons, or

     2.   Meets at least the basic requirement in the definition of an SNF, i.e., it is primarily engaged in providing to inpatients skilled nursing care and related services for patients who require medical or nursing care, or rehabilitation services for the rehabilitation of injured, disabled, or sick persons. All nursing homes that participate in Medicare and/or Medicaid as skilled nursing facilities, and most facilities that participate in Medicaid as intermediate care facilities meet this basic requirement. In addition, many nursing homes which do not choose to participate in Medicare or Medicaid meet this test. Check with your fiscal intermediary or Medicare regional office before serving nursing home patients.

Thus, if an individual is a patient in an institution or distinct part of an institution which provides the services described in (A) or (B) above, he is not entitled to have payment made for home health services under either Part A or Part B since such an institution may not be considered his residence.

When a patient remains in a participating SNF following his discharge from active care, the facility may not be considered his residence for purposes of home health coverage.

204.2   Services Are Provided Under a Plan of Care Established and Approved by a Physician.—

A.   Content of the Plan of Care.—The plan of care must contain all pertinent diagnoses, including the beneficiary's mental status, the types of services, supplies, and equipment ordered, the frequency of the visits to be made, prognosis, rehabilitation potential, functional limitations, activities permitted, nutritional requirements, medications and treatments, safety measures to protect against injury, discharge plans, and any additional items the home health agency or physician choose to include.

NOTE: This manual uses the term "plan of care" to refer to the medical treatment plan established by the treating physician with the assistance of the home health care nurse. The term we used in the past was "plan of treatment." However, the term we used in the past was changed to "plan of care" in the Omnibus Budget Reconciliation Act of 1987 (OBRA'87) without a change in definition. It is anticipated that a discipline-oriented plan of care will be established, where appropriate, by a home health agency nurse regarding nursing and home health aide services and by skilled therapists regarding specific therapy treatment. These plans of care may be incorporated within the physician's plan of care or separately prepared.

B.   Specificity of Orders.—The orders on the plan of care must indicate the type of services to be provided to the beneficiary, both with respect to the professional who will provide them and with respect to the nature of the individual services, as well as the frequency of the services.

EXAMPLE: SN × 7/wk × 1 wk; 3/wk × 4 wk; 2/wk × 3 wk, (skilled nursing visits 7 times per week for 1 week; three times per week for 4 weeks; and two times per week for 3 weeks) for skilled observation and evaluation of the surgical site, for teaching sterile dressing changes and to perform sterile dressing changes. The sterile change consists of . . . (detail of procedure).

Orders for care can indicate a specific range in the frequency of visits to ensure that the most appropriate level of services is provided to home health beneficiaries. When a range of visits is ordered the upper limit of the range is to be considered the specific frequency.

EXAMPLE.   SN × 2-4/wk × 4 wk; 1-2/wk × 4 wk for skilled observation and evaluation of the surgical site. . . .

Example of inappropriate specificity: Skilled nursing visits 3 times per week and PRN as needed. (This order is not specific because: 1) the number of weeks is not specified; 2) "PRN" is open-ended; and 3) the nature of the service is not specified.)

398

C. Who Signs the Plan of Care.   The physician who signs the plan of care must be qualified to sign the physician certification as described in 42 CFR 424 subpart B.

D. Timeliness of Signature.—The plan of care must be signed before the bill is submitted to the intermediary for payment.

E. Use of Verbal Orders.—

(1) Services which are provided from the beginning of the certification period and before the physician signs the plan of care are considered to be provided under a plan of care established and approved by the physician where there is a verbal order for the care prior to rendering the services which is documented in the medical record and where the services are included in a signed plan of care.

EXAMPLE: The HHA acquires a verbal order for venipuncture for a beneficiary to be performed on August 1. The HHA provides the venipuncture on August 1 and evaluates the beneficiary's need for continued care. The physician signs the plan of care for the venipuncture on August 15. Since the HHA had acquired a verbal order prior to the delivery of services, the visit is considered to be provided under a plan of care established and approved by the physician.

(2) Services which are provided in the subsequent certification period are considered to be provided under the subsequent plan of care where there is a verbal order before the services provided in the subsequent period are furnished and the order is reflected in the medical record. However, services which are provided after the expiration of a plan of care, but before the acquisition of a verbal order or a signed plan of care, cannot be considered to be provided under a plan of care.

EXAMPLE 1:   The beneficiary is under a plan of care in which the physician orders venipuncture every 2 weeks. The last day covered by the initial plan of care is July 31. The beneficiary's next venipuncture is scheduled for August 5th, and the physician signs the plan of treatment for the new period on August 1st. The venipuncture on August 5th was provided under a plan of care established and approved by the physician.

EXAMPLE 2:   The beneficiary is under a plan of care in which the physician orders venipuncture every 2 weeks. The last day covered by the plan of care is July 31. The beneficiary's next venipuncture is scheduled for August 5th, and the physician does not sign the plan of treatment until August 6th. The HHA acquires a verbal order for the venipuncture before the August 5th visit, and therefore the visit is considered to be provided under a plan of care established and approved by the physician.

EXAMPLE 3:   The beneficiary is under a plan of care in which the physician orders venipuncture every 2 weeks. The last day covered by the plan of care is July 31. The beneficiary's next venipuncture is scheduled for August 5th, and the physician does not sign the plan of treatment until August 6th. The

HHA <u>does not</u> acquire a verbal order for the venipuncture before the August 5th visit, and therefore the visit cannot be considered to be provided under a plan of care established and approved by the physician. The prior plan of care expired and neither a verbal order nor a signed plan of care was in effect on the date of the service. The visit is not covered.

(3)   Any increase in the frequency of services or addition of new services during a certification period must be authorized by a physician by way of a verbal order or written order prior to the provision of the increased or additional services.

F.   <u>Periodic Review of the Plan of Care</u>.—The plan of care must be reviewed and signed by a physician no less frequently than every 2 months. The physician who reviews and signs the plan of care must be qualified under 42 CFR 424 subpart B to sign the physician certification and plan of care.

204.3   <u>Under the Care of a Physician</u>.—The patient must be under the care of a physician who is qualified to sign the physician certification and plan of care in accord with 42 CFR 424 subpart B.

A beneficiary is expected to be under the care of the physician who signs the plan of care and the physician certification. It is expected, but not required for coverage, that the physician who signs the plan of care will see the patient, but there is no specified interval of time within which the patient must be seen.

240.4   <u>Needs Skilled Nursing Care on an Intermittent Basis, or Physical Therapy or Speech Therapy or Has a Continued Need for Occupational Therapy</u>.—The patient must need one of the following types of services:

- ○   Skilled nursing care which:

    - -   Is reasonable and necessary as defined in §205.1A and B, and

    - -   Is needed on an "intermittent" basis as defined in §205.1C, or

- ○   Physical therapy as defined in §205.2A and B, or

- ○   Speech therapy as defined in §205.2A and C, or

- ○   Have a continuing need for occupational therapy as defined in §205.2A and D.

The beneficiary has a continued need for occupational therapy when:

- ○   The services which the beneficiary requires meet the definition of "occupational therapy" services fo §205.2A and D, and

- ○   The beneficiary's eligibility for home health services has been established by virtue of a prior need for skilled nursing care, speech therapy, or physical therapy in the current or prior certification period.

EXAMPLE: A beneficiary who is recovering from a cerebral vascular accident has an initial plan of care that called for physical therapy, speech therapy, and home health aide services. In the next certification period, the physician orders only occupational therapy and home health aide services because the beneficiary no longer needs the skills of a physical therapist or a speech therapist, but needs the services provided by the occupational therapist. The beneficiary's need for occupational therapy qualifies him or her for home health services, including home health aide services (presuming that all other qualifying criteria are met).

204.5 Physician Certification.—The home health agency must be acting upon a physician certification which is part of the plan of care (HCFA form 485) and which meets the requirements of this section for home health agency services to be covered.

   A. Content of the Physician Certification.—The physician must certify that:

   1. The home health services are or were needed because the beneficiary is or was confined to his home as defined in §204.1;

   2. The beneficiary needs or needed skilled nursing services on an intermittent basis or physical therapy or speech therapy, or continues or continued to need occupational therapy after the need for skilled nursing care or physical therapy or speech therapy ceased;

   3. A plan of care has been established and is periodically reviewed by a physician; and
   4. The services are or were furnished while the individual is or was under the care of a physician.

   B. Periodic Recertification.—The physician certification may cover a period less than but not greater than 62 days (2 months).

   C. Who May Sign the Certification.—The physician who signs the certification must be permitted to do so by 42 CFR 424 subpart B.

205. COVERAGE OF SERVICES WHICH ESTABLISH HOME HEALTH ELIGIBILITY

For any home health services to be covered by Medicare, the beneficiary must meet the qualifying criteria as specified in §204, including having a need for skilled nursing care on an intermittent basis, physical therapy, speech therapy or a continuing need for occupational therapy as defined in this section.

205.1 Skilled Nursing Care.—To be covered as skilled nursing services, the services must require the skills of a registered nurse or a licensed practical nurse under the supervision of a registered nurse, must be reasonable and necessary to the treatment of the beneficiary's illness or injury as discussed in §205.1A and B, and must be intermittent as discussed in §205.1C.

A. <u>General Principles Governing Reasonable and Necessary Skilled Nursing Care.</u>—

1. A skilled nursing service is a service which must be provided by a registered nurse, or a licensed practical nurse or a licensed vocational nurse under the supervision of a registered nurse to be safe and effective. In determining whether a service requires the skills of a nurse, consider both the inherent complexity of the service, the condition of the patient and accepted standards of medical and nursing practice.

Some services may be classified as a skilled nursing service on the basis of complexity alone, e.g., intravenous and intramuscular injections or insertion of catheters, and if reasonable and necessary to the treatment of the beneficiary's illness or injury, would be covered on that basis. However, in some cases the condition of the beneficiary may cause a service which would ordinarily be considered unskilled to be considered a skilled nursing service. This would occur when the beneficiary's condition is such that the service can be safely and effectively provided only by a skilled nurse.

EXAMPLE 1:   The presence of a plaster cast on an extremity generally does not indicate a need for skilled care. However, the patient with a pre-existing peripheral vascular or circulatory condition might need skilled nursing and skilled rehabilitation personnel to observe for complications, to monitor medication administration for pain control and to teach proper ambulation techniques to ensure proper bone alignment and healing.

EXAMPLE 2:   The condition of a beneficiary who has irritable bowel syndrome, or who is recovering from rectal surgery, may be such that he can be given an enema safely and effectively only by a skilled nurse. If the enema is necessary to treat the illness or injury, then the visit would be covered as a skilled nursing visit.

2. A service is not considered a skilled nursing service merely because it is performed by or under the direct supervision of a licensed nurse. Where a service can be safely and effectively performed (or self-administered) by the average nonmedical person without the direct supervision of a licensed nurse, the service cannot be regarded as a skilled nursing service although a skilled nurse actually provides the service. Similarly, the unavailability of a competent person to provide a nonskilled service, notwithstanding the importance of the service to the beneficiary, does not make it a skilled service when the skilled nurse provides it.

EXAMPLE 1:   Giving a bath does not ordinarily require the skills of a licensed nurse and therefore would not be covered as a skilled nursing service unless the beneficiary's condition is such that the bath could be given safely and effectively only by a licensed nurse (as discussed in §205.1.A.1. above).

EXAMPLE 2:   A beneficiary with a well-established colostomy absent complications may require assistance changing the colostomy bag because he cannot do it himself and there is no one else to change it. Notwithstanding the need for the routine colostomy care, the care does not become a skilled nursing service when it is provided by the licensed nurse.

402

205.1 (Cont.)   COVERAGE OF SERVICES   04-89

3. A service which, by its nature, requires the skills of a licensed nurse to be provided safely and effectively continues to be a skilled service even if it is taught to the patient, the patient's family or other caregivers. Where the beneficiary needs the skilled nursing care and there is no one trained, able and willing to provide it, the services of a skilled nurse would be reasonable and necessary to the treatment of the illness or injury.

EXAMPLE: A beneficiary was discharged from the hospital with an open draining wound which requires irrigation, packing and dressing twice each day. The home health agency has taught the family to perform the dressing changes. The home health agency continues to see the patient for the wound care that is needed during the time that the family is not available and willing to provide it. The wound care continues to be skilled nursing care, notwithstanding that the family provides it part of the time, and may be covered as long as it is required by the patient.

4. The skilled nursing service must be reasonable and necessary to the diagnosis and treatment of the beneficiary's illness or injury within the context of the beneficiary's unique medical condition. To be considered reasonable and necessary for the diagnosis or treatment of the beneficiary's illness or injury, the services must be consistent with the nature and severity of the illness or injury, his or her particular medical needs, and accepted standards of medical and nursing practice. A beneficiary's overall medical condition is a valid factor in deciding whether skilled services are needed. A beneficiary's diagnosis should never be the sole factor in deciding that a service the beneficiary needs is either skilled or not skilled.

The determination of whether the services are reasonable and necessary should be made in consideration that a physician has determined that the services ordered are reasonable and necessary. The services must, therefore, be viewed from the perspective of the condition of the patient when the services were ordered and what was, at that time, reasonably expected to be appropriate treatment for the illness or injury throughout the certification period.

EXAMPLE 1:   A physician has ordered skilled nursing visits for a patient with a hairline fracture of the hip. In the absence of any underlying medical condition or illness, nursing visits would not be reasonable and necessary for treatment of the patient's hip injury.

EXAMPLE 2:   A physician has ordered skilled nursing visits for injections of insulin and teaching of self-administration and self management of the medication regimen for a beneficiary with diabetes mellitus. Insulin has been shown to be a safe and effective treatment for diabetes mellitus, and therefore, the skilled nursing visits for the injections and the teaching of self-administration and self management of the treatment regimen would be reasonable and necessary.

The determination of whether a beneficiary needs skilled nursing care should be based solely upon the beneficiary's unique condition and individual needs, without regard to whether the illness or injury is acute, chronic, terminal or expected to extend over a long period of time. In addition, skilled care may, dependent upon the unique condition of the beneficiary, continue to be necessary for beneficiaries whose condition is stable.

EXAMPLE 1:   Following a cerebral vascular accident (CVA), a beneficiary has an in-dwelling foley catheter because of urinary incontinence, and is expected to require the catheter for a long and indefinite period. Periodic visits to change the catheter as needed, to treat the symptoms of catheter malfunction and to teach proper patient care would be covered as long as they are reasonable and necessary, although the beneficiary is stable and there is an expectataion that the care will be needed for a long and indefinite period.

EXAMPLE 2:   A beneficiary with advanced multiple sclerosis undergoing an exacerbation of the illness needs skilled teaching of medications, measures to overcome urinary retention, and the establishment of a program designed to minimize the adverse impact of the exacerbation. The skilled nursing care the benefi-ciary needs for a short period would be covered despite the chronic nature of the illness.

EXAMPLE 3:   A beneficiary with malignant melanoma is terminally ill, and requires skilled observation, assessment, teaching, and treatment. The beneficiary has not elected coverage under Medicare's hospice benefit. The skilled nursing care that the beneficiary requires would be covered, notwithstanding that his condition is terminal, because the services he needs require the skills of a licensed nurse.

    B.   Application of the Principles to Skilled Nursing Services.—The following discus-sion of skilled nursing services applies the foregoing principles to specific skilled nursing services about which questions are most frequently raised.

        1.   Observation and Assessment of Patient's Condition When Only the Specialized Skills of a Medical Professional Can Determine a Patient's Status.—Observation and assessment of the beneficiary's condition by a licensed nurse are reasonable and necessary skilled services when the likelihood of change in a patient's condition requires skilled nursing personnel to identify and evaluate the patient's need for possible modification of treatment or initiation of additional medical procedures until the beneficiary's treatment regimen is essentially stabilized. Where a beneficiary was admitted for home health care for skilled observation because there was a reasonable potential of a complication or further acute episode, but did not develop a further acute episode or complication, the skilled observation services are still covered for 3 weeks or as long as there remains a reasonable potential for such a complication or further acute episode.

404

205.1 (Cont.) COVERAGE OF SERVICES 04-89

Information from the beneficiary's medical history may support the likelihood of a future complication or acute episode and, therefore, may justify the need for continued skilled observation and assessment beyond 3-week period. Moreover, such indications as abnormal/fluctuating vital signs, weight changes, edema, symptoms of drug toxicity, abnormal/fluctuating lab values, and respiratory changes on auscultation may justify skilled observation and assessment. Where these indications are such that it is likely that skilled observation and assessment by a licensed nurse will result in changes to the treatment of the patient, then the services would be covered. There are cases where beneficiaries who are stable continue to require skilled observation and assessment (see example in §205.1. B. 13. d.). However, observation and assessment by a skilled nurse is not reasonable and necessary to the treatment of the illness or injury where these indications are part of a longstanding pattern of the beneficiary's condition, and there is no attempt to change the treatment to resolve them.

EXAMPLE 1: A beneficiary with arteriosclerotic heart disease with congestive heart failure requires close observation by skilled nursing personnel for signs of decompensation, or adverse effects resulting from prescribed medication. Skilled observation is needed to determine whether the drug regimen should be modified or whether other therapeutic measures should be considered until the patient's treatment regimen is essentially stabilized.

EXAMPLE 2: A beneficiary has undergone peripheral vascular disease treatment including a revascularization procedure (bypass). The incision area is showing signs of potential infection (e.g., heat, redness, swelling, drainage); patient has elevated body temperature. Skilled observation and monitoring of the vascular supply of the legs and the incision site is required until the signs of potential infection have abated and there is no longer a reasonable potential of infection.

EXAMPLE 3: A patient was hospitalized following a heart attack and, following treatment but before mobilization, is discharged home. Because it is not known whether exertion will exacerbate the heart disease, skilled observation is reasonable and necessary as mobilization is initiated until the patient's treatment regimen is essentially stabilized.

EXAMPLE 4: A frail 85 year old man was hospitalized for pneumonia. The infection was resolved, but the patient, who had previously maintained adequate nutrition, will not eat or eats poorly. The patient is discharged to the home health agency for monitoring of fluid and nutrient intake, and assessment of the need for tube feeding. Observation and monitoring by skilled nurses of the patient's oral intake, output and hydration status is required to determine what further treatment or other intervention is needed.

405

EXAMPLE 5:   A patient with glaucoma and a cardiac condition has a cataract extraction. Because of the interaction between the eye drops for the glaucoma and cataracts and the beta blocker for the cardiac condition, the patient is at risk for serious cardiac arrhythmias. Skilled observation and monitoring of the drug actions is reasonable and necessary until the patient's condition is stabilized.

EXAMPLE 6:   A patient with hypertension suffered dizziness and weakness. The physician found that the blood pressure was too low and discontinued the hypertension medication. Skilled observation and monitoring of the patient's blood pressure is required until the blood pressure remains stable and in a safe range.

    2.   Management and Evaluation of a Patient Care Plan.—Skilled nursing visits for management and evaluation of the patient's care plan are also reasonable and necessary where underlying conditions or complications require that only a registered nurse can ensure that essential nonskilled care is achieving its purpose. For skilled nursing care to be reasonable and necessary for management and evaluation of the beneficiary's plan of care, the complexity of the necessary unskilled services which are a necessary part of the medical treatment must require the involvement of skilled nursing personnel to promote the patient's recovery and medical safety in view of the beneficiary's overall condition.

EXAMPLE 1:   An aged beneficiary with a history of diabetes mellitus and angina pectoris is recovering from an open reduction of the neck of the femur. He requires among other services, careful skin care, appropriate oral medications, a diabetic diet, a therapeutic exercise program to preserve muscle tone and body condition, and observation to notice signs of deterioration in his condition or complications resulting from his restricted, but increasing mobility. Although any of the required services could be performed by a properly instructed person, that person would not have the capability to understand the relationship among the services and their effect on each other. Since the nature of the patient's condition, his age and his immobility create a high potential for serious complications, such an understanding is essential to ensure the patient's recovery and safety. The management of this plan of care requires skilled nursing personnel until the patient's treatment regimen is essentially stabilized.

EXAMPLE 2:   An aged patient is recovering from pneumonia, is lethargic, is disoriented, has residual chest congestion, is confined to the bed as a result of this debilitated condition and requires restraints at times. To decrease the chest congestion, the physician has prescribed frequent changes in position, coughing, and deep breathing. While the residual chest congestion alone would not represent a high risk factor, the patient's immobility and confusion represent complicating factors which, when coupled with the chest congestion, could create a high probability of a relapse. In this situation, skilled oversight of the nonskilled services would be reasonable and necessary pending the elimination of the chest congestion to ensure the patient's medical safety.

406

Where visits by a licensed nurse are not needed to observe and assess the effects of the nonskilled services being provided to treat the illness or injury, skilled nursing care would not be considered reasonable and necessary to treat the illness or injury.

EXAMPLE: A physician orders one skilled nursing visit every 2 weeks and three home health aide visits each week for bathing and washing hair for a beneficiary whose recovery from a cerebral vascular accident has left him with residual weakness on the left side. The beneficiary's cardiovascular condition is stable, and the beneficiary has reached the maximum restoration potential. There are no underlying conditions which would necessitate the skilled supervision of a licensed nurse in assisting with bathing or hair washing. The skilled nursing visits are not necessary to manage and supervise the home health aide services and would not be covered.

      3.   <u>Teaching and Training Activities</u>.—Teaching and training activities which require skilled nursing personnel to teach a beneficiary, the beneficiary's family or caregivers how to manage his treatment regimen would constitute skilled nursing services. Where the teaching or training is reasonable and necessary to the treatment of the illness or injury, skilled nursing visits for teaching would be covered. The test of whether a nursing service is skilled relates to the skill required to teach and not to the nature of what is being taught. Therefore, where skilled nursing services are necessary to teach an unskilled service, the teaching may be covered. Skilled nursing visits for teaching and training activities are reasonable and necessary where the teaching or training is appropriate to the beneficiary's functional loss, or his illness or injury.

Where it becomes apparent after a reasonable period of time that the patient, family or caregiver will not or is not able to learn or be trained, then further teaching and training would cease to be reasonable and necessary. The reason that the patient, family or caregiver will not or is not able to learn or be trained should be documented in the record. Notwithstanding that the teaching or training was unsuccessful, the services for teaching and training would be considered to be reasonable and necessary prior to the point that it became apparent that the teaching or training was unsuccessful, as long as such services were appropriate to the beneficiary's illness, functional loss or injury.

EXAMPLE 1:   A physician has ordered skilled nursing care for teaching a diabetic who has recently become insulin dependent. The physician has ordered teaching of self injection and management of insulin, signs and symptoms of insulin shock and actions to take in emergencies. The teaching services are reasonable and necessary to the treatment of the illness or injury.

EXAMPLE 2:   A physician has ordered skilled nursing care to teach a beneficiary to follow a new medication regimen (in which there is a significant probability of adverse drug reactions due to the nature of the drug and the beneficiary's condition), signs and symptoms of adverse reactions to new medications and necessary dietary restrictions. After it becomes apparent that the beneficiary remains unable to take the medications properly, cannot demonstrate awareness of potential adverse reactions, and is not following the necessary dietary restrictions, skilled nursing care for <u>further</u> teaching would not be reasonable and necessary, since the beneficiary has demonstrated an inability to be taught.

EXAMPLE 3: A physician has ordered skilled nursing visits to teach self-administration of insulin to a beneficiary who has been self injecting insulin for 10 years and there is no change in the beneficiary's physical or mental status that would require reteaching. The skilled nursing visits would not be considered reasonable and necessary since the beneficiary has a longstanding history of being able to perform the service.

EXAMPLE 4: A physician has ordered skilled nursing visits to teach self-administration of insulin to a beneficiary who has been self injecting insulin for 10 years because the beneficiary has recently lost the use of the dominant hand and must be retrained to use the other hand. Skilled nursing visits to reteach self-administration of the insulin would be reasonable and necessary.

In determining the reasonable and necessary number of teaching and training visits, consideration must be given to whether the teaching and training provided constitutes a reinforcement of teaching provided previously in an institutional setting or in the home or whether it represents the initial instruction. Where the teaching represents initial instruction, the complexity of the activity to be taught and the unique abilities of the beneficiary are to be considered. Where the teaching constitutes a reinforcement, an analysis of the patient's retained knowledge and anticipated learning progress is necessary to determine the appropriate number of visits. Skills taught in a controlled institutional setting often need to be reinforced when the beneficiary returns to his or her home and does not have the advantage of the controlled environment. Where the patient needs reinforcement of the institutional teaching, additional teaching visits in the home are covered.

EXAMPLE 5: A patient recovering from pneumonia is being sent home requiring IV infusion of antibiotics 4 times per day. The patient's spouse has been shown how to administer the drug during the last few days of hospitalization and has been told the signs and symptoms of infection. The physician has also ordered home health services for a skilled nurse to teach the administration of the drug and the signs and symptoms requiring immediate medical attention. Teaching by the skilled nurse in the home would be reasonable and necessary to continue that begun in the hospital, since the home environment, and the nature of the supplies used in the home, differ from that in the hospital.

Reteaching or retraining for an appropriate period may be considered reasonable and necessary where there is a change in the procedure or the beneficiary's condition that requires reteaching, or where the patient, family or caregiver is not properly carrying out the task. The medical record should document the reason that the reteaching or retraining is required.

408

EXAMPLE 6:   A well established diabetic who loses the use of his or her dominant hand would need to be retrained in self-administration of insulin.

EXAMPLE 7:   A spouse who has been taught to perform a dressing change for a post surgical beneficiary may need to be retaught wound care if the spouse demonstrates improper performance of wound care.

NOTE: There is no requirement that the beneficiary, family or other caregiver be taught to provide a service if they cannot or choose not to provide the care.

Teaching and training activities which require the skills of a licensed nurse include, but <u>are not limited to</u> the following:

  ○   Teaching the self-administration of injectable medications, or a complex range of medications;

  ○   Teaching a newly diagnosed diabetic or caregiver all aspects of diabetes management, including how to prepare and to administer insulin injections, to prepare and follow a diabetic diet, to observe foot-care precautions, and to observe for and understand signs of hyperglycemia and hypoglycemia;

  ○   Teaching self-administration of medical gases;

  ○   Teaching wound care where the complexity of the wound, the overall condition of the beneficiary or the ability of the caregiver makes teaching necessary;

  ○   Teaching care for a recent ostomy or where reinforcement of ostomy care is needed;

  ○   Teaching self-catheterization;

  ○   Teaching self-administration of gastrostomy or enteral feedings;

  ○   Teaching care for and maintenance of peripheral and central venous lines and administration of intravenous medications through such lines;

  ○   Teaching bowel or bladder training when bowel or bladder dysfunction exists;

  ○   Teaching how to perform the activities of daily living when the beneficiary or caregiver must use special techniques and adaptive devices due to a loss of function;

  ○   Teaching transfer techniques, e.g., from bed to chair, which are needed for safe transfer;

  ○   Teaching proper body alignment and positioning, and timing techniques of a bed-bound beneficiary;

    ◦   Teaching ambulation with prescribed assistive devices (such as crutches, walker, cane, etc.) that are needed due to a recent functional loss;

    ◦   Teaching prosthesis care and gait training;

    ◦   Teaching the use and care of braces, splints and orthotics and associated skin care;

    ◦   Teaching the proper care and application of any specialized dressings or skin treatments (for example, dressings or treatments needed by beneficiaries with severe or widespread fungal infections, active and severe psoriasis or eczema, or due to skin deterioration from radiation treatments);

    ◦   Teaching the preparation and maintenance of a therapeutic diet; and

    ◦   Teaching proper administration of oral medication, including signs of side-effects and avoidance of interaction with other medications and food.

    4. <u>Administration of Medications</u>.—Although drugs and biologicals are specifically excluded from coverage by the statute (§1816(m)(5) of the Social Security Act), the services of a licensed nurse which are required to administer the medications safely and effectively may be covered if they are reasonable and necessary to the treatment of the illness or injury.

    a. Intravenous, intramuscular, or subcutaneous injections and infusions, and hypodermoclysis or intravenous feedings require the skills of a licensed nurse to be performed (or taught) safely and effectively. Where these services are reasonable and necessary to treat the illness or injury, they may be covered. For these services to be reasonable and necessary, the medication being administered must be accepted as safe and effective treatment of the beneficiary's illness or injury, and there must be a medical reason that the medication cannot be taken orally. Moreover, the frequency and duration of the administration of the medication must be within accepted standards of medical practice, or there must be a valid explanation regarding the extenuating circumstances which justify the need for the additional injections.

    (1) Vitamin B 12 injections are considered specific therapy only for the following conditions:

    - Specified anemias: pernicious anemia, megaloblastic anemias, macrocytic anemias, fish tapeworm anemia

    - Specified gastrointestinal disorders: gastrectomy, malabsorption syndromes such as sprue and idiopathic steatorrhea, surgical and mechanical disorders such as resection of the small intestine, strictures, anastomosis and blind loop syndrome,

    - Certain neuropathies: posterolateral sclerosis, other neuropathies associated with pernicious anemia, during the acute phase or acute exacerbation of a neuropathy due to malnutrition and alcoholism.

410

For an individual with pernicious anemia caused by a B-12 deficiency, intramuscular or subcutaneous injection of vitamin B 12 at a dose of from 100 to 1000 micrograms no more frequently than once monthly is the accepted reasonable and necessary dosage schedule for maintenance treatment. More frequent injections would be appropriate in the initial or acute phase of the disease until it has been determined through laboratory tests that the patient can be sustained on a maintenance dose.

        (2)   <u>Insulin Injections</u>.—Insulin is customarily self-injected by patients or is injected by their families. However, where a beneficiary is either physically or mentally unable to self-inject insulin and there is no other person who is able and willing to inject the beneficiary, the injections would be considered a reasonable and necessary skilled nursing service.

EXAMPLE: A beneficiary who requires an injection of insulin once per day for treatment of diabetes mellitus, also has multiple sclerosis with loss of muscle control in the arms and hands, occasional tremors, and vision loss which cause her not to be able to fill syringes or to self inject the insulin she needs. If there is no able and willing caregiver to inject her insulin, skilled nursing care would be reasonable and necessary for the injection of the insulin.

The prefilling of syringes with insulin (or other medication which is self-injected) does not require the skills of a licensed nurse, and therefore is not considered to be a skilled nursing service. If the beneficiary needs someone only to prefill syringes (and therefore needs no skilled nursing care on an intermittent basis, or physical therapy or speech therapy), the beneficiary, therefore, does not qualify for any Medicare coverage of home health care. Prefilling of syringes for self administration of insulin or other medications is considered to be assistance with medications which are ordinarily self-administered and is an appropriate home health aide service. (See §206.1.) However, where State law requires that a licensed nurse prefill syringes, a skilled nursing visit to prefill syringes is paid as a skilled nursing visit (if the beneficiary otherwise needs skilled nursing care or physical therapy or speech therapy), but is not considered to be a skilled nursing service.

        b.   <u>Oral Medications</u>.—The administration of oral medications by a licensed nurse is not a reasonable and necessary skilled nursing care except in the specific situation in which the complexity of the beneficiary's condition, the nature of the drugs prescribed and the number of drugs prescribed require the skills of a licensed nurse to detect and evaluate side effects or reactions. The medical record must document the specific circumstances that cause administration of an oral medication to require skilled observation and assessment.

        c.   <u>Eye Drops and Topical Ointments</u>.—The administration of eye drops and topical ointments does not require the skills of a licensed nurse. Therefore, even if the administration of eyedrops or ointments is necessary to the treatment of an illness or injury and the patient cannot self-administer them, and there is no one available to administer them, the visits cannot be covered as a skilled nursing service. This section does not eliminate coverage for skilled nursing visits for observation and assessment of the beneficiary's condition. (See §205.1.B.1.)

EXAMPLE 1:   A physician has ordered skilled nursing visits to administer eye drops and ointments for a beneficiary with glaucoma. The administration of eye drops and ointments does not require the skills of a licensed nurse. Therefore, the skilled nursing visits cannot be covered as skilled nursing care, notwithstanding the importance of the administration of the drops as ordered.

EXAMPLE 2:   A physician has ordered skilled nursing visits for a patient with a reddened area under the breast. The physician instructs the beneficiary to wash, rinse, and dry the area daily and apply A and D ointment. Skilled nursing care is not needed to provide this treatment safely and effectively.

5. <u>Tube Feedings</u>.—Nasogastric tube, and percutaneous tube feedings (including gastrostomy and jejunostomy tubes), and replacement, adjustment, stabilization and suctioning of the tubes are skilled nursing services, and if the feedings are required to treat the beneficiary's illness or injury, the feedings and replacement or adjustment of the tubes would be covered as skilled nursing services.

6. <u>Nasopharyngeal and Tracheostomy Aspiration</u>.—Nasopharyngeal and tracheostomy aspiration are skilled nursing services and, if required to treat the beneficiary's illness or injury, would be covered as skilled nursing services.

7. <u>Catheters</u>.—Insertion and sterile irrigation and replacement of catheters, care of a suprapubic catheter, and in selected patients, urethral catheters, are considered to be skilled nursing services. Where the catheter is necessitated by a permanent or temporary loss of bladder control, skilled nursing services which are provided at a frequency appropriate to the type of catheter in use would be considered reasonable and necessary. Absent complications, Foley catheters generally require skilled care once approximately every 30 days and silicone catheters generally require skilled care once every 60-90 days and this frequency of service would be considered reasonable and necessary. However, where there are complications which require more frequent skilled care related to the catheter, such care would, with adequate documentation, be covered.

EXAMPLE: A beneficiary who has a Foley catheter due to loss of bladder control because of multiple sclerosis has a history of frequent plugging of the catheter and urinary tract infections. The physician has ordered skilled nursing visits once per month to change the catheter, and has left a "PRN" order for up to 3 additional visits per month for skilled observation and evaluation and/or catheter changes if the beneficiary or her family reports signs and symptoms of a urinary tract infection or a plugged catheter. During the certification period, the beneficiary's family contacts the HHA because the beneficiary has an elevated temperature, abdominal pain, and scant urine output. The skilled nurse visits the beneficiary and determines that the catheter is plugged and that there are symptoms of a urinary tract infection. The skilled nurse changes the catheter, and contacts the physician to advise him of her findings and to discuss treatment. The skilled nursing visit to change the catheter and to evaluate the beneficiary would be reasonable and necessary to the treatment of the illness or injury.

412

205.1 (Cont.)   COVERAGE OF SERVICES   04-89

    8.   <u>Wound Care</u>.—Care of wounds, (including, but not limited to ulcers, burns, pressure sores open surgical sites, fistulas, tube sites and tumor erosion sites) when the skills of a licensed nurse are needed to provide safely and effectively the services necessary to treat the illness or injury is considered to be a skilled nursing service. For skilled nursing care to be reasonable and necessary to treat a wound, the size, depth, nature of drainage (color, odor, consistency and quantity), condition and appearance of surrounding skin of wound must be documented in the clinical findings so that an assessment of the need for skilled nursing care can be made. Coverage or denial of skilled nursing visits for wound care may not be based solely on the stage classification of the wound, but rather must be based on all of the documented clinical findings. Moreover, the plan of care must contain the specific instructions for the treatment of the wound. Where the physician has ordered appropriate active treatment (e.g. sterile or complex dressings, administration of prescription medications, etc.) of wounds with the following characteristics, the skills of a licensed nurse are usually reasonable and necessary:

    a.   Open wounds which are draining purulent or colored exudate or which have a foul odor present and/or for which the beneficiary is receiving antibiotic therapy;

    b.   Wounds with a drain or T-tube with requires shortening or movement of such drains;

    c.   Wounds which require irrigation or instillation of a sterile cleansing or medicated solution into several layers of tissue and skin and/or packing with sterile gauze;

    d.   Recently debrided ulcers;

    e.   Pressure sores (decubitus ulcers) which present the following characteristics:

      ◦   There is partial tissue loss with signs of infection such as foul odor or purulent drainage, or

      ◦   There is full thickness tissue loss that involves exposure of fat or invasion of other tissue such as muscle or bone;

NOTE: Wounds or ulcers that show redness, edema and induration, at times with epidermal blistering or desquamation do not ordinarily require skilled nursing care.

    f.   Wounds with exposed internal vessels or a mass which may have a proclivity for hemorrhage when a dressing is changed (e.g., post radical neck surgery, cancer of the vulva);

    g.   Open wounds or widespread skin complications following radiation therapy, or which result from immune deficiencies or vascular insufficiencies;

    h.   Post-operative wounds where there are complications such as infection or allergic reaction or where there is an underlying disease which has a reasonable potential to adversely affect healing (e.g., diabetes);

i. Third degree burns, and second degree burns where the size of the burn or presence of complications causes skilled nursing care to be needed;

j. Skin conditions which require application of nitrogen mustard or other chemotherapeutic medication which present a significant risk to the beneficiary; or

k. Other open or complex wounds which require treatment that can only be safely and effectively provided by a licensed nurse.

EXAMPLE 1: A beneficiary has a second-degree burn with full thickness skin damage on his back. The wound is cleansed, followed by an application of Sulfamylon. While the wound requires skilled monitoring for signs and symptoms of infection or complications, the dressing change requires skilled nursing services.

EXAMPLE 2: A beneficiary experiences a decubitus ulcer where the full thickness tissue loss extends through the dermis to involve subcutaneous tissue. The wound involves necrotic tissue with a physician's order to apply a covering of a debriding ointment following vigorous irrigation. The wound is then packed loosely with wet to dry dressings or continuous moist dressing and covered with dry sterile gauze. Skilled nursing care is necessary for a proper treatment and understanding of cellular adherence and/or exudate or tissue healing or necrosis.

NOTE: This section relates to the direct, hands on skilled nursing care provided to beneficiaries with wounds, including any necessary dressing changes on those wounds. While a wound might not require this skilled nursing care, the wound may still require skilled monitoring for signs and symptoms of infection or complication (see §205.1.B.1) or skilled teaching of wound care to the beneficiary or the beneficiary's family (see §205.1.B.3)

9. Ostomy Care.—Ostomy care during the post-operative period and in the presence of associated complications where the need for skilled nursing care is clearly documented is a skilled nursing service. Teaching ostomy care remains skilled nursing care regardless of the presence of complications.

10. Heat Treatments.—Heat treatments which have been specifically ordered by a physician as part of active treatment of an illness or injury and which require observation by a licensed nurse to adequately evaluate the patient's progress would be considered as skilled nursing services.

11. Medical Gasses.—Initial phases of a regimen involving the administration of medical gasses which are necessary to the treatment of the beneficiary's illness or injury, would require skilled nursing care for skilled observation and evaluation of the beneficiary's reaction to the gasses, and to teach the patient and family when and how to properly manage the administration of the gasses.

414

205.1 (Cont.)   COVERAGE OF SERVICES   04-89

12. _Rehabilitation Nursing_.—Rehabilitation nursing procedures, including the related teaching and adaptive aspects of nursing that are part of active treatment (e.g., the institution and supervision of bowel and bladder training programs) would constitute skilled nursing services.

13. _Venipuncture_.—Venipuncture when the collection of the specimen is necessary to the diagnosis and treatment of the beneficiary's illness or injury and when the venipuncture cannot be performed in the course of regularly scheduled absences from the home to acquire medical treatment is a skilled nursing service. The frequency of visits for venipuncture must be reasonable within accepted standards of medical practice for treatment of illness or injury.

For venipuncture to be reasonable and necessary:

-   The physician order for the venipuncture for a laboratory test should be associated with a specific symptom or diagnosis, or the documentation should clarify the need for the test when it is not diagnosis/illness specific. In addition, the treatment must be recognized (in the Physician's Desk Reference, or other authoritative source) as being reasonable and necessary to the treatment of the illness or injury for venipunctures for monitoring the treatment to be reasonable and necessary.

-   The frequency of testing should be consistent with accepted standards of medical practice for continued monitoring of a diagnosis, medical problem or treatment regimen. Even where the laboratory results are consistently stable, periodic venipuncture may be reasonable and necessary because of the nature of the treatment.

Examples of reasonable and necessary venipunctures for stabilized beneficiaries include, but are not limited to those described below. While these guidelines do not preclude a physician from ordering more frequent venipunctures for these laboratory tests, the HHA must present justifying documentation to support the reasonableness and necessity of more frequent testing.

a.   Captopril may cause side effects such as leukopenia and agranulocytosis and it is standard medical practice to monitor the white blood cell count and differential count on a routine basis (every 3 months) when the results are stable and the patient is asymptomatic.

b.   In monitoring phenytoin (e.g., Dilantin) administration, the difference between a therapeutic and a toxic level of phenytoin in the blood is very slight. It is therefore appropriate to monitor the level on a routine basis (every 3 months) when the results are stable and the beneficiary is asymptomatic.

c.   Venipuncture for fasting blood sugar (FBS):

-   An unstable insulin dependent or non-insulin dependent diabetic would require FBS more frequently than once per month if ordered by the physician.

-   Where there is a new diagnosis or where there has been a recent exacerbation, but the beneficiary is not unstable, monitoring once per month would be reasonable and necessary.

- A stable insulin or non-insulin dependent diabetic would require monitoring every 2-3 months.

    d. Venipuncture for prothrombin

- Where the documentation shows that the dosage is being adjusted, monitoring would be reasonable and necessary as ordered by the physician.

- Where the results are stable within the therapeutic ranges, monthly monitoring would be reasonable and necessary.

- Where the results are stable within nontherapeutic ranges, there must be documentation of other factors which would indicate why continued monitoring is reasonable and necessary.

EXAMPLE: A beneficiary with coronary artery disease (CAD) was hospitalized with atrial fibrillation and was subsequently discharged to the home health agency with orders for anticoagulation therapy. Monthly venipunctures as indicated are necessary to report prothrombin (protime) levels to the physician, notwithstanding that the beneficiary's prothrombin time tests indicate essential stability.

    14. Student Nurse Visits.—Visits made by a student nurse may be covered as skilled nursing care when a home health agency participates in training programs in which it utilizes student nurses enrolled in a school of nursing to perform skilled nursing services in a home setting. To be covered, the services must be reasonable and necessary skilled nursing care, and must be performed under the general supervision of a registered or licensed nurse. The supervising nurse need not accompany the student nurse on each visit.

    15. Psychiatric Evaluation and Therapy.—The evaluation and psychotherapy needed by a patient suffering from a diagnosed psychiatric disorder that necessitated active treatment in an institution requires the skills of a psychiatrically trained nurse and the costs of the psychiatric nurse's services may be covered as a skilled nursing care. Psychiatrically trained nurses are nurses who have special training and/or experience beyond the standard curriculum required for an R.N. The services of the psychiatric nurse are to be provided under a plan of care established and reviewed by a psychiatrist. A psychiatrist may also prescribe services of nonpsychiatric nursing such as intramuscular injections of behavior modifying medications.

Because the law precludes agencies that primarily provide care and treatment of mental diseases from participating as home health agencies, psychiatric nursing must be furnished by an agency that does not primarily provide care and treatment of mental diseases.

    C. Intermittent Skilled Nursing Care.—To meet the requirement for "intermittent" skilled nursing care, an individual must have a medically predictable recurring need for skilled nursing services. In most instances, this definition will be met if a patient requires a skilled nursing service at least once every 60 days.

416

Since the need for "intermittent" skilled nursing care makes the individual eligible for other covered home health services, the intermediary should evaluate each claim involving skilled nursing services furnished less frequently than once every 60 days. In such cases, payment should be made only if documentation justifies a recurring need for reasonable, necessary, and medically predictable skilled nursing services. The following are examples of the need for infrequent, yet intermittent, skilled nursing services:

     1.   The patient with an indwelling <u>silicone</u> catheter who generally needs a catheter change only at 90-day intervals;

     2.   The person who experiences a fecal impaction due to the normal aging process (i.e., loss of bowel tone, restrictive mobility, and a breakdown in good health habits) and must be manually disimpacted. Although these impactions are likely to recur, it is not possible to pinpoint a specific timeframe; or

     3.   The blind diabetic who self-injects insulin may have a medically predictable recurring need for a skilled nursing visit at least every 90 days. These visits, for example, would be to observe and determine the need for changes in the level and type of care which have been prescribed, thus supplementing the physician's contacts with the patient. (See Coverage Issues Appendix, §HHA-1.)

Where the need for "intermittent" skilled nursing visits is medically predictable but a situation arises after the first visit making additional visits unnecessary, e.g., the patient is institutionalized or dies, the one visit would be reimbursable. However, a one-time order; e.g., to give gamma globulin following exposure to hepatitis, would not be considered a need for "intermittent" skilled nursing care since a recurrence of the problem which would require this service is not medically predictable.

Although most patients require services no more frequently than several times a week, Medicare will pay for part-time (as defined in §206.7) medically reasonable and necessary skilled nursing care 7 days a week for a <u>short</u> period of time (2-3 weeks). There may also be a few cases involving unusual circumstances where the patient's prognosis indicates the medical need for daily skilled services will extend beyond 3 weeks. As soon as the patient's physician makes this judgment, which usually should be made before the end of the 3-week period, the home health agency must forward medical documentation justifying the need for such additional services and include an estimate of how much longer daily skilled services will be required.

A person expected to need more or less <u>full-time skilled nursing care over an extended period of time</u>; i.e., a patient who requires institutionalization, would usually not qualify for home health benefits.

205.2   Skilled Therapy Services.—

A. General Principles Governing Reasonable and Necessary Physical Therapy, Speech Therapy, and Occupational Therapy.—

1.   The service of a physical, speech or occupational therapist is a skilled therapy service if the inherent complexity of the service is such that it can be performed safely and/or effectively only by or under the general supervision of a skilled therapist. To be covered, the skilled services must also be reasonable and necessary to the treatment of the beneficiary's illness or injury or to the restoration of maintenance of function affected by the beneficiary's illness or injury. It is necessary to determine whether individual therapy services are skilled and whether, in view of the beneficiary's overall condition, skilled management of the services provided is needed although many or all of the specific services needed to treat the illness or injury do not require the skills of a therapist.

2.   The development, implementation management and evaluation of a patient care plan based on the physician's orders constitute skilled therapy services when, because of the beneficiary's condition, those activities require the involvement of a skilled therapist to meet the beneficiary's needs, promote recovery and ensure medical safety. Where the skills of a therapist are needed to manage and periodically reevaluate the appropriateness of a maintenance program because of an identified danger to the patient, such services would be covered, even if the skills of a therapist are not needed to carry out the activities performed as part of the maintenance program.

3.   While a beneficiary's particular medical condition is a valid factor in deciding if skilled therapy services are needed, a beneficiary's diagnosis or prognosis should never be the sole factor in deciding that a service is or is not skilled. The key issue is whether the skills of a therapist are needed to treat the illness or injury, or whether the services can be carried out by nonskilled personnel.

4.   A service that is ordinarily considered nonskilled could be considered a skilled therapy service in cases in which there is clear documentation that, because of special medical complications, skilled rehabilitation personnel are required to perform or supervise the service or to observe the beneficiary. However, the importance of a particular service to a beneficiary or the frequency with which it must be performed does not, by itself, make a nonskilled service into a skilled service.

5.   The skilled therapy services must be reasonable and necessary to the treatment of the beneficiary's illness or injury within the context of the beneficiary's unique medical condition. To be considered reasonable and necessary for the treatment of the illness or injury:

a.   The services must be consistent with the nature and severity of the illness or injury, the beneficiary's particular medical needs, including the requirement that the amount, frequency and duration of the services must be reasonable, and

b.   The services must be considered, under accepted standards of medical practice, to be specific and effective treatment for the patient's condition, and

418

c.   The services must be provided with the expectation, based on the assessment made by the physician of the beneficiary's rehabilitation potential, that:

+   The condition of the beneficiary will improve materially in a reasonable and generally predictable period of time, or

+   The services are necessary to the establishment of a safe and effective maintenance program.

Services involving activities for the general welfare of any beneficiary, e.g., general exercises to promote overall fitness or flexibility and activities to provide diversion or general motivation, do not constitute skilled therapy. Those services can be performed by nonskilled individuals without the supervision of a therapist.

d.   Services of skilled therapists which are for the purpose of teaching the patient or the patient's family or caregivers necessary techniques, exercises or precautions are covered to the extent that they are reasonable and necessary to treat illness or injury. However, visits made by skilled therapists to a beneficiary's home solely to trian other home health agency staff (e.g., home health aides) are not billable as visits since the home health agency is responsible for ensuring that its staff is properly trained to perform any service it furnishes. The cost of a skilled therapist's visit for the purpose of training home health agency staff is an administrative cost to the home health agency.

EXAMPLE: A beneficiary with a diagnosis of multiple sclerosis has recently been discharged from the hospital following an exacerbation of her condition which has left her wheelchair bound and, for the first time, without any expectation of achieving ambulation again. The physician has ordered physical therapy to select the proper wheelchair for her long term use, to teach safe use of the wheelchair and safe transfer techniques to the beneficiary and the family. Physical therapy would be reasonable and necessary to evaluate the beneficiary's overall needs, to make the selection of the proper wheelchair and to teach the beneficiary and/or family safe use of the wheelchair and proper transfer techniques.

B.   Application of the Principles to Physical Therapy Services.—The following discussion of skilled physical therapy services applies the principles in §205.2A to specific physical therapy services about which questions are most frequently raised.

1.   Assessment.—The skills of a physical therapist to assess a beneficiary's rehabilitation needs and potential or to develop and/or implement a physical therapy program are covered when they are reasonable and necessary because of the beneficiary's condition. Skilled rehabilitation services concurrent with the management of a patient's care plan include objective tests and measurements such as, but not limited to, range of motion, strength, balanced coordination endurance or functional ability.

2. <u>Therapeutic Exercises</u>.—Theapeutic exercises which must be performed by or under the supervision of the qualified physical therapist to ensure the safety of the beneficiary and the effectiveness of the treatment, due either to the type of exercise employed or to the condition of the beneficiary, constitute skilled physical therapy.

3. <u>Gait Training</u>.—Gait evaluation and training furnished a beneficiary whose ability to walk has been impaired by neurological, muscular or skeletal abnormality require the skills of a qualified physical therapist and constitute skilled physical therapy and are considered reasonable and necessary if they can be expected to improve materially the beneficiary's ability to walk.

Gait evaluation and training which is furnished to a beneficiary whose ability to walk has been impaired by a condition other than a neurological, muscular or skeletal abnormality would nevertheless be covered where physical therapy is reasonable and necessary to restore the lost function.

EXAMPLE 1:   A physician has ordered gait evaluation and training for a beneficiary whose gait has been materially impaired by scar tissue resulting from burns. Physical therapy services to evaluate the beneficiary's gait, to establish a gait training program and to provide the skilled services necessary to implement the program would be covered.

EXAMPLE 2:   A beneficiary who has had a total hip replacement is ambulatory but demonstrates weakness, and is unable to climb stairs safely. Physical therapy would be reasonable and necessary to teach the beneficiary to safely climb and descend stairs.

Repetitive exercises to improve gait, or to maintain strength and endurance and assistive walking are appropriately provided by nonskilled persons and ordinarily do not require the skills of a physical therapist. Where such services are performed by a physical therapist as part of the initial design and establishment of a safe and effective maintenance program, the services would, to the extent that they are reasonable and necessary, be covered.

EXAMPLE: A beneficiary who has received gait training has reached his maximum restoration potential, and the physical therapist is teaching the beneficiary and family how to safely perform the activities which are a part of the maintenance program being established. The visits by the physical therapist to demonstrate and teach the activities (which by themselves do not require the skills of a therapist) would be covered since they are needed to establish the program.

4. <u>Range of Motion</u>.—Only a qualified physical therapist may perform range of motion tests and therefore such tests are skilled physical therapy.

420

Range of motion exercises constitute skilled physical therapy only if they are part of an active treatment for a specific disease state, illness, or injury, which has resulted in a loss or restriction of mobility (as evidenced by physical therapy notes showing the degree of motion lost and the degree to be restored). Range of motion exercises which are not related to the restoration of a specific loss of function often may be provided safely and effectively by nonskilled individuals. Passive exercises to maintain range of motion in paralyzed extremities that can be carried out by nonskilled persons do not constitute skilled physical therapy.

However, as indicated in section 205.2A4, where there is clear documentation that, because of special medical complications (e.g., susceptible to pathological bone fractures), the skills of a therapist are needed to provide services which ordinarily do not need the skills of a therapist, then the services would be covered.

      5.   <u>Maintenance Therapy</u>.—Where repetitive services which are required to maintain function involve the use of complex and sophisticated procedures, the judgement and skill of a physical therapist might be required for the safe and effective rendition of such services. If the judgement and skill of a physical therapist is required to safely and effectively treat the illness or injury, the services would be covered as physical therapy services.

EXAMPLE: Where there is an unhealed, unstable fracture which requires regular exercise to maintain function until the fracture heals, the skills of a physical therapist would be needed to ensure that the fractured extremity is maintained in proper position and alignment during maintenance range of motion exercises.

Establishment of a maintenance program is a skilled physical therapy service where the specialized knowledge and judgement of a qualified physical therapist is required for the program to be safely carried out and the treatment aims of the physician achieved.

EXAMPLE: A Parkinson's patient or a patient with rheumatoid arthritis who has not been under a restorative physical therapy program may require the services of a physical therapist to determine what type of exercises are required for the maintenance of his present level of function. The initial evaluation of the patient's needs, the designing of a maintenance program which is appropriate to the capacity and tolerance of the patient and the treatment objectives of the physician, the instruction of the beneficiary, family or caregivers to safely and effectively carry out the program and such reevaluations as may be required by the beneficiary's condition, would constitute skilled physical therapy.

While a patient is under a restorative physical therapy program, the physical therapist should regularly reevaluate his condition and adjust any exercise program the patient is expected to carry out himself or with the aid of supportive personnel to maintain the function being restored. Consequently, by the time it is determined that no further restoration is possible (i.e., by the end of the last restorative session) the physical therapist will already have designed the maintenance program required and instructed the beneficiary or caregivers in carrying out the program.

6. <u>Ultrasound, Shortwave, and Microwave Diathermy Treatments</u>.—These treatments must always be performed by or under the supervision of a qualified physical therapist and are skilled therapy.

7. <u>Hot Packs, Infra-Red Treatments, Paraffin Baths and Whirlpool Baths</u>.—Heat treatments and baths of this type ordinarily do not require the skills of a qualified physical therapist. However, the skills, knowledge and judgment of a qualified physical therapist might be required in the giving of such treatments or baths in a particular case, e.g., where the patient's condition is complicated by circulatory deficiency, areas of desensitization, open wounds, fractures or other complications.

C. <u>Application of the General Principles to Speech Language Pathology Services</u>.— Speech pathology services are those services necessary for the diagnosis and treatment of speech and language disorders which result in communication disabilities and for the diagnosis and treatment of swallowing disorders (dysphagia), regardless of the presence of a communication disability. The following discussion of skilled speech language pathology services applies the principles to specific speech language pathology services about which questions are most frequently raised.

1. The skills of a speech language pathologist are required for the assessment of a beneficiary's rehabilitation needs (including the causal factors and the severity of the speech and language disorders), and rehabilitation potential. Reevaluation would only be considered reasonable and necessary if the beneficiary exhibited a change in functional speech or motivation, clearing of confusion or the remission of some other medical condition that previously contraindicated speech language pathology services. Where a beneficiary is undergoing restorative speech language pathology services, routine reevaluations are considered to be a part of the therapy and could not be billed as a separate visit.

2. The services of a speech language pathologist would be covered if they are needed as a result of an illness, or injury and are directed towards specific speech/voice production.

3. Speech language pathology would be covered where the service can only be provided by a speech language pathologist and where it is reasonably expected that the service will materially improve the beneficiary's ability to independently carry out any one or combination of communicative activities of daily living in a manner that is measurably at a higher level of attainment than that prior to the initiation of the services.

4. The services of a speech language pathologist to establish a hierarchy of speech-voice-language communication tasks and cueing that directs a beneficiary toward speech-language communication goals in the plan of care would be covered speech language pathology.

422

205.2 (Cont.)   COVERAGE OF SERVICES   08-89

5. The services of a speech language pathologist to train the beneficiary, family or other caregivers to augment the speech-language communication, treatment or to establish an effective maintenance program would be covered speech therapy.

6. The services of a speech language pathologist to assist beneficiaries with aphasia in rehabilitation of speech and language skills is covered when needed by a beneficiary.

7. The services of a speech therapist to assist individuals with voice disorders to develop proper control of the vocal and respiratory systems for correct voice production are covered when needed by a beneficiary.

D. Application of the General Principles to Occupational Therapy.—The following discussion of skilled occupational therapy services applies the principles to specific occupational therapy services about which questions are most frequently raised.

1. Assessment.—The skills of an occupational therapist to assess and reassess a beneficiary's rehabilitation needs and potential or to develop and/or implement an occupational therapy program are covered when they are reasonable and necessary because of the beneficiary's condition.

2. Planning, Implementing and Supervision of Therapeutic Programs.—The planning, implementing and supervision of therapeutic programs including, but not limited to those listed below are skilled occupational therapy services, and if reasonable and necessary to the treatment of the beneficiary's illness or injury would be covered.

a. Selecting and teaching task oriented therapeutic activities designed to restore physical function.

EXAMPLE: Use of woodworking activities on an inclined table to restore shoulder, elbow and wrist range of motion lost as a result of burns.

b. Planning, implementing and supervising therapeutic tasks and activities designed to restore sensory-integrative function.

EXAMPLE: Providing motor and tactile activities to increase sensory output and improve response for a stroke patient with functional loss resulting in a distorted body image.

c. Planning, implementing and supervising of individualized therapeutic activity programs as part of an overall "active treatment" program for a patient with a diagnosed psychiatric illness.

EXAMPLE: Use of sewing activities which require following a pattern to reduce confusion and restore reality orientation in a schizophrenic patient.

d. Teaching compensatory techniques to improve the level of independence in the activities of daily living.

EXAMPLE: Teaching a beneficiary who has lost use of an arm how to pare potatoes and chop vegetables with one hand.

EXAMPLE: Teaching a stroke patient new techniques to enable him to perform feeding, dressing and other activities of daily living as independently as possible.

     e.   The designing, fabricating and fitting of orthotic and self-help devices.

EXAMPLE: Construction of a device which would enable an individual to hold a utensil and feed himself independently.

EXAMPLE: Construction of a hand splint for a patient with rheumatoid arthritis to maintain the hand in a functional position.

     f.   Vocational and prevocational assessment and training which is directed toward the restoration of function in the activities of daily living lost due to illness or injury would be covered. Where vocational or prevocational assessment and training is related solely to specific employment opportunities, work skills or work settings, such services would not be covered because they would not be directed toward the treatment of an illness or injury.

     3.   Illustration of Covered Services.—

EXAMPLE 1:   A physician orders occupational therapy for a patient who is recovering from a fractured hip and who needs to be taught compensatory and safety techniques with regard to lower extremity dressing, hygiene, toileting and bathing. The occupational therapist will establish goals for the beneficiary's rehabilitation (to be approved by the physician), and will undertake the teaching of the techniques necessary for the patient to reach the goals. Occupational therapy services would be covered at a duration and intensity appropriate to the severity of the impairment and the beneficiary's response to treatment.

EXAMPLE 2:   A physician has ordered occupational therapy for a beneficiary who is recovering from a CVA. The beneficiary has decreased range of motion, strength and sensation in both the upper and lower extremities on the right side. In addition, the beneficiary has perceptual and cognitive deficits resulting from the CVA. The beneficiary's condition has resulted in decreased function in activities of daily living (specifically bathing, dressing, grooming, hygiene and toileting). The loss of function requires assistive devices to enable the beneficiary to compensate for the loss of function and to maximize safety and independence. The beneficiary also needs equipment such as hlmi-slings to prevent shoulder subluxation and a hand splint to prevent joint contracture and deformity in the right hand.

The services of an occupational therapist would be necessary to assess the beneficiary's needs, develop goals (to be approved by the physician), to manufacture or adapt the needed equipment to the beneficiary's use, to teach compensatory techniques, to strengthen the beneficiary as necessary to permit use of compensatory techniques, to provide activities which are directed towards meeting the goals governing increased perceptual and cognitive function. Occupational therapy services would be covered at a duration and intensity appropriate to the severity of the impairment and the beneficiary's response to treatment.

206. COVERAGE OF OTHER HOME HEALTH SERVICES

206.1   Skilled Nursing Care, Physical Therapy, Speech Therapy, and Occupational Therapy.—Where the beneficiary meets the qualifying criteria in 204, Medicare covers skilled nursing services which meet the requirements of 205.1 A and B and 206.7, physical therapy which meets the requirements of 205.2 A and B, speech therapy which meets the requirements of 205.2 A and C, and occupational therapy which meets the requirements of 205.2 A and D.

206.2   Home Health Aide Services.—For home health aide services to be covered, the beneficiary must meet the qualifying criteria as specified in §204, the services which are provided by the home health aide must be part-time or intermittent as discussed in §206.7; the services must meet the definition of home health aide services of this section; and the services must be reasonable and necessary to the treatment of the beneficiary's illness or injury.

The reason for the visits by the home health aide must be to provide hands-on personal care of the beneficiary or services which are needed to maintain the beneficiary's health or to facilitate treatment of the beneficiary's illness or injury.

The physician's order should indicate the frequency of the home health aide services required by the beneficiary. These services may include but are not limited to:

    a.   Personal Care.—Personal care means:

        ◦   Bathing, dressing, grooming, caring for hair, nail and oral hygiene which are needed to facilitate treatment or to prevent deterioration of the beneficiary's health, changing the bed linens of an incontinent beneficiary, shaving, deodorant application, skin care with lotions and/or powder, foot care, and ear care.

        ◦   Feeding, assistance with elimination (including enemas unless the skills of a licensed nurse are required due to the patient's condition, routine catheter care and routine colostomy care), assistance with ambulation, changing position in bed, assistance with transfers.

EXAMPLE 1:   A physician has ordered home health aide visits to assist the beneficiary in personal care because the beneficiary is recovering from a stroke and continues to have significant right side weakness which causes him to be unable to bathe, dress or perform hair and oral care. The plan of care established by the home health agency nurse sets forth the specific tasks with which the beneficiary needs assistance. Home health aide visits at an appropriate frequency would be reasonable and necessary to assist in these tasks.

EXAMPLE 2:   A physician ordered four home health aide visits per week for personal care for a multiple sclerosis patient who is unable to perform these functions because of increasing debilitation. The home health aide gave the beneficiary a bath twice per week and washed hair on the other two visits each week. Only two visits are reasonable and necessary since the services could have been provided in the course of two visits.

EXAMPLE 3:   A physician ordered seven home health aide visits per week for personal care for a bed-bound, incontinent patient. All visits are reasonable and necessary because the patient has extensive personal care needs.

EXAMPLE 4:   A beneficiary with a well established colostomy forgets to change the bag regularly and has difficulty changing it. Home health aide services at an appropriate frequency to change the bag would be considered reasonable and necessary to the treatment of the illness or injury.

Other services which may be covered when provided by home health aides include, but are not limited to:

    b.   Simple dressing changes which do not require the skills of a licensed nurse.

EXAMPLE: A beneficiary who is confined to the bed has developed a small reddened area on the buttocks. The physician has ordered home health aide visits for more frequent repositioning, bathing and the application of a topical ointment and a gauze 4 × 4. Home health aide visits at an appropriate frequency would be reasonable and necessary.

    c.   Assistance with medications which are ordinarily self-administered and which do not require the skills of a licensed nurse to be provided safely and effectively.

NOTE: Prefilling of insulin syringes is ordinarily performed by the diabetic as part of the self-administration of the insulin and, unlike the injection of the insulin, does not require the skill of a licensed nurse to be performed properly. Therefore, if the prefilling of insulin syringes is performed by home health agency staff, it is considered to be a home health aide service. However, where State law precludes the provision of this service by other than a licensed nurse or

426

206.2 (Cont.)   COVERAGE OF SERVICES   04-89

physician, Medicare will make payment for this service, when covered, as though it were a skilled nursing service. Where the beneficiary needs only prefilling of insulin syringes and does not need skilled nursing care on an intermittent basis, or physical therapy or speech therapy or have a continuing need for occupational therapy, then Medicare cannot cover any home health services to the beneficiary (even if State law requires that the insulin syringes be filled by a licensed nurse).

    d.   Assistance with activities which are directly supportive of skilled therapy services but do not require the skills of a therapist to be safely and effectively performed such as routine maintenance exercises, and repetitive speech routines to support speech therapy.

    e.   Routine care of prosthetic and orthotic devices.

When a home health aide visits a patient to provide a health related service as discussed above, the home health aide may also perform some incidental services which do not meet the definition of a home health aide service (e.g., light cleaning, preparation of a meal, taking out the trash, shopping). However, the purpose of a home health aide visit may not be to provide these incidental services since they are not health related services, but rather are necessary household tasks that must be performed by anyone to maintain a home.

EXAMPLE 1:   A home health aide visits a recovering stroke patient whose right side weakness and poor endurance cause her to be able to leave the bed and chair only with extreme difficulty. The physician has ordered physical therapy and speech therapy for the beneficiary and has ordered home health aide services three or four times per week for personal care, assistance with ambulation as mobility increases, and assistance with repetitive speech exercises as her impaired speech improves. The home health aide also provides incidental household services such as preparation of meals, light cleaning and taking out the trash. The beneficiary lives with an elderly frail sister who is disabled and who cannot perform either the personal care or the incidental tasks. The home health aide visits at a frequency appropriate to the preformance of the health related services would be covered, notwithstanding the incidental provision of noncovered services (i.e., the household services) in the course of the visits.

EXAMPLE 2:   A physician orders home health aide visits 3 times per week. The only services provided are light housecleaning, meal preparation and trash removal. The home health aide visits cannot be covered, notwithstanding their importance to the beneficiary, because the services provided do not meet Medicare's definition of "home health aide services."

206.3   <u>Medical Social Services</u>.—Medical social services which are provided by a qualified medical social worker or a social work assistant under the supervision of a qualified medical social worker may be covered as home health services where the beneficiary meets the qualifying criteria specified in §204, and:

    ◦   The services of these professionals are necessary to resolve social or emotional problems which are or are expected to be an impediment to the effective treatment of the beneficiary's medical condition or his or her rate of recovery, and

    ◦   The plan of care indicates how the services which are required necessitate the skills of a qualified social worker or a social work assistant under the supervision of a qualified medical social worker to be performed safely and effectively.

Where both of these requirements for coverage are met, services of these professionals which may be covered include, but are not limited to:

    ◦   Assessment of the social and emotional factors related to the beneficiary's illness, need for care, response to treatment and adjustment to care,

    ◦   Assessment of the relationship of the beneficiary's medical and nursing requirements to the individual's home situation, financial resources and availability of community resources,

    ◦   Appropriate action to obtain available community resources to assist in resolving the beneficiary's problem. (Note: Medicare does not cover the services of a medical social worker to complete or assist in the completion of an application for Medicaid because Federal regulations require the State to provide assistance in completing the application to anyone who chooses to apply for Medicaid.), and

    ◦   Counseling services which are required by the beneficiary. Counseling of beneficiaries' families is covered only when such services are incidental to other covered medical social services being provided to the beneficiary, and when they are reasonable and necessary to treat the beneficiary's illness or injury. Visits by a medical social worker are not covered when the only reason for the visit is to counsel the beneficiary's family.

NOTE: Participating in the development of the plan of treatment, preparing clinical and progress notes, participating in discharge planning and inservice programs, and acting as a consultant to other agency personnel are appropriate administrative costs to the home health agency.

EXAMPLE 1:   The physician has ordered a medical social worker assessment of a diabetic beneficiary who has recently become insulin dependent and is not yet stabilized. The skilled nurse, who is providing skilled observation and evaluation to try to restabilize the beneficiary notices during her visits that the supplies left in the home for the bebneficiary's use appear to be frequently missing, and that the beneficiary is not compliant with the regimen although she refuses to discuss the matter. The assessment by a medical social worker would be reasonable and necessary to determine if there are underlying social or emotional problems which are impeding the beneficiary's treatment.

428

EXAMPLE 2:   A physician ordered an assessment by a medical social worker for a multiple sclerosis patient who was unable to move anything but her head and who had an indwelling catheter. The beneficiary had experienced recurring urinary tract infections and multiple infected ulcers. The physician ordered medical social services after the home health agency indicated to him that the home was not well cared for, and that the beneficiary appeared to be neglected much of the time and that the relationship between the beneficiary and family was very poor. The physician and home health agency were concerned that social problems created by family caregivers were impeding the treatment of the recurring infections and ulcers. The assessment and follow-up for counseling both the beneficiary and the family by a medical social worker were reasonable and necessary.

EXAMPLE 3:   A physician is aware that a beneficiary with arteriosclerosis and hypertension is not taking medications as ordered and is not adhering to dietary restrictions because he is unable to afford the medication and is unable to cook. The physician orders several visits by a medical social worker to assist in resolving these problems. The visits by the medical social worker to review the beneficiary's financial status, to discuss options and to make appropriate contacts with social services agencies or other community resources to arrange for medications and meals would be a reasonable and necessary medical social service.

EXAMPLE 4:   A physician has ordered counseling by a medical social worker for a beneficiary with cirrhosis of the liver who has recently been discharged from a 28-day inpatient alcohol treatment program to her home which she shares with an alcoholic and neglectful adult child. The physician has ordered counseling several times per week to assist the beneficiary in remaining free of alcohol and in dealing with the adult child. The services of the medical social worker would be covered until the beneficiary's social situation ceased to impact on her recovery and/or treatment.

EXAMPLE 5:   A physician has ordered medical social services for a beneficiary who is worried about her financial arrangements and payment for medical care. The services ordered are to arrange Medicaid if possible and resolve unpaid medical bills. There is no evidence that the beneficiary's concerns are adversely impacting recovery or treatment of her illness or injury. Medical social services cannot be covered.

EXAMPLE 6:   A physician has ordered medical social services for a beneficiary of extremely limited income who has incurred large unpaid hospital and other medical bills following a significant illness. The beneficiary's recovery is adversely affected because the beneficiary is not maintaining a proper therapeutic diet, and cannot leave the home to acquire the medication necessary to treat his/her illness. The medial social worker reviews the beneficiary's financial status, arranges meal service to resolve the dietary problem, arranges for home delivered medications, gathers the information necessary for application to Medicaid to acquire coverage for the medications the beneficiary needs, files the application on behalf of the beneficiary, and follows up repeatedly with the Medicaid State agency.

The medical social services which are necessary to review the financial status of the beneficiary, to arrange for meal service, to arrange for the medications to be delivered to the home, and to arrange for the Medicaid State agency to assist the beneficiary with the application for Medicaid are covered. The services related to the assistance in filing the application for Medicaid, and the followup on the application are not covered since they are provided by the State agency free of charge, and hence the beneficiary has no obligation to pay for such assistance.

206.4   Medical Supplies (Except for Drugs and Biologicals) and the Use of Durable Medical Equipment.—

A.   Medical Supplies.—Medical supplies are items which, due to their therapeutic or diagnostic characteristics, are essential in enabling HHA personnel to carry out effectively the care which the physician has ordered for the treatment or diagnosis of the patient's illness or injury. Certain items which, by their very nature, are designed only to serve a medical purpose are obviously considered medical supplies; e.g., catheters, needles, syringes, surgical dressings and materials used for dressings such as cotton gauze and adhesive bandages, and materials used for aseptic techniques. Other medical supplies include, but are not limited to, irrigating solutions, and intravenous fluids.

Consider other items which are often used by persons who are not ill or injured to be medical supplies only where (1) the item is recognized as having the capacity to serve a therapeutic or diagnostic purpose in a specific situation, and (2) the item is required as a part of the actual physician-prescribed treatment of a patient's existing illness or injury. For example, items which generally serve a routine hygienic purpose, e.g., soaps and shampoos, and items which generally serve as skin conditioners, e.g., baby lotion, baby oil, skin softeners, powders, lotions, are not considered medical supplies unless the particular item is recognized as serving a specific therapeutic purpose in the physician's prescribed treatment of the patient's existing skin (scalp) disease or injury.

Limited amounts of medical supplies may be left in the home between visits where repeated applications are required and rendered by the patient or by family members. Do not leave such supplies as needles, syringes, and catheters which require administration by a nurse in the home between visits.

430

C. _Drugs and Biologicals_.—Drugs and biologicals are excluded from coverage as items or services administered by Hoise under Medicare. In certain cases, they are covered under medical insurance when administered by a physician as a part of his/her professional service, and are not capable of being self-administered.

D. _Durable Medical Equipment_.—Durable medical equipment which meets the requirements of §220ff is covered under the home health benefit, with the beneficiary responsible for payment of a 20 percent coinsurance.

206.5 _Services of Interns and Residents_.—Home health services include the medical services of interns and residents-in-training under an approved hospital teaching program (if the agency has an affiliation with or is under common control of a hospital providing such medical services). Approved means approved by the Council on Medical Education of the American Medical Association, or in the case of an osteopathic hospital, the Committee on Hospitals of the Bureau of Professional Education of the American Osteopathic Association and, in the case of an intern or resident-in-training in the field of dentistry, the Council on Dental Education of the American Dental Association. Payment is provided under Part B for other services hospital interns and residents furnish to beneficiaries receiving home health services.

The services of interns and residents-in-training in the field of podiatry, under a teaching program approved by the Council on Podiatric Medical Education of the American Podiatric Medical Association, are covered under Part A on the same basis as the services of other interns and residents-in-training in approved teaching programs.

206.6 _Outpatient Services_.—Outpatient services include any of the items or services described above which are provided under arrangements on an outpatient basis at a hospital, SNF rehabilitation center, or outpatient department affiliated with a medical school, and (1) which require equipment not readily available at the patient's place of residence, or (2) which are furnished while the patient is at the facility to receive the services. The hospital, SNF, or outpatient department affiliated with a medical school must be qualified providers of services. However, there are special provisions for the use of the facilities of rehabilitation centers. (See §200.3.) The cost of transporting an individual to a facility cannot be paid.

206.7 _Part-time or Intermittent Home Health Aide and Skilled Nursing Services_.—Where a beneficiary qualifies for coverage of home health services, Medicare covers either part-time or intermittent home health aide services and skilled nursing services.

A. _Definition of Part-Time_.—Part-time means any number of days per week:

° Up to and including 28 hours per week of skilled nursing and home health aide services combined for less than 8 hours per day; or

    ° Up to 35 hours per week of skilled nursing and home health aide services combined for less than 8 hours per day subject to review by fiscal intermediaries on a case by case basis, based upon documentation justifying the need for and reasonableness of such additional care.

    B. Definition of "Intermittent".—"Intermittent" means:

    ° Up to and including 28 hours per week of skilled nursing and home health aide services combined provided on a less than daily basis;

    ° Up to 35 hours per week of skilled nursing and home health aide services combined which are provided on a less than daily basis, subject to review by fiscal intermediaries on a case by case basis, upon documentation justifying the need for and reasonableness of such additional care; or

    ° Up to and including full-time (i.e., 8 hours per day) skilled nursing and home health aide services combined which are provided and needed 7 days per week for temporary, but not indefinite, periods of time of up to 21 days with allowances for extensions in exceptional circumstances where the need for care in excess of 21 days is finite and predictable.

    C. Impact on Care Provided in Excess of "Intermittent" or "Part-Time" care.—Home health aide and/or skilled nursing care in excess of the amounts of care which meet these definitions of part time or intermittent may be provided to a home care beneficiary or purchased by other payers without bearing on whether the home health aide and skilled nursing care meets the Medicare definitions of part time or intermittent.

EXAMPLE: A beneficiary needs skilled nursing care monthly for a catheter change and the home health agency also renders needed daily home health aide services 24 hours per day which will be needed for a long and indefinite period of time. The HHA bills Medicare for the skilled nursing and home health aide services which were provided before the 35th hour of service each week and bills the beneficiary (or another payer) for the remainder of the care. If the intermediary determines that the 35 hours of care are reasonable and necessary, Medicare would therefore cover the 35 hours of skilled nursing and home health aide visits.

    D. Application of This Policy Revision.—A beneficiary must meet the longstanding and unchanged qualifying criteria for Medicare coverage of home health services, before this policy revision becomes applicable to skilled nursing services and/or home health aide services. The definition of "intermittent" with respect to the need for skilled nursing care where the beneficiary qualifies for coverage based on the need for "skilled nursing care on an intermittent basis" remains unchanged. Specifically:

    ° This policy revision always applies to home health aid services when the beneficiary qualifies for coverage;

432

206.7 (Cont.) COVERAGE OF SERVICES 04-89

° This policy revision applies to skilled nursing care only when the beneficiary needs physical therapy or speech therapy or continued occupational therapy, and also needs skilled nursing care; and

° If the beneficiary needs skilled nursing care but does not need physical therapy or speech therapy or occupational therapy, the beneficiary must still meet the longstanding and unchanged definition of "intermittent" skilled nursing care in order to qualify for coverage of any home health services.

(next page is 18.5)

GUIDELINES FOR FILING PAYMENT: COMPLETION OF THE PLAN OF CARE (485 SERIES FORMS)

medicare
Home Health Agency Manual

Department of Health
and Human Services

Health Care Financing
Administration

Transmittal No. 272   Date SEPTEMBER 1994

REVISED MATERIAL	REVISED PAGES	REPLACED PAGES
Table of Contents		
Chapter II	11-12.2 (4 pp.)	11-12.2 (4 pp.)
Secs. 234.5-234.13	24m3-24m4x (26 pp.)	24m3-24m4y (35 pp.)
Exhibits I-VI	24m4x.1-24m4x.9 (9 pp.)	24m4y.1-24m4z.3 (7 pp.)

REVISED PROCEDURES—EFFECTIVE DATE: 10/17/94

Section 234.6, Data Elements Needed to Render a Home Health Coverage Determination, is revised to reflect new guidelines for submitting the HCFA-485 and for completion of the HCFA-486. These forms are no longer submitted routinely with the initial claim or other subsequent claim. The completed HCFA-485, signed by the physician, is retained in your files and a copy submitted to your intermediary when requested by them. The HCFA-486 needs to be completed and submitted only upon request by the intermediary. All references to the HCFA-485 are amended to reflect the change in the title of the form to "Home Health Certification and Plan of Care."

Section 234.7, HCFA-485—Home Health Certification and Plan of Care, is revised to reflect the new guidelines for submitting the HCFA-485.

Item 2 is amended to read Start of Care Date rather than the acronym SOC Date.

The provider's telephone number is added to Item 7, Provider Name and Address, as a convenience for physicians.

The check boxes are removed from Item 26, Physician Certification, and the statement is reworded for clarity.

Item 28, Penalty Statement, is added to the form.

434

COVERAGE OF SERVICES

Section 234.8, HCFA-486 Medical Update and Patient Information, is amended to reflect the change in guidelines for use of the form. You need to complete the form only when it is specifically requested by the intermediary for MR.

Item 13, Specific Services and Treatments, is deleted since this information is no longer keyed by the intermediary and used for automatic screening of the plan of care.

Items 14 through 22 are renumbered 13 through 21.

Subsection B instructions for completion of the HCFA-486 for submission with an interim claim when a plan of care is modified are deleted. Completion and routine submission of an updated plan is no longer required.

Use your supply of the old forms through December 31, 1994.

Filing for Payment

436

233.   FILING A REQUEST FOR PAYMENT AND CLAIM FOR PAYMENT

Medicare payment of reasonable costs may not be made for provider services furnished under Part A or Part B, unless the beneficiary or his representative files a timely written request for payment and the provider files a timely claim. (See §§ 235-239.4 for an explanation of time limits.)

The home health agency should ask the patient to complete the request for payment at the time the covered services begin, if he is or may be a Medicare beneficiary, i.e., he is at least age 65 or there is other reason to believe he may be a beneficiary. If the beneficiary does not file his request upon start of care, he may file it later with the HHA. Once the patient or his representative has filed his request for payment with the HHA, the HHA must file a claim for payment (billing) with its intermediary. (See § 236 for HHA and beneficiary liability where a claim is not filed timely.)

An HHA has filed a claim for an item or service reimbursable on a cost basis if it submits to its intermediary a HCFA billing form that includes the item or service.

233.1   Establishing Date of Filing a Claim for Payment.—Whenever the last day for timely filing of a claim for payment falls on a Saturday, Sunday, legal holiday, or other day all or part of which is a non-workday for Federal employees because of Federal statute or executive order, the claim will be considered timely if it is filed on the next workday.

233.2   Use of Postmark to Establish Filing Date of a Claim for Payment.—Where a claim is submitted by mail, the claim can be considered filed on the day the envelope was postmarked in the United States.

234.   REQUEST FOR PAYMENT

234.1   Billing Form as Request for Payment.—Each of the billing forms (Provider Billing for Medical and Other Health Services, Form HCFA-1483; Home Health Agency Report and Billing, Form HCFA-1487; HCFA-1450 (UB82); and Request for Medicare Payment, Form HCFA-1490) contains a patient's signature line incorporating the patient's request for payment of benefits, authorization to release information, and assignment of benefits. When the billing form is used as the request for payment, it must be signed. (See § 234.2 for request on agency records.) The request for payment will then be forwarded to the intermediary (Part B carrier in the case of the HCFA-1490) or to HCFA where the provider deals directly with the Government.

When the home health agency billing form is used as the request for payment, a single signed request ordinarily suffices for each plan. However, a subsequent signed request for payment is required if the patient's care is transferred from one home health agency to another.

234.2   Request for Payment on Provider Record.—In place of signatures on the billing forms, a home health agency may use a procedure under which the signature of the patient (or his representative under §234.4) on its records will serve as the request for payment for services of the agency and for physician services for which the agency is authorized to bill under §427. In the case of physician services, claims may be submitted on either an assigned or unassigned basis.

To implement the procedure, the home health agency must incorporate language to the following effect in its records:

Statement to Permit Payment
of Medicare Benefits to Provider,
Physicians and Patient

NAME OF BENEFICIARY   HI CLAIM NUMBER

I request payment of authorized Medicare benefits to me or on my behalf for any services furnished me by or in (name of home health agency), including physician services. I authorize any holder of medical and other information about me to release to Medicare and its agents any information needed to determine these benefits or benefits for related services.

The request is effective until revoked. If a patient objects to part of the request for payment, the agency should annotate the statement accordingly and notify any physician affected.

The home health agency submitting claims under this procedure indicates on the claim form that it has obtained the patient's signature, by checking the block "Signature contained in the provider record," or, if the form does not contain such a block, by entering "Patient's request for payment in file" on the patient's signature line of the claim. A physician or medical group submitting claims under this procedure indicates that the agency has obtained the patient's signature, by entering on the patient signature line of the claim, "Patient's request for payment on file in (name of home health agency)."

In using this procedure, the home health agency, physician or medical group undertakes:

    1.   To complete and submit promptly the appropriate Medicare billing form whenever it furnishes services to a Medicare beneficiary—even in those cases in which assignment is not accepted for the physician services.

438

2. To incorporate, by stamp or otherwise, information to the following effect on any bills it sends to Medicare patients: "Do not use this bill for claiming Medicare benefits. A claim has been or will be submitted to Medicare on your behalf." This requirement is necessary to prevent patients from submitting duplicate claims.

The home health agency also undertakes to make the patient signature files available for carrier and intermediary inspection on request.

The intermediary and carrier must make periodic audits of signature files selected on a random basis. The carrier may arrange with the intermediary for the latter to perform this function on its behalf.

234.4   Signature on the Request for Payment by Someone Other Than the Patient.—If at all practical, the patient should sign the request whether on the billing form or on the provider's record at the time of start of care.

In certain circumstances, it is impractical for an individual to sign the request for payment himself because when he first receives home health services, he is incompetent, or otherwise in such condition that he cannot transact any business. In such a situation, his representative payee (i.e., a person designated by the Social Security Administration to receive monthly benefits on the patient's behalf), a relative, legal guardian, a representative of an institution (other than the agency) usually responsible for his care, or a representative of a governmental entity providing welfare assistance, if present at time of start of services, should be asked to sign on behalf of the individual.

A.   Provider Signs Request.—If, at the time of start of care, the patient cannot be asked to sign the request for payment and there is no person present exercising responsibility for him, an authorized official of the agency may sign the request. However, the agency should not routinely sign the request on behalf of any patient. If experience reveals an unusual frequency of such agency-filed requests from a particular agency, the matter will be subject to review by the intermediary.

If it is impractical to obtain the patient's signature because a home health agency does not make a visit to his home (e.g., the physician certifies that the patient needs a certain item of durable medical equipment but no visits are certified), the agency may furnish the equipment and need not obtain the patient's signature. An agency representative should sign on behalf of the patient and write in Item 12 of the HCFA-1483 "Patient not visited."

B.   Patient Dies Before Signing Request for Payment.—If the patient dies before the request for payment is signed, it may be signed by the legal representative of his estate, or by any of the persons or institutions (including an authorized official of the agency) who could have signed it had he been alive and incompetent.

C. Need for Explanation of Signer's Relationship to Patient.—When someone other than the patient signs the request for payment, the signer submits a brief statement explaining his/her relationship to the patient and the circumstances which made it impracticable for the patient to sign. Retain it in your files if the signature is obtained on your own record.

234.5   Refusal by Patient to Request Program Payment.—A patient may refuse to request Medicare payment and agree to pay for services with his/her own funds or from other insurance. Such patients may have a philosophical objection to Medicare or may feel that they will receive better care if they pay themselves or are paid under another insurance policy. The patient's impression that another insurer will pay for the services may or may not be correct, as some contracts expressly disclaim liability for services covered under Medicare. Where the patient refuses to request Medicare payment, obtain his/her signed refusal wherever possible. If the patient (or his/her representative) is unwilling to sign, record that the patient refused to file a request for payment but was unwilling to sign the statement of refusal.

In any event, there is no provision which requires a patient to have covered services he/she receives paid for under Medicare if he/she refuses to request payment. Therefore, you may bill an insured patient who positively and voluntarily declines to request Medicare payment. However, if such a person subsequently changes his/her mind (because he/she finds his/her other insurance will not pay or for another reason) and requests payment under the program within the prescribed time limit, bill the intermediary. Refund any amounts the patient paid in excess of the permissible charges.

Where a patient who had declined to request payment dies, his/her right to request payment may be exercised by the legal representative of his/her estate, by any of the persons or institutions mentioned in §234.4B, by a person or institution which paid part or all of the bill, or in the event a request could not otherwise be obtained, by an authorized official of your agency. This permits payment to you for services which would not otherwise be paid for and allows a refund to the estate or to a person or institution which paid the bill on behalf of the deceased.

See §236 for effect on beneficiary and provider of refusal to file.

234.6   Data Elements Needed to Render a Home Health Coverage Determination.— Standardized data collection forms promote more consistent coverage decisions and minimize payment for noncovered services.

   ∘   The HCFA-485, Home Health Certification and Plan of Care, contains the data necessary to meet regulatory and national survey requirements for the physician's plan of care and certification.

   ∘   The HCFA-486, Medical Update and Patient Information, contains data needed by intermediaries to make coverage determinations.

   ∘   The HCFA-487, Addendum to the Plan of Treatment/Medical Update and Patient information, may be used to provide additional documentation of any elements on the HCFA-485/486.

   ∘   The HCFA-488, Intermediary Medical Information Request, contains supplemental data which may be required on a case-by-case basis where the HCFA-485, 486, and/or 487 do not provide sufficient information.

440

Only the HCFA-485/486/487/488 may be required by intermediaries as medical information forms.

HCFA requires you to obtain a signed certification as soon as practicable after the start of care and prior to submitting a claim to the intermediary. You may provide services prior to obtaining the physician's written plan of care based on documented verbal orders. If care continues beyond the certification period, you must obtain a recertification from the physician. The signed HCFA-485 must be retained in your files and available upon request by the intermediary. The HCFA-486 is completed upon request of the intermediary when it is needed for MR. Complete the forms in their entirety. Do not leave any items blank. However, there are items where "not applicable" (N/A) is acceptable. These items are specified.

If you submit the HCFA 485/486 via electronic media, retain the hardcopy versions and submit them to the intermediary upon request. Specifications for electronic transmissions are in Addenda A and D. If you choose to use the abbreviated format for electronic submission, complete those items identified in the Addenda with an asterisk.

Where the information on the HCFA-485/486/487 is not sufficient to make a coverage decision, the HCFA-488 is used to request additional information and/or the medical record. It is also used to request medical information on interim claims which require development prior to payment because the HCFA-485/486 was not required. Routine submission of medical records will be requested only when absolutely necessary (e.g., you had been identified as a poor performer based on denial statistics or postpayment audits).

The intermediary may pay or deny visits/services based upon information provided on the forms. However, additional information must be requested (via the HCFA-488 or a copy of the medical record) when objective clinical evidence needed to support a decision is not clearly present. (See §203.1.) Claims will not be denied because a field necessary on the HCFA-485/486 has not been completed. If the missing information is needed to make a coverage determination, a HCFA-488 will request the necessary information. The claim will be denied if the missing information is not submitted within 30 days of the date of the request for documentation or if you indicate that the information is not available. Intermediaries follow the procedures below for the items noted.

    ◦   Missing or Incomplete Physician's Orders - (HCFA-485, Item 21; HCFA-486, Item 16; HCFA-487, Addendum).

    1.   Visits for a discipline are billed but there is no physician order or the physician's order is present but is not specific or there is no frequency.

    —   The physician's order for the services is requested. A documented verbal order or signed written order is accepted. (See below for acceptable verbal orders.) Orders signed after the service(s) is rendered are not acceptable unless there is evidence of a pre-existing verbal order. If you furnish services without a physician's order, the services are denied. Such findings may be reported to the State survey office.

Services documented on the HCFA-486, Item 13 will not be accepted in lieu of physician's orders in the appropriate fields on the HCFA-485/486/487.

441

234.6 (Cont.)   COVERAGE OF SERVICES   09-94

   2. Physician order for discipline and frequency is present but there is no duration of visits.

   —   The duration is requested if a discipline(s) is visiting at different frequencies during the certification period.

   —   Where you consistently omit duration, claims and the HCFA-485/486 may be returned for proper completion.

   °   You provide fewer visits than the physician orders.

   —   Visits will not be denied because you provide fewer visits. However, report the decrease to the physician. Where you consistently decrease visits without reporting to the physician, the State survey office may be notified.

   °   Documentation of Physician's Verbal Orders. Any of the following are acceptable:

   —   Receipt of verbal orders is identified by the nurse's signature and date in Item 23 of the HCFA-485 and the form is signed by the physician;

   —   The HCFA-485 is signed by the physician and contains the verbal order(s) which has been written, signed and dated by agency staff in the clinical record;

   —   The form on which the verbal order is written, signed or dated by agency staff is countersigned by the physician;

   —   A document signed by the physician contains the written signed and dated verbal order in the clinical record.

There is no required form or format for documentation or confirmation of verbal orders.

   °   Physician Certification/Recertification:

   —   The intermediary is requried to investigate whether the physician certifying the need for home health services has a financial interest or ownership in your agency.

   —   Submit a listing of physicians associated with your agency who have such an interest or relationship. For each physician, identify their UPIN. (See §475.)

   —   Once a year, the intermediary will ask you to verify and update the listing. Notify the intermediary of any changes in ownership in the interim.

   —   The intermediary automates the list and establishes edits to match the list against the UPIN. The intermediary denies claims that show a matching UPIN.

442

234.7   <u>HCFA-485 - Home Health Certification and Plan of Care.</u>—Meets the regulatory requirements (State and Federal) for both the physician's home health plan of care and home health certification and recertification requirements. HCFA requires you to obtain a signed certification as soon as practicable after the start of care and prior to submitting a claim to the intermediary. You may provide services prior to obtaining the physician's written plan of care based on documented verbal orders. If care continues beyond the certification period, you must obtain a recertification from the physician. The signed HCFA-485 must be retained in your files and a copy of the signed form made available upon request by the intermediary.

Complete the following:

     1.   <u>Patient's HICN.</u>—Enter the HICN (numeric plus alpha indicator(s)) as shown on the patient's health insurance card, certificate award, utilization notice, temporary eligibility notice, or as reported by the SSO.

     2.   <u>Start of Care Date.</u>—Enter the 6 digit month, day, year on which covered home health services began, i.e., MMDDYY (e.g., 101593). The start of care date is the first Medicare billable visit. This date remains the same on subsequent plans of treatment until the patient is discharged. Home health may be suspended and later resumed under the same start of care date in accordance with your internal procedures.

     3.   <u>Certification Period.</u>—Enter the 2 digit month, day, year, MMDDYY (e.g., 101593-121593), which identifies the period covered by the physician's plan of care. The "From" date for the initial certification must match the start of care date. The "To" date can be <u>up to</u>, but never exceed, two calendar months later and mathematically never exceed 62 days. Always repeat the "To" date on a subsequent recertification as the next sequential "From" date. Services delivered on the "To" date are covered in the next certification period.

EXAMPLE: Initial certification "From" date 101593
                   Initial certification "To" date 121593

                   Recertification "From" date 121593
                   Recertification "To" date 121594

     4.   <u>Medical Record Number.</u>—Enter the patient's medical record number that you assign. This is an <u>optional</u> item. If not applicable, enter "N/A."

     5.   <u>Provider number.</u>—Enter your 6-digit number issued by Medicare. It contains 2 digits, a hyphen, and 4 digits (e.g., 00-7000).

     6.   <u>Patient's Name and Address.</u>—Enter the patient's last name, first name, and middle initial as shown on the health insurance card followed by the street address, city, State, and ZIP code.

     7.   <u>Provider's Name, Address and Telephone No.</u>—Enter your name and/or branch office (if applicable), street address (or other legal address), city, State, and ZIP code and telephone number.

     8.   <u>Date of Birth.</u>—Enter the date (6 digit month, day, year) in numerics (MMDDYY, e.g., 040120).

443

234.7 (Cont.)   COVERAGE OF SERVICES   09-94

9. Sex.—Check the appropriate box.

10. Medications: Dose/Frequency/Route.—Enter all physicians orders for all medications, including the dosage, freqency and route of administration for each.

    ◦ Use the addendum HCFA-487 for drugs which cannot be listed on the plan of treatment.

    ◦ Use the letter "N" after the medication(s) which are "new" orders.

    ◦ Use the letter "C" after the medication(s) which are "change" orders either in dose, frequency or route of administration.

"New" orders refer to medications which the patient has not taken recently, i.e., within the last 30 days. "Change" orders for medications include dosage, frequency or route of administration changes within the last 60 days.

11. Principal Diagnosis, ICD-9-CM Code and Date of Onset/Exacerbation.— Enter the principal diagnosis on all HCFA-485 forms. The principal diagnosis is the diagnosis most related to the current plan of treatment. It may or may not be related to the patient's most recent hospital stay, but must relate to the services you rendered. If more than one diagnosis is treated concurrently, enter the diagnosis that respresents the most acute condition and requires the most intensive services.

Enter the appropriate ICD-9-CM code in the space provided. The code must be the full ICD-9-CM diagnosis code including all digits. V codes are acceptable as both primary and secondary diagnosis. In many instances, the V code more accurately reflects the care provided. However, do not use the V code when the acute diagnosis code is more specific to the exact nature of the patient's condition. A list of V codes is in Exhibit VI.

EXAMPLES: Patient is surgically treated for a subtrochanteric fracture (Code 820.22). Admission to home care is for rehabilitation services (V57.1). Use 820.22 as the primary diagnosis since V57.1 does not specify the type or location of the fracture.

Patient is surgically treated for a malignant neoplasm of the colon (Code 153.2) with exteriorization of the colon. Admission to home care is for instruction in care of colostomy (V 55.3). Use V 55.3 as the primary diagnosis since it is more specific to the nature of the services.

The principal diagnosis may change on subsequent forms only if the patient develops an acute condition or an exacerbation of a secondary diagnosis requiring intensive services different than those on the established plan of care.

List the actual _medical_ diagnostic term next to the ICD-9-CM code. Do not describe in narrative format any symptoms or explanations. Do not use surgical procedure codes.

444

The <u>date</u> is always represented by six digits (MMDDYY); if the exact day is not known, use 00. The date of onset is specific to the medical reason for home health care services. If a condition is chronic or long term in nature, use the date of exacerbation. Use one or the other, not both. Always use the latest date. Enter all dates as close as possible to the actual date, to the best of your knowledge.

12. <u>Surgical Procedure, Date, ICD-9-CM Code.</u>—Enter the surgical procedure relevant to the care rendered. For example, if the diagnosis in Item 11 is "Fractured Left Hip", note the ICD-9-CM Code, the surgical procedure, and date (e.g., 81.62, Insertion of Austin Moore Prosthesis, 060987). If a surgical procedure was not performed or is not relevant to the plan of care, do not leave the box blank. Enter N/A. Use the addendum (HCFA-487) for additional relevant surgical procedures. At a minimum, the month and year must be present for the date of surgery. Use 00 if the day is unknown.

13. <u>Other Pertinent Diagnoses: Dates of Onset/Exacerbation, ICD-9-CM Code.</u>— Enter all pertinent diagnoses, both narrative and ICD-9-CM codes, relevant to the care rendered. Other pertinent diagnoses are all conditions that coexisted at the time the plan of care was established or which developed subsequently. Exclude diagnoses that relate to an earlier episode which have no bearing on this plan of care. These diagnoses can be changed to reflect changes in the patient's condition.

In listing the diagnoses, place them in order to best reflect the seriousness of the patient's condition and to justify the disciplines and services provided. If there are more than four pertinent diagnoses, use the addendum (HCFA-487) to list them. Enter N/A if there are no pertinent secondary diagnoses.

The date reflects either the date of onset, if it is a new diagnosis, or the date of the most recent exacerbation date of a previous diagnosis. Note the date of onset or exacerbation as close to the actual date as possible. If the date is unknown, note the year and place 00s in the month or day if not known.

14. <u>DME and Supplies.</u>—All nonroutine supplies must be specifically ordered by the physician or the physician's order for services must require the use of the specific supplies. Enter in this item, nonroutine supplies that you are billing to Medicare that are not specifically required by the order for services. For example, an order for foley insertion requires specific supplies, i.e., foley catheter tray. Therefore, these supplies are not required to be listed. Conversely, an order for wound care may require the use of nonroutine supplies which would vary by patient. Therefore, list the nonroutine supplies.

If you use a commonly used commercially packaged kit, you are not required to list the individual components. However, if there is a question of cost or content, the intermediary can request a breakdown of kit components.

Refer to the Provider Reimbursement Manual, §2115 for a definition of nonroutine supplies.

List DME ordered by the physician that will be billed to Medicare. Enter N/A if no supplies or DME are billed.

15. <u>Safety Measures.</u>—Enter the physician's instructions for safety measures.

445

234.7 (Cont.) COVERAGE OF SERVICES 11-94

16. <u>Nutritional Requirements</u>.—Enter the physician's order for the diet. This includes specific therapeutic diets and/or any specific dietary requirements. Record fluid needs or restrictions. Total Parenteral Nutrition (TPN) can be listed, and if more room is needed, place additional information under medications. If more space is necessary, use the HCFA-487.

17. <u>Allergies</u>.—Enter medications to which the patient is allergic and other allergies the patient experiences (e.g., foods, adhesive tape, iodine). "No known allergies" may be an appropriate response.

18A. <u>Functional Limitations</u>.—Check all items which describe the patient's current limitations as assessed by the physician and you.

18B. <u>Activities Permitted</u>.—Check the activity(ies) which the physician allows and/or for which physician orders are present.

If you check "Other" under either the "Functional Limitations" or "Activities Permitted" category, provide a narrative explanation in Item 17 of the HCFA-486.

19. <u>Mental Status</u>.—Check the block(s) most appropriate to describe the patient's mental status. If you check "Other" specify the conditions.

20. <u>Prognosis</u>.—Check the box which specifies the most appropriate prognosis for the patient: poor, guarded, fair, good or excellent.

21. <u>Orders for Discipline and Treatments (Specify amt/freq/dura)</u>.—The physician must specify the frequency and the expected duration of the visits for each discipline. The duties/treatments to be performed by each discipline must be stated. A discipline may be one or more of the following: skilled nursing (SN), physical therapy (PT), speech therapy (ST), occupational therapy (OT), medical social services (MSS), or home health aid (AIDE).

Orders must include all disciplines and treatments, even if they are not billable to Medicare. In general, the narrative explanation for applicable treatment codes is acceptable to the order when that narrative is sufficiently descriptive of the services to be furnished. (See §234.9.) However, additional explanation is required in this item to describe specific services, i.e., A1, A4, A5, A6, A7, A22, A23, A28, A29, A32, B15, C9, D11, E4, E6, and F15. Refer to treatment codes Exhibit V. Additional explanation is also required where the physician has ordered specific treatment, medications, or supplies. When aide services are needed to furnish personal care, an order for "personal care" is sufficient. See example of orders below.

Frequency denotes the number of visits per discipline to be rendered, stated in days, weeks, or months. Duration identifies the length of time the services are to be rendered and may be expressed in days, weeks, or months.

A range of visits may be reflected in the frequency (e.g., 2 to 4 visits per week). When a range is used, consider the upper limit of the range the specific frequency. An agency may use ranges if acceptable to the physician without regard to diagnosis or other limits.

EXAMPLE OF PHYSICIAN'S ORDERS; Certification Period is 101593 to 121593.

OT-	Eval., ADL training fine motor coordination	$3 \times$/wk $\times$ 6 wks
ST-	Eval., increase articulation of single syllable words, all motor exercises following 2-step verbal directions	$3 \times$/wk $\times$ 4 wks
SN-	Skilled observation of C/P and neuro status; instruct meds and diet/hydration, instruct wound care-wash, betadine to affected area, cover w/DSD; Foley catheter care	QD $\times$ 5 days $3 \times$/wk $\times$ 2 wks $2 \times$/wk $\times$ 2 wks $1 \times$/wk $\times$ 4 wks
MSS-	Assessment of emotional and social factors related to response to treatment	$1 \times$/mo. $\times$ 2 mos
AIDE-	Assist with personal care; complete bed bath, shave, catheter care	3-$5 \times$/wk $\times$ 9 wks

Specific services rendered by physical, speech and occupational therapists may involve different modalities. The "AMOUNT" is necessary when a discipline is providing a specific modality for therapy. Modalities usually mentioned are for heat, sound, cold, and electronic stimulation.

EXAMPLE: PT - To apply hot packs to the C5-C6 $\times$ <u>10 minutes</u> $3 \times$/wk $\times$ 2 wks

PRN visits may be ordered on a plan of care only where they are qualified in a manner that is specific to the patient's potential needs. Both the nature of the services and the number of PRN visits to be permitted for each type of service must be specified. Open-ended, unqualified PRN visits do not constitute physician orders since neither their nature nor their frequency is specified.

EXAMPLE: Skilled nursing visits 1xmx2m for Foley change and PRNx2 for emergency Foley irrigations and/or changes.

Skilled nursing visits 1xmx2m to draw blood sugar and PRNx2 to draw emergency blood sugar if blood sugar level is above 400.

22.   <u>Goals/Rehabilitation Potential/Discharge Plans</u>.—Enter information which reflects the physician's description of the achievable goals and the patient's ability to meet them as well as plans for care after discharge.

Examples of realistic goals:

- ○   Independence in transfers and ambulation with walker.

- ○   Healing of leg ulcer(s).

- ○   Maintain patency of Foley catheter. Decrease risk of urinary infection.

- ○   Achieve optimal level of cardiovascular status. Medication and diet compliance.

- ○   Ability to demonstrate correct insulin preparation/administration.

447

234.7 (Cont.)   COVERAGE OF SERVICES   09-94

Rehabilitation potential addresses the patient's ability to attain the goals and an estimate of the time needed to achieve them. This information is pertinent to the nature of the patient's condition and ability to respond. The words "Fair", or "Poor" alone, are not acceptable. Add descriptors.

EXAMPLE: Rehabilitation potential good for partial return to previous level of care, but patient will probably not be able to perform ADL independently.

Where daily care has been ordered, be specific as to the goals and when the need for daily care is expected to end.

EXAMPLE: Granulation of wound with daily wound care is expected to be achieved in 4 weeks. Skilled nursing visits will be decreased to $3 \times$ week at that time.

Discharge plans include a statement of where, or how, the patient will be cared for once home health services are not provided.

23.   Verbal Start of Care, Nurse's Signature and Date.—This verifies for surveyors, HCFA representatives, and intermediaries that a nurse spoke to the attending physician and has received verbal authorization to visit the patient. This date may precede the SOC date in Item 2, and may precede the "From" date in Item 3. This field may be used to document verbal orders to begin care, modify care or continue care at recertification.

The item is signed by the nurse receiving the verbal orders, by the nurse responsible for completion of the form or by a nonclerical agency representative responsible for review. The date is necessary. If the nurse who received the orders does not prepare the HCFA-485, then the orders must be transcribed to a form, signed and dated by her/him and retained in your files. Document the initial and ongoing communications with the physician.

Enter N/A if the physician has signed and dated the HCFA-485 on or before the SOC or recertification date, or has submitted a written order to start, modify or continue care on a document other than the HCFA-485.

24.   Physician's Name and Address.—Print the physician's name and address. The attending physician is the physician who established the plan of care and who certifies and recertifies the medical necessity of the visits and/or services. Mention supplemental physicians involved in a patient's care only on the HCFA-486. The physician must be qualified to sign the certification and plan of care in accordance with 42 CFR 424, Subpart B. Physicians who have significant ownership interest in, or a significant financial or contractual relationship with an HHA may not establish or review a plan of care or certify or recertify the need for home health services. (See §234.6 Physician Certification/Recertification.)

25.   Date HHA Received Signed POT.—Enter the date you received the signed POT from the attending/referring physician. Enter N/A if Item 27 DATE is completed.

26.   Physician Certification.—This statement serves to verify that the physician has reviewed the plan of care and certifies to the need for the services.

27. Attending Physician's Signature and Date Signed.—The attending physician signs and dates the plan of treatment/certification prior to your submitting the claim. Rubber signature stamps are not acceptable. The form may be signed by another physician who is authorized by the attending physician to care for his/her patient in his/her absence.

Do not predate the orders for the physician, nor write the date in this field. If the physician left it blank, enter the date you received the signed POT under Item 25. Do not enter "N/A." Submit an unsigned copy of the HCFA-485. Retain the signed copy.

28. Penalty Statement.—This statement specifies the penalties imposed for misrepresentation, falsification or concealment of essential information on the HCFA-485.

234.8   HCFA-486–Medical Update and Patient Information.—Contains data needed by your intermediary to make coverage determinations. The intermediary requests the form and/or medical records if the claim is selected for MR.

Complete the HCFA-486 as follows:

1. Patient's HICN.—See §234.7 Item 1.

2. SOC Date.—See §234.7, Item 2.

3. Certification Period.—See §234.7, Item 3.

4. Medical Record Number.—See §234.7, Item 4.

5. Provider Number.—See §234.7, Item 5.

6. Patient's Name.—See §234.7, Item 6.

7. Provider's Name.—See §234.7, Item 7.

8. Medicare Covered.—This is your agency's opinion as to whether the patient's care is covered or noncovered. Check the appropriate box. Check the "noncovered" box when you believe the care is noncovered but the claim is submitted "at the patient's request" or to establish other third party eligibility.

9. Date Physician Last Saw Patient.—Enter the date the physician last saw the patient if this information can be obtained during the home visit. If you are unable to determine this date, enter "Unknown."

NOTE: It is not intended that you contact the physician's office to account for patient's visits. It is expected but not required for coverage, that the physician who signs the plan of care will see the patient, but there is no specified interval of time within which the patient is expected to be seen. Your intermediary evaluates the patient's medical condition. Visits will not be denied solely on the basis that the physician does not see the patient.

449

234.8 (Cont.)   COVERAGE OF SERVICES   09-94

10.   Date Last Contacted Physician.—Note the date MMDDYY (e.g., 121093) of your most recent physician contact (verbal or written) regarding the status or problems encountered with the patient during the last 60 days. Briefly state the purpose of your contact under Item 16 (Updated Information).

11.   Is Patient Receiving Care in an 1861(j)(1) SNF or Equivalent?.—Check the appropriate block. Since a requirement for eligibility for the home health benefit is that services be provided at the patient's residence, if the patient is residing in a nursing home which meets at least the requirements of §1861(J)(1), the facility cannot be considered the patient's residence. (See §208.5.)

12.   Certification Recertification Modified.—Check one of the blocks to identify this plan of care as a certification, recertification or modification. Modified, refers to the HCFA-486 submitted with an interim claim to report changes in the disciplines or numbers of visits ordered, or to obtain a Medicare denial letter.

13.   Dates of Last Inpatient Stay.—Enter the admission and discharge dates (month, day and year: e.g., 100293 - 101293) of the last inpatient stay relevant to the care provided. Enter N/A if not applicable.

14.   Type of Facility.—Identify the type of facility. If Locator 13 has been completed recording a stay relevant to care being provided, this locator must also be completed. Enter N/A if not applicable.

The responses for this locator are:

- A = Acute Hospital
- S = SNF
- R = Rehabilitation Hospital
- I = ICF
- O = Other
- U = Unknown

15.   Updated Information: New Orders/Treatments/Clinical Facts/Summary From Each Discipline.—Record any new orders, treatments or changes and associated date(s) from the time the HCFA-485 is completed to the time the HCFA-486 is completed.

On certifications, enter the clinical findings of the initial assessment visit for all disciplines involved in the care plan. Describe the clinical facts about the patient that require skilled home health services. Include specific dates.

On recertifications, record significant clinical findings for each discipline incorporating all symptoms and changes in the patient's condition during the last 60 days of service. Include specific dates. Document progress and nonprogress for each discipline.

Include any pertinent information on a patient's inpatient stay and the purpose of any agency contact with the physician, if applicable.

450

16. <u>Functional Limitations (Expand From HCFA-485 and ADL)/Reason Homebound/Prior Functional Status.</u>—Provide a narrative description of the patient's prior functional status and current limitations and activities permitted. Elaborate on the information in the checklist (HCFA-485 Items 18A and 18B) and provide any other information needed to describe the patient. Clearly reflect the restrictions imposed by the physician. Include a description of ADL limitations and indicate the type and scope of assistance needed. Include a brief statement of why the patient is homebound. Include a description of the home environment, if it is relevant to the homebound determination, e.g., patient lives in a third floor walk-up apartment and is recovering from congestive heart failure.

17. <u>Supplementary Plan of Care (POC) on File From Physician Other Than the Referring Physician? (If Yes, Specify Giving Goals/Rehabilitation Potential/Discharge Plan).</u>—Provide this information if more than one POC is being used to provide services. If so, document the specialty, the type of service, duties, goals, rehabilitation potential, discharge plans here or attach a copy of the written plan to the HCFA-486. Give the reasons necessitating a supplemental plan.

18. <u>Unusual Home/Social Environment (Optional).</u>—Use this block to include information which would enhance the reviewer's concept of the home situation and help to justify the need for services in the home, e.g., patient lives with retarded son who is unable to provide any assistance or to comprehend instructions. The information may explain the rationale for medical social services by documenting the problems which are or will be an impediment to the effective treatment of the patient's medical condition or rate of recovery.

19. <u>Indicate Any Time When You Made a Visit and Patient Was Not Home and Reasons Why if Ascertainable.</u>—Indicate when and why this occurred. For example: 11/03/93 - Patient was taken to the emergency room for evaluation and treatment after a fall at home.

20. <u>Specify Any Known Medical and/or Nonmedical Reasons the Patient Regularly Leaves Home and Frequency of Occurrence.</u>—Obtain information from the patient, family or caretaker for the patient's absences from the home and whether they were for medical or nonmedical reasons. For example, the patient goes to the barber shop $1 \times$ a month and to the doctor's $2/\times$ a month.

21. <u>Signature of Nurse or Therapist Completing or Reviewing Form/Date (MO, DAY, YR).</u>—The nurse or therapist responsible for the completion of the form or a nonclerical agency representative or supervisor responsible for the review signs and dates the form.

234.9 <u>Treatment Codes for Home Health Services.</u>—The agency may use the narrative explanation for the treatment codes which represent the services to be furnished. The narrative is entered in Item 21 of the HCFA-485. Additional narrative is required under Item 21 of the HCFA-485 to describe specific services, i.e., A1, A4, A5, A6, A7, A22, A23, A28, A29, A32, B15, C9, D11, E4, E6, and F15. (See asterisked items/services in Exhibit V.) Non-asterisked items/services do not require additional narrative unless the physician has ordered specific treatment and/or use of prescription medications and/or nonroutine supplies.

Listing of a code for a particular service is not intended to imply coverage. The codes are to ease identification of services ordered by the physician whether or not these services are payable individually by Medicare. Physician's orders reflect a narrative description of treatment and services to be furnished.

451

234.9 (Cont.)   COVERAGE OF SERVICES   09-94

   A.   Skilled Nursing (SN).—These represent the services to be performed by the nurse. Services performed by the patient or other person in the home without the teaching or supervision of the nurse are not coded. The following is a further explanation for each service:

   °   A1. Skilled Observation (Inc. V.S., Response to Med., etc.)—Include all skilled observation and assessment of the patient where the physician determines that the patient's condition is such that a reasonable probability exists that significant changes may occur which require the skills of a licensed nurse to supplement the physician's personal contacts with the patient. (See §3117.4.A.)

   °   A2. Foley Insertion—Insertion and/or removal of the Foley catheter by nurse.

   °   A3. Bladder Instillation—Instilling medications into the bladder.

   °   A4. Wound Care/Dressing—Includes irrigation of open post-surgical wounds, application of medication and/or dressing changes. Does not include decubitus care. Describe dimension of wound (size and amount and type of drainage) in Item 16 on the HCFA 486. See A28 for observation of uncomplicated surgical incision.

   °   A5. Decubitus Care—Includes irrigation, application of medication and/or dressing changes to decubitus. The agency describes size (depth and width) and appearance in Item 16 of the HCFA-486. Use this code only if the decubitus presents the following characteristics:

      °   Partial tissue loss with signs of infection as foul odor or purulent drainage; and

      °   Full thickness tissue loss involves exposure of fat or invasion of other tissue such as muscle or bone.

For decubitus care not meeting this definition, see A29.

   °   A6. Venipuncture—Specify the test and frequency to be performed under physician's orders.

   °   A7. Restorative Nursing—Includes exercises, transfer training, carrying out of restorative program ordered by the physician. This may or may not be established by a physical therapist. Do not use this code to describe nonskilled services (e.g., routine range of motion exercises).

   °   A8. Post Cataract Care—Includes observation, dressings, teaching, etc., of the immediate postoperative cataract patient. (See §3117.4.A.)

   °   A9. Bowel/Bladder Training—Includes training of patients who have neurological or muscular problems or other conditions where the need for bowel or bladder training is clearly identified. (See §3114.4.E.1.)

   °   A10. Chest Physio (Inc. postural drainage)—Includes breathing exercises, postural drainage, chest percussion, conservation techniques, etc.

452

    °   __A11. Adm. of Vitamin B/12__–Administration of vitamin B/12 preparation by injection for conditions identified in Medicare guidelines. (See §3117.4.)

    °   __A12. Prep/Adm. Insulin__–Preparation of insulin syringes for administration by the patient or other person, or the administration of the insulin by the nurse.

    °   __A13. Adm. Other IM/Subq.__–Administration of any injection other than vitamin B/12 or insulin ordered by the physician.

    °   __A14. Adm. IVs/Clysis__–Administration of intravenous fluids or clysis or intravenous medications.

    °   __A15. Teach. Ostomy or Ileo Conduit Care__–Teaching the patient or other person to care for a colostomy, ileostomy or ileoconduit or nephrostomy.

    °   __A16. Teach. Nasogastric Feeding__–Teaching the patient or other person to administer nasogastric feedings. Includes teaching care of equipment and preparation of feedings.

    °   __A17. Reinsertion Nasogastric Feeding Tube__–Includes changing the tube by the nurse.

    °   __A18. Teach. Gastrostomy Feeding__–Teaching the patient or other person to care for gastrostomy and administer feedings. Includes teaching care of equipment and preparation of feedings.

    °   __A19. Teach. Parenteral Nutrition__–Teaching the patient and/or family to administer parenteral nutrition. Includes teaching aseptic technique for dressing changes to catheter site. Your documentation must specify that this service is necessary and does not duplicate other teaching.

    °   __A20. Teach. Care of Trach.__–Teaching the patient or other person to care for a tracheostomy. This includes care of equipment.

    °   __A21. Adm. Care of Trach.__–Administration of tracheostomy care by the nurse, including changing the tracheostomy tube and care of the equipment.

    °   __A22. Teach. Inhalation Rx__–Teaching patient or other person to administer therapy and care for equipment.

    °   __A23. Adm. Inhalation Rx__–Administration of inhalation treatment and care of equipment by the nurse.

    °   __A24. Teach. Adm. of Injection__–Teaching patient or other person to administer an injection. Does not include the administration of the injection by the nurse (see A11, A13) or the teaching/administration of insulin. (See A12, A25.)

    °   __A25. Teach. Diabetic Care__–Includes all teaching of the diabetic patient (i.e., diet, skin care, administration of insulin, urine testing).

453

234.9 (Cont.)   COVERAGE OF SERVICES   09-94

    °   __A26. Disimpaction/Follow-up Enema__—Includes nursing services associated with removal of an impaction. Enema administration in the absence of a fecal impaction only if a complex condition exists—e.g., immediate postoperative rectal surgery.

    °   __A27. Other (Spec. under orders)__—Includes any SN or teaching ordered by the physician and not identified above. Specify what is being taught in Item 21 (HCFA-485).

    °   __A28. Wound Care/Dressing__—Skilled observation and care of surgical incision/ suture line including application of DSD. (See A4.)

    °   __A29. Decubitus Care__—Includes irrigation, application of medication and/or dressing changes to decubitus/other skin ulcer or lesion, which is other than that described in A5. Describe size (depth and width) and appearance in Item 16 of the HCFA-486.

    °   __A30. Teaching Care of Any Indwelling Catheter__—Teaching patient or other person to care for indwelling catheter.

    °   __A31. Management and Evaluation of a Patient Care Plan__—The complexity of necessary unskilled services require skilled management by a registered nurse to ensure that these services achieve their purpose, and to promote the beneficiary's recovery and medical safety.

    °   __A32. Teaching and Training (Other)__—Specify under physician orders.

    B. __Physical Therapy.__—These codes represent all services to be performed by the physical therapist. If services are provided by a nurse, they are included under A7. The following is a further explanation of each service:

    °   __B1. Evaluation__—Visit(s) made to determine patient's condition, physical therapy plans and rehabilitation potential. Also to evaluate home environment to eliminate structural barriers and improve safety to increase functional independence (ramps, adaptive wheelchair, bathroom aides).

    °   __B2. Therapeutic Exercise__—Exercises designed to restore function. Specific exercise techniques (e.g., Proprioceptive Neuromuscular Facilitation (PNF), Rood, Brunstrom, Codman's, William's) should be specified in the plan of care. The exercise technique should be listed in the medical record specific to the patient's condition. Also, manual therapy techniques which include soft tissue and joint mobilization to reduce joint deformity and increase functional range of motion.

    °   __B3. Transfer Training__—Evaluate and instruct safe transfers (bed, bath, toilet, sofa, chair, commode) using appropriate body mechanics, and equipment (sliding board, Hoyer lift, trapeze, bath bench, wheelchair). Instruct patient, family, and caregivers in appropriate transfer techniques.

    °   __B4. Establish or Upgrade Home Program__—To improve the patient's functional level by instruction to patient and other responsible individuals in exercise which may be used in adjunct to PT programs.

454

    ◦   B5. Gait Training—Includes gait evaluation and ambulation training of a patient whose ability to walk has been impaired. Gait training is the selection and instruction in use of various assistive devices (orthotic appliances, crutches, walker, cane, etc.).

    ◦   B6. Pulmonary Physical Therapy—Includes breathing exercises, postural drainage, etc., designed for patients with acute or severe pulmonary dysfunction.

    ◦   B7. Ultra Sound—Mechanism to produce heat or micro-massage in deep tissues for conditions in which relief of pain, increase in circulation, and increase in local metabolic activity are desirable.

    ◦   B8. Electro Therapy—Includes treatment for neuromuscular dysfunction and pain through use of electrotherapeutic devices (electromuscular stimulation, TENS, Functional Electrical Stimulation (FES), biofeedback, high voltage galvanic stimulation (HVGS) etc.).

    ◦   B9. Prosthetic Training—Includes stump conditioning (shrinking, shaping, etc.), range of motion, muscle strengthening and gait training with or without the prosthesis and appropriate assistive devices.

    ◦   B10. Fabrication Temporary Devices—Includes fabrication of temporary prostheses, braces, splints, and slings.

    ◦   B11. Muscle Reeducation—Includes therapy designed to restore function due to illness disease or surgery affecting neuromuscular function.

    ◦   B12. Management and Evaluation of a Patient Care Plan—The complexity of necessary unskilled services require skilled management by a qualified physical therapist to ensure that these services achieve their purpose, and to promote the beneficiary's recovery and medical safety.

    ◦   B13. through B14.—Reserved.

    ◦   B15. Other (Spec. Under Orders)—Include all PT services not identified above. Identify specific therapy services under physician's orders (HCFA-485 Item 21).

   C. Speech Therapy (ST).—These codes represent all services to be performed by the speech therapist. Following is a further explanation of each.

    ◦   C1. Evaluation—Visit made to determine the type, severity and prognosis of a communication disorder, whether speech therapy is reasonable and necessary and to establish the goals, treatment plan, and estimated frequency and duration of treatment.

    ◦   C2. Voice Disorders Treatments—Procedures and treatment for patients with an absence or impairment of voice caused by neurologic impairment, structural abnormality, or surgical procedures affecting the muscles of voice production.

455

234.9 (Cont.)   COVERAGE OF SERVICES   09-94

    ◦   C3. Speech Articulation Disorders Treatments–Procedures and treatment for patients with impaired intelligibility (clarity) of speech–usually referred to as anarthria or dysarthria and/or impaired ability to initiate, inhibit, and/or sequence speech sound muscle movements–usually referred to as apraxia/dyspraxia.

    ◦   C4. Dysphagia Treatments–Includes procedures designed to facilitate and restore a functional swallow.

    ◦   C5. Language Disorders Treatments–Includes procedures and treatment for patients with receptive and/or expressive aphasia/dysphasia, impaired reading comprehension, written language expression, and/or arithmetical processes.

    ◦   C6. Aural Rehabilitation–Procedures and treatment for patients with communication problems related to impaired hearing acuity.

    ◦   C7. Reserved

    ◦   C8. Nonoral Communications–Includes any procedures designed to establish a nonoral or augmentive communication system.

    ◦   C9. Other (Spec. Under Orders)–Speech therapy services not included above. Specify service to be rendered under physician's orders (HCFA-485 Item 21).

    D. Occupational Therapy.—These codes represent all services to be rendered by the occupational therapist. Following is a further explanation:

    ◦   D1. Evaluation–Visit made to determine occupational therapy needs of the patient at the home. Includes physical and psychosocial testing, establishment of plan of treatment, rehabilitation goals, and evaluating the home environment for accessibility and safety and recommending modifications.

    ◦   D2. Independent Living/Daily Living Skills (ADL training)—Refers to the skills and performance of physical cognitive and psychological/emotional self care, work, and play/leisure activities to a level of independence appropriate to age, life-space, and disability.

    ◦   D3. Muscle Re-education–Includes therapy designed to restore function lost due to disease or surgical intervention.

    ◦   D4. Reserved.

    ◦   D5. Perceptual Motor Training–Refers to enhancing skills necessary to interpret sensory information so that the individual can interact normally with the environment. Training designed to enhance perceptual motor function usually involves activities which stimulate visual and kinesthetic channels to increase awareness of the body and its movement.

    ◦   D6. Fine Motor Coordination–Refers to the skills and the performance in fine motor and dexterity activities.

456

  ° __D7. Neurodevelopmental Treatment__—Refers to enhancing the skills and the performance of movement through eliciting and/or inhibiting stereotyped, patterned, and/or involuntary responses which are coordinated at subcortical and cortical levels.

  ° __D8. Sensory Treatment__—Refers to enhancing the skills and performance in perceiving and differentiating external and internal stimuli such as tactile awareness, stereognosis, kinesthesia, proprioceptive awareness, ocular control, vestibular awareness, auditory awareness, gustatory awareness, and olfactory awareness necessary to increase function.

  ° __D9. Orthotics/Splinting__—Refers to the provision of dynamic and static splints, braces, and slings for relieving pain, maintaining joint alignment, protecting joint integrity, improving function, and/or decreasing deformity.

  ° __D10. Adaptive Equipment (fabrication and training)__—Refers to the provision of special devices that increase independent functions.

  ° __D11. Other__—Occupational therapy services not quantified above.

  E. __Medical Social Services (MSS).__—These codes represent all services to be rendered by the medical social service worker. Following is a further explanation:

  __E1. Assessment of Social and Emotional Factors__—Skilled assessment of social and emotional factors related to the patient's illness, need for care, response to treatment and adjustment to care; followed by care plan development.

  ° __E2. Counseling for Long-Range Planning and Decision Making__—Assessment of patient's needs for long term care including: evaluation of home and family situation; enabling patient/family to develop an in-home care system exploring alternatives to in-home care; arrangement for placement.

  ° __E3. Community Resource Planning__—The promotion of community centered service(s) including education, advocacy, referral and linkage.

  ° __E4. Short Term Therapy__—Goal oriented intervention directed toward management of terminal illness; reaction/adjustment to illness; strengthening family/support system; conflict resolution related to chronicity of illness.

  ° __E5. Reserved__.

  ° __E6. Other (Specify Under Orders)__—Include other medical social services related to the patient's illness and need for care. Problem resolution associated with high risk indicators endangering patient's mental and physical health including: abuse/neglect, inadequate food/medical supplies; high suicide potential. The service to be performed must be written under doctor's orders (HCFA-485 Item 21).

457

234.9 (Cont.)   COVERAGE OF SERVICES   09-94

F. Home Health Aide.—These codes represent all services to be rendered by the home health aide. Specific personal care services to be provided by the home health aide must be determined by a registered professional nurse. Services are given under the supervision of the nurse, and if appropriate, a physical, speech or occupational therapist. Following is a further explanation:

○ F1. Tub/Shower Bath—Assistance with tub or shower bathing.

○ F2. Partial/Complete Bed Bath—Bathing or assisting the patient with bed bath.

○ F3. Reserved

○ F4. Personal Care—Includes shaving the patient or shampooing the hair.

○ F5. Reserved

○ F6. Catheter Care—Care of catheter site and/or irrigations under nursing supervision.

○ F7. Reserved

○ F8. Assist with Ambulation—Assisting the patient with ambulation as determined necessary by the nursing care plan.

○ F9. Reserved

○ F10. Exercises—Assisting the patient with exercises in accordance with the plan of care.

○ F11. Prepare Meal—May be furnished by the aide during a visit for personal care.

○ F12. Grocery Shop—May be furnished as an adjunct to a visit for personal care to meet the patient's nutritional needs in order to prevent or postpone the patient's institutionalization.

○ F13. Wash Clothes—This service may be provided as it relates to the comfort and cleanliness of the patient and the immediate environment.

○ F14. Housekeeping—Household services incidental to care and which do not substantially increase the time spent by the home health aide.

○ F15. Other (Specify under Orders)—Include other home health aide services in accordance with determination made by a registered professional nurse. Specify in Item 21 of the HCFA-485.

458

234.10 <u>HCFA-487–Addendum to the Plan of Treatment/Medical Update</u>.—Use the HCFA-487 only as an addendum to the HCFA-485/486 when additional space is needed to complete the fields on those forms. The data for each field must be initiated on the HCFA-485 or 486. Use a separate addendum for the plan of care and the medical update. If the addendum is used to continue items on the plan of care, forward the HCFA-487 to the physician with the HCFA-485 for his signature.

To provide additional documentation of items on the plan of care or medical information, check the appropriate block. Identify the item being addressed under Item 8. For example, if the plan of treatment block is checked and Item 10 (medications) requires additional space, specify Item (10) on the left margin of column 8. Upon completion of Item 10, note the next item number, e.g., Item 14, (DME) then complete that item.

      1. <u>Patient's HICN</u>.—See §234.7, Item 1.

      2. <u>Start of Care Date</u>.—See §234.7, Item 2.

      3. <u>Certification Period</u>.—See §234.7, Item 3.

      4. <u>Medical Record Number</u>.—See §234.7, Item 4.

      5. <u>Provider Number</u>.—See §234.7, Item 5.

      6. <u>Patient's Name</u>.—See §234.7, Item 6.

      7. <u>Provider Name</u>.—See §234.7, Item 7.

      8. <u>Item Number</u>.—Indicate the item number for which you are providing additional information.

      9. <u>Signature of Physician</u>.—If the certification/plan of treatment block is checked, the physician's signature or an annotation is required on the HCFA-485 which indicates that the physician is aware that he is signing for information contained on additional pages (e.g., page 1 of 2). Retain the signed copy in your files.

      10. <u>Date</u>.—The physician enters the date he signed the addendum in this space.

      11. <u>Optional Name/Signature of Nurse/Therapist</u>.—If the medical update/patient information block is checked, the Nurse/Therapist filling the form signs.

      12. <u>Date</u>.—The date the nurse/therapist filled out the addendum appears in this space.

234.11 <u>HCFA-488—Intermediary Medical Information Request</u>.—The intermediary uses only the HCFA-488 when necessary to obtain additional medical information. All requests for subsequent medical information are limited to the items listed below. The intermediary completes Items 1 through 9 and checks the item(s) it is requesting you to complete. Provide the requested information as timely as possible. Use the HCFA-488 to respond as space allows. Return the HCFA-488 as a cover sheet for identification of requested information.

459

234.11 (Cont.)   COVERAGE OF SERVICES   09-94

1. <u>Initial Request Date</u>.—The date on which the request was initiated.

2. <u>Final Request Date</u>.—Not applicable. The intermediary sends only one request.

3. <u>Provider Number</u>.—Your six digit number.

4. <u>Document Control Number</u>.—The number used to identify individual claims. This number is an internal processing number determined by the intermediary.

5. <u>Patient Name</u>.—The last name, first name, middle initial.

6. <u>HICN</u>.—The patient's Medicare number including alpha designator.

7. <u>Medical Record Number</u>.—The medical record number you assigned and located in Item 4 on the HCFA-485.

8. <u>Period of Claim</u>.—The 6 digit month, day, year dates from Item 22 on the HCFA-1450. Include "From" and "To" dates.

9. <u>SOC Date</u>.—The 6 digit month, day, year on which covered home health services began. The date remains the same on subsequent plans of treatment until the patient is discharged.

When pertinent to a coverage decision, the intermediary requests one or more of the following:

10. <u>HCFA-485/486–Period Covered</u>.—This item is used to request a copy of the applicable POT/MIF forms (HCFA-485/486) on interim claims where you were not required to submit these forms with the claim. The intermediary enters the month, day, year, dates (i.e., 60 day period) that incorporates the date of the claim. Forward the applicable HCFA-485 and an updated HCFA-486 with Items 1-3, 5-10, 12-16, and 22 completed.

11. <u>HCFA-486–Period Covered</u>.—This item is checked to request only an updated HCFA-486 by entering the dates of the claim; month, day and year. Complete only Items 1-3, 5-10, 12-16 and 22.

12. <u>Frequency of Doctor's Visits</u>.—This item is checked if information is needed regarding the frequency that the patient is seen by the physician.

13. <u>Status of Chronic Condition</u>.— This item is checked if a narrative statement is needed to explain the status of a chronic condition that is not adequately addressed on the HCFA-485/486.

14. <u>List Primary Need for: SN, PT, ST, OT, MSS, AIDE, Other Visits</u>.—If one or more of the above services is in question as to the need for the services that have been billed, the intermediary checks the appropriate box(es). Submit a narrative statement listing the reason(s) the patient required the service(s).

15. <u>List Dates of Visits for: SN, PT, ST, OT, MSS, AIDE, Other Visits</u>.—If one or more of the above services is in question as to the dates that the services were provided, the intermediary checks the appropriate box(es). Submit a list of all dates on which the services were provided by that discipline for the period covered, including PRN visits.

460

16. _Laboratory Tests (frequency, types, results)._—This box is checked and the intermediary circles one or more items as needed.

17. _Other tests (frequency, types, results)._—The intermediary checks this box and enters the name of the tests it is requesting.

18. _Diet._—The intermediary checks this item and the box(es) that represents the requested information.

19. _Date(s) on Which Frequency of SN or AIDE Increased or Decreased._—The intermediary checks this box and writes on the service and the frequency in question.

20. _Specific Progress Notes for: SN, PT, ST, OT, MSS, AIDE, Other Visits._—The intermediary checks this item and the box(es) specifying the type of progress notes requested.

21. _Reason for Continued Medicare Coverage._—This item is checked if the HCFA-485/486 information raises a question for continued coverage of services.

22. _Doctor's Orders, Signed by the Physician._—This item is checked where a copy of the physician's orders or specific change of orders is requested.

23. _Supplemental Plans of Care, if Applicable._—The intermediary uses this item to request supplemental plans of care when necessary to make a coverage decision. This item corresponds to Item 18 on the HCFA-486.

24. _Signature of FI Representative._—The signature of the intermediary's representative appears.

234.12 _Coverage Compliance Review._—The intermediary performs coverage compliance reviews by reviewing medical records onsite or in-house. The purpose of the review is to assure that services meet Medicare program requirements and to verify that the information on the 485/486 matches that in the medical record and claim.

A. _Selection of HHAs._—The intermediary may select HHAs for review based on a number of factors (e.g., denial rates, provider profiling, problem areas identified during prepayment review, failure on prior compliance review, new HHAs).

B. _Coverage Compliance Review._—

1. _Sample Selection._—Claims will be selected with recent service dates or those reviewed and paid within the last 120 days.

The intermediary will select enough beneficiaries (a minimum of 15), to review a minimum of 100 visits or a maximum of 5 percent of your average monthly visits billed. Visits can be reduced if your volume is low.

Claims that have been fully denied will be excluded.

    2.   File Compilation.—The intermediary will establish an audit trail which identifies the claims and beneficiaries selected, sample size, the period of review for medical records, the records reviewed and the review findings.

    3.   HHA Onsite vs. In-House (at the Intermediary) Reviews.—The intermediary will determine whether to conduct a review onsite at the HHA or in-house at the intermediary.

    4.   Notification of Selection for Coverage Compliance Review.—

        a.   In-House.—You will be notified in writing when an in-house coverage compliance review is scheduled. The intermediary will furnish a list of beneficiaries for whom medical documentation is needed. Submit documentation within 30 days of the notification.

        b.   On-Site at HHA.—You will be advised by telephone of the visit 24 working hours in advance, followed with a written confirmation. The intermediary will advise you which records will be reviewed at the start of the review.

    5.   Review.—Points which will be addressed:

    ◦   Was the physician certification requirement met?

    ◦   Were the services rendered medically necessary?

    ◦   Were visits billed only when appropriate?

    ◦   Were visits billed actually furnished?

    ◦   Did skilled nursing and aide visits meet part-time or intermittent requirements?

    ◦   Were medical appliances and/or medical supplies appropriately ordered and/or supplied?

    ◦   Do the records support the evidence submitted originally? What information, or lack thereof, influenced the prepayment coverage decision?

    ◦   Is the certifying physician qualified to establish and certify a plan of care? (See 42 CFR §424.22.)

    ◦   Is the patient homebound?

    ◦   Is the patient's residence an §1819(a)(l) facility?

    ◦   Were the services furnished under a plan of care?

    ◦   Was the plan put into writing timely?

    ◦   Is the plan complete?

    ◦   Were plan of care changes or extensions made in accord with policy?

○ Compare home health aide tasks ordered with those furnished to assure tasks are accomplished.

NOTE: If you have obviously omitted a part of the data needed for review, e.g., home health aide notes, the intermediary will alert you to correct the problem.

Services prior to the period of the selected claims will not be reviewed unless the issue is homebound status. Where that question is raised, all previous records will be reviewed to determine when the patient ceased to meet that criterion. Where applicable, you will be asked to submit the actual hours spent in the home for all skilled nursing and aide visits. Coverage criteria in effect at the time services were rendered will be applied if changes have occurred in the interim which make coverage more restrictive.

6. Special On-Site Requirements.—

a. Staff.—Only intermediary staff who have authority to deny claims will perform the review. This process intends that if denials occur, they occur during the onsite review. The pertinent records will be photocopied for the physician's review only where a question arises which requires physician consultation. In these cases, the final decision to deny the claim is made by the physician reviewer, based upon information gathered at the onsite review.

b. Copying Records.—The intermediary will photocopy the pertinent records when the on-site reviewer has denied services, where physician consultation is needed, or where records may have been altered.

c. Entrance and Exit Interviews.—The intermediary will hold both entrance and exit interviews. It will explain in the entrance interview the scope and purpose of the review. You will be given an opportunity to produce documents during the review process.

The tentative findings of the review will be discussed during the exit interview. You will be provided with sufficient information to enable you to provide comments on the cases involved.

Physician review will be completed within 7 days of the date of the interview. You will be notified in writing of any additional services which are noncovered.

You may submit written comments on the denied services within 2 weeks of the exit conference, or receipt of the letter regarding the physician's findings, whichever is later.

The intermediary must finalize its findings within 6 weeks after the exit conference.

d. Beneficiary Home Visits.—Home visits may occur. This will be decided by the intermediary with RO approval.

463

234.12 (Cont.)   COVERAGE OF SERVICES   09-94

     7.   Distribution of Findings.—The intermediary will advise you in writing of the results within 6 weeks after the on-site review including:

     ◦   Written findings of the review;

     ◦   Specifics of denied care for educational purposes;

     ◦   Impact on prepayment review or documentation requirements; and

     ◦   Overpayments resulting from denials that are not payable under waiver of liability.

For denied services, the intermediary will send the beneficiary a notice if one would have been sent in the course of prepayment review. The intermediary will send you a copy of these denial notices since the beneficiary will be contacting you about the letter(s).

For in-house reviews, 14 days from the date of the report of findings will be allowed for your rebuttal or response.

     8.   Impact of Adverse Review Findings.—

     a.   Impact Upon Payment.—The intermediary will apply the waiver of liability provision where applicable. (See §§262-265 where you are determined to be liable.)

Where care is not covered for a reason for which waiver of liability provisions do not apply (e.g., lack of physician certification) the claim will be denied. In these cases, the amount of overpayment will be determined and recovered. (See §§262-265.) Payment will be made for cases which were previously denied and now covered. The intermediary will credit the denial rate for these visits.

     b.   Impact on Prepayment Review.—Where appropriate, prepayment review will be intensified until identified problems are corrected. A denial rate exceeding 15 percent, calculated by the total number of visits denied (medical and technical) divided by the total number of visits reviewed for this audit, may indicate a need for intensified review. When looking at denial rates, the reasons for denials will be considered. For example, denial of dependent services may disproportionately increase the denial rate and may not be indicative of a problem. The level and length of intensified review will be determined by the RHHI, in consultation with the RO.

     9.   Other Impact.—As a result of the coverage compliance audit, your intermediary may implement actions to improve your performance. For example, if the audit identifies problems with the accuracy of the information, i.e., you did not include pertinent information on HCFA-485/486, the intermediary advises you of corrective action to be taken. In another example, where cases contain erroneous or insufficient information, but the coverage decision remains the same, they will discuss with the appropriate HHA personnel. If a trend is noted where the documentation does not support the information submitted on the forms, corrective action is indicated. This could include an additional coverage compliance review within 3 months to determine if the problems have been corrected. Training will be provided to HHA staff on identified problem areas through bulletins, correspondence and teleconferences, etc.

When the lack of documentation or inaccurate information results in inappropriate payment, the intermediary will identify the reason, conduct educational training, usually on coverage and documentation, and evaluate the further need for intensified review. The intermediary will pursue corrective action where the audit results in inappropriate payment. At a minimum, it must recoup the inappropriate payments.

234.13 <u>Documentation of Skilled Nursing and Home Health Aide Hours.</u>—To document that SN and aide services are part-time or intermittent, you must maintain records which show the entrance and exit times of skilled nurse's and aide's visits and total hours spent in the home by each discipline. Exclude travel time.

Intermediaries may request this information when a question arises as to whether services are part-time or intermittent under §206.7.

○ When actual hours per day are full-time (up to and including 8 hours per day) 7 days per week, document their need. Document the medical complications, safety needs, condition of the beneficiary and reasons for the intensive full-time care. Document the specific services provided.

○ Extension beyond 21 days of full-time services for a finite and predictable period of time may be approved on an exception basis only when you have clearly documented the need, or the justification, for this frequency. Document the medical complications, safety needs, and/or other individual care needs that warrant your services. Stress the inherent complexity of services provided, the medical condition of the patient, functional losses and/ or other reasons that the beneficiary's condition is such that the service(s) can only be safely and effectively provided through skilled nursing care.

Department of Health and Human Services Health Care Financing Administration	**EXHIBIT I**	Form Approved OMB No. 0938-0357

HOME HEALTH CERTIFICATION AND PLAN OF TREATMENT

1. Patient's HI Claim No.	2. SOC Date	3. Certification Period		4. Medical Record No.	5. Provider No.
		From:	To:		

6. Patient's Name and Address	7. Provider's Name and Address

8. Date of Birth:	9. Sex	M	F	10. Medications: Dose/Frequency/Route (N)ew (C)hanged

11. ICD-9-CM	Principal Diagnosis	Date	
12. ICD-9-CM	Surgical Procedure	Date	
13. ICD-9-CM	Other Pertinent Diagnoses	Date	

14. DME and Supplies	15. Safety Measures:
16. Nutritional Req.	17. Allergies:

18. A. Functional Limitations

1	Amputation	5	Paralysis	9	Legally Blind
2	Bowel/Bladder (Incontinence)	6	Endurance	A	Dyspnea with Minimal Exertion
3	Contracture	7	Ambulation	B	Other (Specify)
4	Hearing	8	Speech		

18. B. Activities Permitted

1	Complete Bedrest	6	Partial Weight Bearing	A	Wheelchair
2	Bedrest BRP	7	Independent At Home	B	Walker
3	Up as Tolerated	8	Crutches	C	No Restrictions
4	Transfer Bed/Chair	9	Cane	D	Other (Specify)
5	Exercise Prescribed				

19. Mental Status:

1	Oriented	3	Forgetful	5	Disoriented	7	Agitated
2	Comatose	4	Depressed	6	Lethargic	8	Other

20. Prognosis

1	Poor	2	Guarded	3	Fair	4	Good	5	Excellent

21. Orders for Discipline and Treatments (Specify Amount/Frequency/Duration)

22. Goals/Rehabilitation Potential/Discharge Plans

23. Nurse's Signature and Date of Verbal SOC Where Applicable:	25. Date HHA Received Signed POT

24. Physician's Name and Address	26. I certify/recertify that this patient is confined to his/her home and needs intermittent skilled nursing care, physical therapy and/or speech therapy or continues to need occupational therapy. The patient is under my care, and I have authorized the services on this plan of care and will periodically review the plan.
27. Attending Physician's Signature and Date Signed	28. Anyone who misrepresents, falsifies, or conceals essential information required for payment of Federal funds may be subject to fine, imprisonment, or civil penalty under applicable Federal laws.

Form HCFA-485 (C-4) (02-94)   PROVIDER

466

Privacy Act Statement

Sections 1812, 1814, 1815, 1816, 1861, and 1862 of the Social Security Act authorize collection of this information. The primary use of this information is to process and pay Medicare benefits to or on behalf of eligible individuals. Disclosure of this information may be made to: Peer Review Organizations and Quality Review Organizations in connection with their review of claims, or in connection with studies or other review activities, conducted pursuant to Part B of Title XI of the Social Security Act; State Licensing Boards for review of unethical practices or nonprofessional conduct; A congressional office from the record of an individual in response to an inquiry from the congressional office at the request of that individual.

Where the individual's identification number is his/her Social Security Number (SSN), collection of this information is authorized by Executive Order 9397. Furnishing the information on this form, including the SSN, is voluntary, but failure to do so may result in disapproval of the request for payment of Medicare benefits.

Paper Work Burden Statement

Public reporting burden for this collection of information is estimated to average 15 minutes per response and recordkeeping burden is estimated to average 15 minutes per response. This includes time for reviewing instructions, searching existing data sources, gathering and maintaining data needed, and completing and reviewing the collection of information. Send comments regarding this burden estimate or any other aspect of this collection of information, including suggestions for reducing the burden, to Health Care Financing Administration, P.O. Box 26684, Baltimore, Maryland 21207, and to the Office of Information and Regulatory Affairs, Office of Management and Budget, Washington, D.C. 20503. Paperwork Reduction Project 0938-0357.

| Department of Health and Human Services
Health Care Financing Administration | **EXHIBIT II** | Form Approved
OMB No. 0938-0357 |

MEDICAL UPDATE AND PATIENT INFORMATION

1. Patient's HI Claim No.	2. SOC Date	3. Certification Period		4. Medical Record No.	5. Provider No.
		From:	To:		

6. Patient's Name and Address	7. Provider's Name

8. Medicare Covered: [ ] Y [ ] N	9. Date Physician Last Saw Patient:	10. Date Last Contacted Physician:

11. Is the Patient Receiving Care in an 1861 (JJ)(1) Skilled Nursing Facility or Equivalent? [ ] Y [ ] N [ ] Do Not Know	12. [ ] Certification [ ] Recertification [ ] Modified

13. Dates of Last Inpatient Stay: Admission	Discharge	14. Type of Facility:

15. Updated information: New Orders/Treatments/Clinical Facts/Summary from Each Discipline

16. Functional Limitations (Expand From 485 and Level of ADL) Reason Homebound/Prior Functional Status

17. Supplementary Plan of Care of File from Physician Other than Referring Physician:
(If Yes, Please Specify Giving Goals/Rehab. Potential/Discharge Plan)   [ ] Y [ ] N

18. Unusual Home/Social Environment

19. Indicate Any Time When the Home Health Agency Made a Visit and Patient was Not Home and Reason Why if Ascertainable	20. Specify Any Known Medical and/or Non-Medical Reasons the Patient Regularly Leaves Home and Frequency of Occurrence

21. Nurse or Therapist Completing or Reviewing Form	Date (Mo., Day, Yr.)

Form HCFA-486 (C3) (02-94)   PROVIDER

Privacy Act Statement

Sections 1812, 1814, 1815, 1816, 1861, and 1862 of the Social Security Act authorize collection of this information. The primary use of this information is to process and pay Medicare benefits to or on behalf of eligible individuals. Disclosure of this information may be made to: Peer Review Organizations and Quality Review Organizations in connection with their review of claims, or in connection with studies or other review activities, conducted pursuant to Part B of Title XI of the Social Security Act; State Licensing Boards for review of unethical practices or nonprofessional conduct; A congressional office from the record of an individual in response to an inquiry from the congressional office at the request of that individual.

Where the individual's identification number is his/her Social Security Number (SSN), collection of this information is authorized by Executive Order 9397. Furnishing the information on this form, including the SSN, is voluntary, but failure to do so may result in disapproval of the request for payment of Medicare benefits.

Paper Work Burden Statement

Public reporting burden for this collection of information is estimated to average 15 minutes per response and recordkeeping burden is estimated to average 15 minutes per response. This includes time for reviewing instructions, searching existing data sources, gathering and maintaining data needed, and completing and reviewing the collection of information. Send comments regarding this burden estimate or any other aspect of this collection of information, including suggestions for reducing the burden, to Health Care Financing Administration, P.O. Box 26684, Baltimore, Maryland 21207, and to the Office of Information and Regulatory Affairs, Office of Management and Budget, Washington, D.C. 20503. Paperwork Reduction Project 0938-0357.

Department of Health and Human Services Health Care Financing Administration		EXHIBIT III		Form Approved OMB No. 0938-0357	
ADDENDUM TO:		**PLAN OF TREATMENT**		**MEDICAL UPDATE**	
1. Patient's HI Claim No. No.	2. SOC Date	3. Certification Period From: To:		4. Medical Record No.	5. Provider
6. Patient's Name Name			7. Provider		

8. Item
No.

9. Signature of Physician

10. Date

11. Optional Name/Signature of Nurse/Therapist

12. Date

Form HCFA-487 (C4) (4-87)

470

| DEPARTMENT OF HEALTH AND HUMAN SERVICES
HEALTH CARE FINANCING ADMINISTRATION | **EXHIBIT IV** | FORM APPROVED
OMB NO. 0938-0357 |

HOME HEALTH AGENCY
INTERMEDIARY MEDICAL INFORMATION REQUEST

1. Initial Request Date:	2. Final Request Date:	
3. Provider Number:	4. Document Control Number:	
5. Patient Name:	6. HI Claim Number	
7. Medical Record Number:	8. Period of Claim: From: To:	9. SOC Date

☐ 10. HCFA-485/486:
     Period Covered:

☐ 11. HCFA-486:
     Period Covered:

☐ 12. Frequency of doctors visits:

☐ 13. Status of chronic condition:

☐ 14. List primary need for:
   ☐ SN   ☐ PT   ☐ ST   ☐ OT   ☐ MSS   ☐ HHA   ☐ Other Visits

☐ 15. List dates of visits for:
   ☐ SN   ☐ PT   ☐ ST   ☐ OT   ☐ MSS   ☐ HHA   ☐ Other Visits

☐ 16. Laboratory tests (frequency, types, results):

☐ 17. Other tests (frequency, types, results):

☐ 18. Diet   ☐ Type   ☐ Compliance   ☐ Teaching Duration   ☐ Length of time on the diet

☐ 19. Date(s) on which frequency of SN or HHA increased or decreased:

☐ 20. Specific progress notes for:
   ☐ SN   ☐ PT   ☐ ST   ☐ OT   ☐ MSS   ☐ HHA   ☐ Other Visits

☐ 21. Reason for continued Medicare coverage:

☐ 22. Doctor's orders, signed by physician

☐ 23. Supplemental Plans of Treatment, if applicable:	24. Signature of F.I. Representative

Form HCFA-488 (C4) (4-87)

EXHIBIT V

TREATMENT CODES FOR PROFESSIONAL SERVICES REQUIRED
Skilled Nursing

A1*	Skilled Observation and Assessment (Inc. V.S., Response to Med., etc.)	A15	Teach Ostomy or Ileo conduit care
A2	Foley Insertion	A16	Teach Nasogastric Feeding
A3	Bladder Instillation	A17	Reinsertion Nasogastric Feeding Tube
A4*	Open Wound Care/Dressing	A18	Teach Gastrostomy Feeding
A5*	Decubitus Care (Partial tissue loss with signs of infection or full thickness tissue loss etc.)	A19	Teach Parenteral Nutrition
		A20	Teach Care of Trach
		A21	Adm. Care of Trach
A6*	Venipuncture	A22*	Teach Inhalation Rx
A7*	Restorative Nursing	A23*	Adm. Inhalation Rx
A8	Post Cataract Care	A24	Teach Adm. of Injection
A9	Bowel/Bladder Training	A25	Teach Diabetic Care
A10	Chest Physio (Inc. Postural drainage)	A26	Disimpaction/F.U. Enema
		A27*	Other (Spec. under Orders)
A11	Adm. of Vitamin B/12	A28*	Wound Care/Dressing–Closed Incision/Suture Line
A12	Adm. Insulin		
A13	Adm. Other IM/Subq.	A29*	Decubitus Care (Other than A5)
A14	Adm. IVs/Clysis	A30	Teaching Care of Any Indwelling Catheter
		A31	Management and Evaluation of Patient Care Plan
		A32*	Teaching and Training (other) (spec. under order)

Physical Therapy

B1	Evaluation	B7	UltraSound
B2	Therapeutic Exercise	B8	ElectroTherapy
B3	Transfer Training	B9	Prosthetic Training
B4	Home Program	B10	Fabrication Temporary Devices
B5	Gait Training	B11	Muscle Re-education
B6	Pulmonary Physical Therapy	B12	Management and Evaluation of a Patient Care Plan
		B13-14	Reserved
		B15*	Other (Specify under orders)

Speech Therapy

C1	Evaluation	C6	Aural Rehabilitation
C2	Voice Disorders Treatments	C7	Reserved
C3	Speech Articulation Disorders Treatments	C8	Nonoral Communication
		C9*	Other (Specify under Orders)
C4	Dysphagia Treatments		
C5	Language Disorders Treatments		

* Code which requires a more extensive descriptive narrative for physician's orders.

Occupational Therapy

D1	Evaluation
D2	Independent Living/Daily Living Skills (ADL Training)
D3	Muscle Re-education
D4	Reserved
D5	Perceptual Motor Training
D6	Fine Motor Coordination
D7	Neuro-developmental Treatment
D8	Sensory Treatment
D9	Orthotics/Splinting
D10	Adaptive Equipment (fabrication and training)
D11*	Other (Specify Under Orders)

Medical Social Services

E1	Assessment of Social and Emotional Factors
E2	Counseling for Long Range Planning and Decision Making
E3	Community Resource Planning
E4*	Short Term Therapy
E5	Reserved
E6*	Other (Specify Under Orders)

Home Health Aide

F1	Tub/Shower Bath		F8	Assist with Ambulation
F2	Partial/Complete Bed Bath		F9	Reserved
F3	Reserved		F10	Exercises
F4	Personal Care		F11	Prepare Meal
F5	Reserved		F12	Grocery Shop
F6	Catheter Care		F13	Wash Clothes
F7	Reserved		F14	Housekeeping
			F15*	Other (Spec. under Orders)

* Code which requires a more extensive descriptive narrative for physician's orders.

EXHIBIT VI

ACCEPTABLE V CODES

V45.6	States following surgery of eye and adnexa
V45.81	Postsurgical status, aortocoronary bypass status
V45.89	Postsurgical status, presence of neuropacemaker or other electronic device
V46.0	Dependence on Aspirator
V46.1	Dependence on Respirator
V52.0	Fitting and adjustment of artificial arm
V52.1	Fitting and adjustment of artificial leg
V53.5	Fitting and adjustment ileostomy or other intestinal appliance
V53.6	Fitting and adjustment urinary devices
V54.0	Orthopedic aftercare involving removal of internal fixation device
V54.8	Orthopedic aftercare kirschner wire, plaster cast, external splint, external fixation device or traction device
V54.9	Unspecified orthopedic aftercare
V55.0	Attention to tracheostomy
V55.1	Attention to gastrostomy
V55.2	Attention to ileostomy
V55.3	Attention to colostomy
V55.4	Attention to other artificial opening of digestive tract
V55.5	Attention to cystostomy
V55.6	Attention to other artificial opening of urinary tract
V58.3	Attention to surgical dressing and sutures
V58.4	Other aftercare following surgery

PART EIGHT

HOME CARE DEFINITIONS, ROLES, AND ABBREVIATIONS

KEY HOME HEALTH CARE
DEFINITIONS AND ROLES

Case management: This is the supervision of the care given to a specific patient or caseload population. In home health care, this is often a primary care model with the RN case manager rendering the skilled care, supervising, or collaborating with other ordered professional services. Communication among the services and disciplines involved in the care must be documented in the clinical record. In these care conferences, input is given to the RN case manager to assist the ''intradisciplinary'' team in reaching the patient's goals.

Chaplaincy services: The chaplain serves a population that spans the life continuum from birth through death. The chaplain, like the professional nurse, interfaces with patients and their families and friends at some of the most difficult times of their lives. This struggle with the meaning of life, experienced by many who have significant health concerns, is the work of the chaplain, regardless of any formal religious beliefs. The role varies, based on the setting, the patient and family, or other needs. It may include bereavement counseling, serving on ethics committees, hospice staff support, or performing the sacrament of the sick. The chaplain facilitates the patient's movement toward his or her own resolution of life's questions.

Patients who may benefit from chaplaincy services include those for whom the NANDA nursing diagnosis, *spiritual distress* (distress of the human spirit), has been identified as an appropriate nursing diagnosis. Other patients may have a need for spiritual care based on their health problems. For example, the elderly patient, who is temporarily homebound due a recent fall and fracture and misses going to church services on Sunday morning, may need a call made to her priest or minister to arrange visits to her home.

Daily Care: Medicare patients meet eligibility requirements when skilled nursing care is needed 4 or fewer days per week. This is regardless of the duration of the care. When nursing care is needed 5, 6, or 7 days per week (daily), eligibility is established only when the service is not needed indefinitely. This means that the home care nurse needs a projected endpoint for daily visits. These patients who need daily nursing care for an unspecified amount of time or indefinitely do not receive coverage under Medicare.

When admitting a patient who needs daily wound care or other daily care such as calcimar injection administration, the documentation needs to support medical necessity and assure the meeting of intermittent requirements. Remember that for the purposes of qualifying the patient for home health services, daily is defined as 5 or more days per week. Specify this projected endpoint in #22 of the form 485. It must be specific, not ''when the wound is healed.'' This finite and estimated endpoint needs to be stated as a specific date. For example, daily RN visits until MD reevaluates patient for further wound surgery on 2/22/9_. Another example is daily for 3 months, 10/01/9_ to 01/01/9_.

When determining the projected date, it should be realistically based on the patient's unique medical condition. After your projected date, the visits should decrease to less than daily (4 or less visits per week). If the patient has had a wound for 2 years and is referred to your HHA, it is not realistic that the wound will now heal. In this case, the patient may not be appropriate for home care because this patient may need a level of care (full time) that the Medicare program does not cover. Such cases need to be discussed with your manager.

If your patient had 3-times-per-week skilled wound care orders initially and the MD increases these to daily, be sure to discuss and obtain a supplemental or telephone order with a projected endpoint in either a date format or specific number of days or weeks. Be certain to include this updated order in the clinical record. Remember that it is only for daily visits that a finite, projected endpoint is needed.

Document progress or lack of progress and the specific clinical findings related to the wound and other problems having an impact on the care provided. For wound-care patients, this includes accurate size, drainage, amount, character, presence of odor, etc.

Insulin administration is the exception to daily intermittent care. In unusual circumstances, where the patient is physically or mentally unable to self-inject and there is no available able and willing caregiver, the HHA can give these visits daily, while trying to locate a caregiver. These are the only daily visits that usually do not need a projected ending date.

Dietitian: The role of the professional, registered dietitian in home care is expanding as more patients are cared for in the community setting. Many home health agencies and hospices have professional dietitians available to make home visits and provide consultative services to promote optimal patient nutrition. Another important component of the dietitian's role is as in-service educator for the home health and hospice team.

Often, after being hospitalized, patients will receive instructions on nutrition in relation to their unique needs and medical condition. Some of the common reasons home care patients consult with a dietitian are for enteral/parenteral nutrition, diabetes, AIDS, and other chronic diseases, as well as assessment and monitoring of nutritional needs. Malnutrition in the elderly is also cared for by the professional dietitian.

More innovative insurers are reimbursing for this care if the HHA can clearly articulate the patient's need and justify the visits as part of the comprehensive plan.

Enterostomal therapy nurse: Some HHAs have an ET nurse available to their nurses as a consultant and clinical specialist. This role is particularly important in the HHA and in hospice settings with a high volume of patients with ostomy and wound problems. The clinical specialist role is also important in that the educational needs of the clinical visiting staff and community are served.

Evaluation visit (assessment visit): This is the first or initial home visit to determine whether the patient meets the HHA's criteria for admission. It is often the first skilled visit, made when the nurse already has specific physician's orders and is providing a skilled service to the patient.

Homebound: Synonymous with *confined primarily to the home as a result of medical reasons,* the term connotes that it is a ''considerable and taxing effort'' to leave the home. Please refer to Part Seven for specific descriptions and examples of homebound.

Home health aide (HHA): The HHA's primary, supportive function is to provide personal care and ADL assistance. This role and the associated functions are very important. The HHA usually spends more actual time with the patient and family than any other team member. The HHA's contribution is invaluable to both the team process and positive patient outcomes.

Hospice care: Hospice care is sometimes appropriate for patients with a terminal illness. Hospice care focuses on the comfort and quality of life to assist the patient and family in making every remaining day the best that it can be. Hospice is a philosophy and can be provided in any setting, such as home or an inpatient hospice unit. Palliative care, emotional support, and control of pain and other symptoms are some of the areas of expertise addressed by the hospice team. Through team meetings and individual visits, the physician, the spiritual counselor, the primary nurse, the hospice volunteers, the social worker, the hospice clinical specialist, and others assist the patient and family in meeting their unique needs.

After death, bereavement support services are provided to the family as a key component of continued hospice care.

Management and Evaluation of the Patient Plan of Care (POC): This Medicare service is called various things, including skilled management, skilled planning and assessment, skilled management and planning, case management, and M and E of the patient POC.

Before this became a covered service by Medicare, nurses practicing in home health had limited exposure to this level of care. Many times patients were kept on the service by HHAs with no reimbursement because the patient had an extensive medical history of multifaceted problems, no caregivers, or multiple needs that the caregiver could not safely and effectively meet. However, they were frequently readmitted when they fell and refractured their hip or had an acute exacerbation of CHF or COPD that necessitated hospitalization.

In discussing this skilled service, the Medicare manual states: "Skilled nursing . . . where underlying conditions or complications require that only a registered nurse can ensure that essential nonskilled care is achieving its purpose. . . . The complexity of the necessary unskilled services which are a necessary part of the medical treatment must require the involvement of skilled nursing personnel to promote the patient's recovery and medical safety in view of the beneficiary's overall condition."

The following are typical issues that need to be addressed when determining if the patient is appropriate for management. Evaluation and documentation may support these services: (1) the patient's medical history; (2) the caregiver's support system; (3) current or highly probable medical concerns, based on past history; (3) multiple medications listed on the POC; (4) functional limitations that effect care; (5) safety or other high-risk factors identified; (6) unusual home/environment; (7) ordered disciplines and interventions; (8) diagnoses and underlying pathologies that effect the plan; and (9) the patient's mental status. The nurse needs to assess and document why the skills of an RN are needed to promote the patient's recovery (document evidence of movement toward patient goals) and assure medical safety.

Revision 222 of the HHA manual on page 14.11 explains the skilled nursing service, "Management and Evaluation of the Patient Plan of Care." Please refer to this section in Part Seven, for further clarification and examples of the kinds of patients that may be appropriate for management and evaluation.

Medical Social Services (MSS): The social services used in HHC are directly related to the treatment of the patient's medical condition. When social concerns impede the effective implementation of the POC, a social worker is appropriate. The social problems seen in HHC include finances, housing, and caregiver concerns. The services must be documented to focus on the patient, even though the social worker also assists the family, in conjunction with the patient in HHC.

Occupational therapy (OT): OT assists the patient to attain the maximum level of physical and psychosocial independence. Areas of expertise include fine motor coordination, perceptual-motor skills, sensory testing, adaptive/assistive equipment, ADLs, and specialized upper extremity/hand therapies. The kinds of problems frequently seen in HHC, which require OT include CVAs, amputations, and lung processes for conservation of energy skills. Please refer to the Medicare coverage guidelines in Part Seven for specific details regarding OT coverage. Remember that for Medicare, OT is not a qualifying skilled service that can begin HHC services. However, when a patient has already been receiving another skilled service, such as nursing or physical therapy, and the patient no longer needs these services, the occupational therapist can provide continued services.

Occupational Safety and Health Administration (OSHA): Nurses have heard much in recent years about the need for the practice of universal precautions. The Labor Department's OSHA released its final rule to prevent occupational transmission of bloodborne pathogens and infections. Nurses are well aware of the dangers of hepatitis B and HIV. Employees must create infection control policies that support universal precautions. In addition, nurses, home health aides, and other staff members must be educated about the policy. In practice, this means that hepatitis B immunizations are available when the job requires exposure to blood or other potentially infectious body fluids. The HHA must also provide protective equipment and supplies. This includes, gloves, face masks or other protective shields, aprons that are fluidproof, gowns, and other needed protection. These should be provided by the agency, free of charge to the home care nurses and staff. There are also guidelines on blood or other body fluid transport, blood spill clean up, and the safe disposal of infectious waste.

Personal emergency response systems (PERS): PERS are a unique technology that links the frail or elderly with community resources, neighbors, or a friend at the push of a button or through voice-activated mechanisms. Although there are different types, all are telephone-service dependent. PERS may be appropriate for single patients returning home after surgery, patients who live alone or spend many hours at home alone, or for patients at risk from falls. PERS signal for help at the push of a button, which is worn by the PERS subscriber. For the system to be effective, the emergency device must be worn at all times. Home care and hospice nurses are in a unique position to identify this safety need in the community setting, so a referral can be initiated.

Pharmacist: The role of the clinical pharmacist in home care is growing, as the emphasis on quality and addressing patient needs from an ''intradisciplinary'' model continues. In practice, nurses are acutely aware of many patients who are inappropriately or overmedicated. It is the nurse in the community who sees the whole picture and the shoeboxes full of medications given to patients from multiple physicians. It is in this instance that the nurse addresses safety concerns, acts as the patient's advocate, and consults with the pharmacist who can effectively evaluate the multiple medication regimens.

Traditionally, the pharmacist has been considered the provider of a product, drugs. While this is certainly true, there are many services that the pharmacist can offer to the home care team.

Many, if not most, home care patients are elderly and have multiple risk factors for therapeutic misadventures, secondary to drug therapy. They may have multiple pathologies, different prescribers, exhibit polypharmacy (both prescription and nonprescription medications), and are at a greater risk for adverse effects from medications due to altered physiology, secondary to aging and disabilities (i.e., poor eyesight, impaired hearing, arthritic fingers). Don't forget that a pharmacist can offer more than the provision of drugs; the pharmacist is the drug expert. This discipline is in an excellent position to review medication regimens and screen for drug interactions (drug-drug, drug-disease, drug-food), adverse drug reactions, incorrect doses or dosage forms, and make recommendations. The pharmacist can suggest simplifying the patient's medication regimen, by altering drug delivery systems, medication administration scheduling, or by suggesting how to monitor and assess the therapeutic or toxic effect of drugs. Home care providers can always turn to a pharmacist for drug information, to provide inservice education, or to participate in case conferences and home care/hospice rounds.

Physical therapy (PT): PT services usually are based on patient need and diagnosis. PT, like OT and S-LP, should have a restorative function. This usually means that the patient has a good or fair rehabilitation potential. The PT documentation must show progression toward a goal. The most common kinds of patient problems in HHC, which require PT include CVAs, hip fractures or surgery, knee replacements, and acute exacerbations of osteoarthritis. One of the primary PT skills focuses on teaching the patient and family the home exercise regimens. For specific information, see the Medicare guidelines in Part Seven related to PT coverage.

Psychiatric nurse: The role of the psychiatric nurse in home care has been expanding as more care is provided in the community setting. With the Medicare manual revision of 1989, the role of the psychiatric nurse was clarified to assist the agency in obtaining payment for patients that meet the criteria for coverage. (The specific coverage of services related to psychiatric evaluation and therapy are listed on page 15 of Revision 222, which can be found in Part Seven.) The kinds of problems seen in home care by specially trained psychiatric nurses include depression and therapy, bipolar disorder, evaluation of medication therapeutic levels and effectiveness, as well as many geriatric affective disorders.

The social worker may also be involved in counseling, while the psychiatric nurse is primarily needed for the skills of medication evaluation, observation and assessment, and evaluation and therapy.

Remember that sometimes, it may be appropriate for cases to be shared. The psychiatric nurse visit, which is a skilled nursing visit, may be covered for that expertise. For example, the patient with medical-surgical problems and depression or manipulative behavior may also be seen by the psychiatric nurse; the same way the primary nurse may arrange for the ET nurse to see a patient with specialized wound problems. The psychiatric nurse would set up the POC in conjunction with the primary nurse and other team members to establish a behavioral plan for the team. The documentation needs to focus on the psychiatric needs, as documented by the psychiatric data base, such as a mental status exam and other interventions.

Please refer to ''Depression and Other Psychiatric Home Care'' for specific care, nursing diagnoses, and International Classification of Diseases (ICD-9) codes.

Rehabilitative services: In HHC, this includes the services of PT, OT, and S-LP therapy; all of which should be restorative in focus. When any of these services are indicated, based on patient need, diagnosis, and patient rehabilitation potential status, there must be sufficient documentation of communication among all services. This multidisciplinary case conferencing should be reflected in the progress notes at least every 4 to 6 weeks.

Skilled nursing: Skilled nursing occurs when an RN uses knowledge as a professional nurse to execute skills, render judgments, and evaluate process and outcome. If a nonprofessional can perform a particular function, it is probablly not a skilled function. Teaching, assessment, and evaluation skills are some of the many areas of expertise that are classified as skilled services. As the length of inpatient facility stays have decreased, so has the amount of teaching before discharge. To justify teaching visits, always document and describe specific knowledge deficits that are assessed on admission. Explain that patient teaching was incomplete or was not effective in the inpatient setting. For example, a patient discharged from the hospital on April 2 began a new medication regimen on April 1. Admission to HHC would evaluate the medication effectiveness; however, the dates should be documented clearly to justify medication effectiveness and teaching visits.

Speech-language pathology (S-LP): S-LP services are a vital rehabilitative service indicated for various speech pathologies. Patients that frequently need home health S-LP services have the following problems: CVAs, tracheostomy, laryngectomy, and various neuromuscular diseases. Progress must be noted in the clinical documentation, and case conferencing must occur. It is important that the reason for homebound status be clearly and regularly identified in the clinical record.

Supervisory visit: A supervisory visit at least every 2 weeks (484.36) is a Condition of Participation in the Medicare program. This is not a covered service and may be an administrative expense. A supervisory visit becomes billable when a skilled service is performed during the same visit. For example, a bedridden patient has a decubitus ulcer and the nurse changes the dressing after observing the HHA completing the bed/bath and reviewing the HHA assignment sheet.

KEY HOME HEALTH
CARE ABBREVIATIONS

The following abbreviations are among those most commonly used in the practice of home care. Please refer to your agency's own designated list of approved abbreviations for daily use in documentation.

ADL	Activities of daily living
ALS	Amyotrophic lateral sclerosis (Lou Gehrig's disease)
AMI	Acute myocardial infarction
APHA	American Public Health Association
ASCVD	Arteriosclerotic cardiovascular disease
ASD	Atrial septal defect
ASHD	Arteriosclerotic heart disease
BP	Blood pressure
BPH	Benign prostatic hypertrophy
BRP	Bathroom privileges
BS	Blood sugar
CA	Cancer
CABG	Coronary artery bypass graft
CBC	Complete blood count
CDC	Centers for Disease Control and Prevention
CHF	Congestive heart failure
CNS	Clinical nurse specialist
COPD	Chronic obstructive pulmonary disease
COPS	(Medicare) Conditions of Participation
CPM	Continuous passive motion
CPR	Cardiopulmonary resuscitation
C/S	Cesarian section
CVA	Cerebral vascular accident
CXR	Chest X ray
DJD	Degenerative joint disease
DM	Diabetes mellitus
DOE	Dyspnea on exertion
DRG	Diagnosis Related Group
DX	Diagnosis
EDC	Estimated date of confinement
ET	Enterostomal therapist
FBS	Fasting blood sugar
FHR	Fetal heart rate

FX	Fracture
HCFA	Health Care Financing Administration
HEP	Home exercise program
HHA	Home health agency or Home health aide
HHC	Home health care
HIM	Health Insurance Manual
HME	Home medical equipment
HVGS	High voltage galvanic stimulation
IDDM	Insulin dependent diabetes mellitus
IM	Intramuscular
IPPB	Intermittent positive pressure breathing
IV	Intravenous
JCAHO	Joint Commission on Accreditation of Healthcare Organizations
LLE	Left lower extremity
LLL	Left lower lung
LUE	Left upper extremity
MI	Myocardial infarction
MOW	Meals on Wheels
MSS	Medical Social Services
NHP	Nursing home placement
NIDDM	Non-insulin dependent diabetes mellitus
NIH	National Institutes of Health
OBS	Organic brain syndrome
OSHA	Occupational Safety and Health Administration
OT	Occupational therapy
PCA	Patient-controlled analgesia
PERLA	Pupils equal, react to light and accommodation
PICC (line)	Peripherally inserted central catheter
PKU	Phenylketonuria
PO	By mouth (orally)
POC	Plan of care
PRE	Progressive resistive exercises
PRN	As needed
PT	Physical therapy
PVD	Peripheral vascular disease
RHHI	Regional Home Health Intermediary
RLE	Right lower extremity
RLL	Right lower lung
ROM	Range of motion
RUE	Right upper extremity
S-LP	Speech-language pathology
SNV	Skilled nursing visit

SOB	Shortness of breath
S/P	Status post
SQ	Subcutaneous
SX	Symptoms
TENS	Transcutaneous electrical nerve stimulation
TIA	Transient ischemic attack
Title XVIII	The Medicare section of the Social Security Act
Title XIX	The Medicaid section of the Social Security Act
Title XX	The Social Services section of the Social Security Act
TKR	Total knee replacement
TO	Telephone order
TPN	Total parenteral nutrition
TPR	Temperature, pulse, and respiration
TUR	Transurethral resection
TURP	Transurethral resection of prostate
TX	Treatment
UA/C&S	Urinalysis/culture and sensitivity
UE	Upper extremity
URI	Upper respiratory infection
UTI	Urinary tract infection
VO	Verbal order
WIC	Women, Infants, and Children Program
WNL	Within normal limits

PART NINE

NANDA-APPROVED
NURSING DIAGNOSES

NANDA-APPROVED
NURSING DIAGNOSES

Activity intolerance
Activity intolerance, high risk for
Adjustment, impaired
Airway clearance, ineffective
Anxiety
Aspiration, high risk for
Body image disturbance
Body temperature, altered, high risk for
Bowel incontinence
Breast-feeding, effective
Breast-feeding, ineffective
Breast-feeding, interrupted
Breathing pattern, ineffective
Cardiac output, decreased
Caregiver role strain
Caregiver role strain, high risk for
Communication, impaired verbal
Constipation
Constipation, colonic
Constipation, perceived
Coping, defensive
Coping, family: potential for growth
Coping, ineffective family: compromised
Coping, ineffective family: disabling
Coping, ineffective individual
Decisional conflict (specify)
Denial, ineffective
Diarrhea
Disuse syndrome, high risk for
Diversional activity deficit
Dysreflexia
Family processes, altered
Fatigue
Fear
Fluid volume deficit (1)
Fluid volume deficit (2)
Fluid volume deficit, high risk for
Fluid volume excess

Gas exchange, impaired
Grieving, anticipatory
Grieving, dysfunctional
Growth and development, altered
Health maintenance, altered
Health-seeking behaviors (specify)
Home maintenance management, impaired
Hopelessness
Hyperthermia
Hypothermia
Incontinence, functional
Incontinence, reflex
Incontinence, stress
Incontinence, total
Incontinence, urge
Infant feeding pattern, ineffective
Infection, high risk for
Injury, high risk for
Knowledge deficit (specify)
Management of therapeutic regimen (individuals), ineffective
Mobility, impaired physical
Noncompliance (specify)
Nutrition, altered: high risk for more than body requirements
Nutrition, altered: less than body requirements
Nutrition, altered: more than body requirements
Oral mucous membrane, altered
Pain
Pain, chronic
Parental role conflict
Parenting, altered
Parenting, altered, high risk for
Peripheral neurovascular dysfunction, high risk for
Personal identity disturbance
Poisoning, high risk for
Posttrauma response
Powerlessness
Protection, altered
Rape-trauma syndrome
Rape-trauma syndrome: compound reaction
Rape-trauma syndrome: silent reaction
Relocation stress syndrome
Role performance, altered
Self-care deficit, bathing/hygiene

Self-care deficit, dressing/grooming
Self-care deficit, feeding
Self-care deficit, toileting
Self-esteem, chronic low
Self-esteem disturbance
Self-esteem, situational low
Self-mutilation, high risk for
Sensory/perceptual alterations (specify) (visual, auditory, kinesthetic, gustatory, tactile, olfactory)
Sexual dysfunction
Sexuality patterns, altered
Skin integrity, impaired
Skin integrity, impaired, high risk for
Sleep pattern disturbance
Social interaction, impaired
Social isolation
Spiritual distress (distress of the human spirit)
Suffocation, high risk for
Swallowing, impaired
Thermoregulation, ineffective
Thought processes, altered
Tissue integrity, impaired
Tissue perfusion, altered (specify type) (renal, cerebral, cardipulmonary, gastrointestinal, peripheral)
Trauma, high risk for
Unilateral neglect
Urinary elimination, altered
Urinary retention
Ventilation, inability to sustain spontaneous
Ventilatory weaning process, dysfunctional
Violence, high risk for: self-directed or directed at others

PART TEN

GUIDELINES FOR HOME MEDICAL EQUIPMENT AND SUPPLY CONSIDERATIONS

GUIDELINES FOR HOME MEDICAL EQUIPMENT AND SUPPLY CONSIDERATIONS

The most common home medical equipment (HME) for patients in the home setting is listed here. Please consult an HME manual or equipment company representative for any specific coverage or documentation requirements. Medicare has made many changes relating to HME and this is why you need to consult the HME representative. Most private insurers have a HME benefit. The specific rules and coverage depend on the insurance program. Physician's orders are needed for all of these items. The HME and supplies used by your patient should be documented in item #14 of form 485.

The term *covered* means that generally, with the appropriate physician documentation and patient documented need, this item would be covered for some reimbursement.

Equipment	Indications/guidelines
Alternating pressure pad and pump (covered)	Patient is bedridden and has (or is prone to) decubitus ulcers
Apnea monitor (covered)	Physician documentation needs to be supportive of high-risk history necessitating monitoring for coverage of equipment
Bathtub lifts/seat safety rails (not covered)	Convenience or comfort item, though may be an appropriate safety item
Bedpan (covered)	Bedridden patient
Bedside commode (covered)	Impaired ambulation, patient confined to room or bed
Blood glucose monitoring machine (patient dependent)	Usually insulin dependent DM with documentation of poor control history
Cane (covered)	Impaired ambulation condition
Commode (covered)	Patient confined to room or bed
Crutches (covered)	Impaired ambulation

Electric hospital bed with rails (covered)	Condition requires frequent change in position, usually cardiac or lung processes and the patient can self-operate the controls, otherwise some payers see this as a convenience item for the caregiver (note: overbed table usually not covered; can be rented privately)
Food pumps, enteral feedings (patient dependent)	Diagnosis dependent, usually via G-tube or nasogastric tube
Geriatric chair (covered)	Medical need justified by diagnosis in lieu of a wheelchair
High-tech specialty beds including low air-loss beds/mattresses, Clinitrons, etc. (patient dependent)	Supportive physician documentation of decubitus ulcer in bedbound patient; refer to HME representative for specific coverage and documentation requirements
Home phototherapy (covered)	Physician documentation supportive of increased bilirubin as documented by venipuncture results
Hospital bed (nonelectric) with rails (covered)	Patient usually confined to bed and chair. Need for bed must be clearly evident in documentation
Hydraulic lift (covered)	Condition requires movement in chair/bedridden patient
Infusion pump (covered)	Ordered in conjunction with a course of treatment by physician that is appropriate to patient diagnosis
IPPB machine (covered)	Severely impaired respiratory status
Lamb's wool (covered)	Patient is usually bed/chair bound and is prone to decubitus ulcers
Nebulizer (covered)	Severely impaired respiratory status/system

Oxygen therapy equipment (patient dependent, if meets diagnostic requirements of blood gas)	Covered conditions include most severe lung disease processes. For ranges of acceptable laboratory values refer to specific HME requirements.
Personal emergency response system (not generally covered)	Not seen as therapeutic, although often indicated for patients with history of falls or at risk for falls
Postural drainage board(s) (covered)	Impaired pulmonary status
Quad-cane (covered)	Impaired ambulation condition
Raised toilet seat (not covered)	Seen as primarily a convenience item, though frequently indicated S/P hip surgery
Siderails	Not covered when attached to patient's own bed
	Covered when attached to hospital bed and patient qualifies for hospital bed
Suction machine (covered)	Based on diagnosis, clinical need, and physician documentation
Telephone alert systems (not generally covered)	Not seen as therapeutic in purpose, though often indicated for elderly patients at risk for falls
TENS unit (covered)	Extensive physician documentation of pain, usually an orthopedic or neurologic diagnosis
Traction equipment (covered)	Orthopedic impairment documented, describing need for equipment by physician
Trapeze (covered)	Bed confinement, need for body position change, or respiratory condition
Walker (covered)	Impaired ambulation condition
Water pressure pads/ mattress (covered)	Patient is usually chair/ bedbound and has (or is prone to) decubitus ulcers

Wheelchair (covered)

Bedbound or chairbound, specialty wheelchair (note: special sizes or features are based on physician documentation and patient condition)

GUIDELINES FOR HOME MEDICAL EQUIPMENT AND SUPPLY CONSIDERATIONS

The most common home medical equipment (HME) for patients in the home setting is listed here. Please consult an HME manual or equipment company representative for any specific coverage or documentation requirements. Medicare has made many changes relating to HME and this is why you need to consult the HME representative. Most private insurers have a HME benefit. The specific rules and coverage depend on the insurance program. Physician's orders are needed for all of these items. The HME and supplies used by your patient should be documented in item #14 of form 485.

The term *covered* means that generally, with the appropriate physician documentation and patient documented need, this item would be covered for some reimbursement.

Equipment	Indications/guidelines
Alternating pressure pad and pump (covered)	Patient is bedridden and has (or is prone to) decubitus ulcers
Apnea monitor (covered)	Physician documentation needs to be supportive of high-risk history necessitating monitoring for coverage of equipment
Bathtub lifts/seat safety rails (not covered)	Convenience or comfort item, though may be an appropriate safety item
Bedpan (covered)	Bedridden patient
Bedside commode (covered)	Impaired ambulation, patient confined to room or bed
Blood glucose monitoring machine (patient dependent)	Usually insulin dependent DM with documentation of poor control history
Cane (covered)	Impaired ambulation condition
Commode (covered)	Patient confined to room or bed
Crutches (covered)	Impaired ambulation

PART ELEVEN

RESOURCES

DIRECTORY OF RESOURCES

Accent on Information: (309) 378-2961

Agency for Health Care Policy and Research (AHCPR): 1-800-358-9295. (AHCPR has a congressional mandate for developing clinical practice guidelines. Free copies of released guidelines are available.)

AIDS Adult and Pediatric Clinical Trials Information Services: 1-800-874-2572 or 1-800-TRIALS-A

AIDS Hotline, National: 1-800-342-2437 or 1-800-342-AIDS

AIDS Hotline, National, Spanish: 1-800-344-7432

AIDS Medical Foundation: (212) 206-0670

AIDS, National Information Clearinghouse, CDC: 1-800-458-5231

Alliance for Aging Research: (202) 293-2856

Alzheimer's Disease and Other Related Disorders Association: 1-800-621-0379

Alzheimer's Disease Educational and Referral Center (NIH, National Institute on Aging): 1-800-438-4380

American Association of Kidney Patients: (813) 254-2558

American Association of Retired Persons (AARP): (202) 872-4700

American Brain Tumor Association: 1-800-886-2282 or (312) 286-5571

American Cancer Society: 1-800-ACS-2345

American Cancer Society: 1-800-395-LOOK. ("Look Good . . . Feel Better" program for women undergoing chemotherapy or radiation)

American Cleft Palate Association: (412) 681-9620

American Council of the Blind: 1-800-424-8666 or (202) 833-1251

American Diabetes Association: 1-800-232-6366 or (212) 683-7444

American Dietetic Association: (313) 280-5012

American Fertility Association: (205) 251-9764

American Federation of Home Health Agencies: (301) 588-1454

American Foundation for the Blind: 1-800-232-5463

American Foundation for Urologic Disease: 1-800-828-7866

American Heart Association: 1-800-242-8721 or (214) 750-5300

American Lung Association: 1-800-232-5864

American Hospital Association: (312) 280-6000

American Nurses Association: (202) 554-4444

American Occupational Therapy Association: 1-800-426-2547

American Physical Therapy Association: (703) 684-2782

American Red Cross: (202) 737-8300

American Society on Aging: (415) 543-2617

American Speech-Language-Hearing Association: 1-800-638-8255

Arthritis Foundation: (404) 872-7100

Association of Nurses in AIDS Care: (215) 321-2371

Association for Retarded Citizens (ARC) of the United States: (817) 640-0204

Breast Cancer Patient Resource: 1-800-221-2141. (The Y-Me Hotline for women who want to talk with other women with breast cancer)

Cancer Federation, Inc.: 1-800-982-3270

Cancer Care, Inc.: (212) 221-3300

Cancer Information Service (CIS): 1-800-4-CANCER

Canadian Nurses Association, 50 The Driveway, Ottawa, Ontario K2P1E2

CDC National AIDS Clearinghouse: 1-800-458-5231

Children with AIDS Project of America: 1-800-866-2437

Continence Restored, Inc.: (212) 879-3131

Council of Community Health Services, National League for Nursing: (212) 582-1022 or (301) 881-9130

Cystic Fibrosis Foundation: 1-800-FIGHT-CF

Elder Care Locator Services: 1-800-677-1116

Environmental Protection Agency: Send for the following free brochures: (1) *Disposal Tips for Home Health Care: Educating Your Patients;* (2) *Disposal Tips for Home Health Care;* and (3) *Handle with Care, How to Throw Out Used Insulin Syringes and Lancets at Home, a Booklet for Young People with Diabetes and Their Families.*

FDA's ''Product Problem Reporting Program'': 1-800-638-6725

Foundation for Hospice and Home Care: (202) 547-7424

Gray Panthers: (212) 382-3300

Head and Neck Cancer Information Service: 1-800-368-1422

Help for Incontinent People (HIP): 1-800-252-3337 or 1-800-BLADDER

Hospice Association of America: (202) 546-4759

Hospice Nurses Association, P.O. Box 8166, Van Nuys, CA 91409

International Center for Social Gerontology: (202) 479-2642

La Leche League: (312) 455-7730

Leukemia Society of America, Inc.: 1-800-955-4LSA or (212) 573-8484

Make-A-Wish Foundation of America: 1-800-722-9474 or (602) 240-6060

March of Dimes Birth Defects Foundation: (914) 428-7100

Medic Alert Foundation International: 1-800-344-3226 or (209) 668-3333

Muscular Dystrophy Association: (212) 586-0808

National Association for Home Care (NAHC): (202) 547-7424

National Association for the Deaf: (301) 587-1788

National Association of Area Agencies on Aging: (202) 484-7520

National Association of Physically Handicapped, Inc.: (614) 852-1664

National Brain Tumor Foundation: 1-800-934-CURE or (415) 296-0404

National Cancer Institute: (301) 496-5583

National Coalition for Cancer Research: (202) 544-1880

National Council of Senior Citizens: (202) 347-8800

National Council on Patient Information and Education: (202) 347-6711

National Council on the Aging: (202) 479-1200

National Easter Seal Society: (312) 243-8400

National Foundation for Ileitis and Colitis: 1-800-343-3637

National Hemophiliac Foundation: (212) 431-8541

National Hospice Organization: 1-800-658-8898 or (703) 243-5900

National Institute on Aging: (301) 496-1752

National Institute of Mental Health: (301) 443-2403

National Kidney and Urologic Diseases Information Clearinghouse: (301) 468-6345

National Kidney Foundation: 1-800-622-9010 or (212) 889-2210

National Library of Congress Referral Center: (202) 287-5670. (This is a free referral service that can help the professional nurse locate information or identify needed services.)

National Lymphedema Network: 1-800-541-3259

National Multiple Sclerosis Society: (212) 986-3240

National Rehabilitation Association: (703) 836-0850

National Spinal Cord Injury Association: (617) 964-0521

Oncology Nursing Society: (412) 921-7373

People with AIDS Coalition: 1-800-828-3280

Prostate Cancer Support Group (Us Too): 1-800-82-US-TOO or 1-800-828-7866

Skin Cancer Foundation: (212) 725-5176

Spina Bifida Association of America (SBAA): (301) 770-SBAA

United Cerebral Palsy Association: (212) 481-6316

United Ostomy Association: (714) 660-8624 or (213) 413-5510 or 1-800-826-0826

Visiting Nurse Association of America: 1-800-426-2547

Y-Me National Organization for Breast Cancer Information and Support: (708) 799-8338

CLINICAL NEWSLETTERS
AND JOURNALS

The American Journal of Hospice and Palliative Care, 470 Boston Post Road, Weston, MA 02193, 1-800-869-2700.

Caring magazine is published monthly by the National Association for Home Care. Inquiries for subscription and/or membership can be directed to: The National Association for Home Care at 519 C Street, NE, Washington, DC, 20002-5809.

Home Health Care Nurse is published bimonthly by J.B. Lippincott Company, 12107 Insurance Way, Hagerstown, MD 21740.

Home Health Care Pharmacy and Therapeutics Update is a monthly newsletter that addresses updates on new drugs, reviews therapeutic issues, and has ''Drug Information'' and ''Hospice Happenings'' columns. This newsletter, which answers questions submitted by HHA and hospice staff, is $20 for an annual subscription. Written inquiries should be directed to: Sinai Home Care-Hospice Program, Attn: Dr. Lynn McPherson, 21 Crossroad Drive, Suite 450, Owings Mills, MD 21117 or the newsletter can be ordered by calling (410) 356-9112.

The Hospice Journal is published by The Haworth Press, Inc., 10 Alice Street, Bingingham, NY 13904, 1-800-342-9678.

Journal of Home Health Care Practice is published quarterly by Aspen Publishers, Inc., 7201 McKinney Circle, Frederick, MD 21781, 1-800-638-8437.

FOR FURTHER READING

Albrecht M et al: The Albrecht nursing model for home healthcare, *Journal of Nursing Administration* 23:1, 1993.

American Nurses Association: *A statement on the scope of home health nursing practice,* Washington, DC, 1992, American Nurses Association.

American Nurses Association: *Standards and scope of hospice nursing practice,* Washington, DC, American Nurses Association.

American Nurses Association: *Standards of community health nursing practice,* Kansas City, Missouri, 1986, American Nurses Association.

American Nurses Association: *Standards of home health nursing practice,* Kansas City, Missouri, 1986, American Nurses Association.

Bobnet N et al: Continuous quality improvement, improving quality in your home care organization, *Journal of Nursing Administration* 23:2, 1993.

Bradshaw Matz L, Gary G: Patient outcomes measure home health care accomplishments, *Nursing Management* 24:5, 1993.

Chromiak D: Referral sources in home healthcare, *Journal of Nursing Administration* 22:12, 1992.

Cookfair J: *Nursing process and practice in the community,* St. Louis, 1991, Mosby Year Book.

Crigger BJ, Campbell C, editors: The ethics of home care: autonomy and accommodation, *Hastings Center Report,* March/April, 1990.

Culbertson L: A comparison of foley catheter types in home care use, *Home Healthcare Nurse* 10:6, 1993.

Cyr L: The clinical nurse specialist in a home healthcare setting, *Home Healthcare Nurse* 8:1, 1990.

Erickson G: Ethical dilemmas in home care of chronically ill elderly persons, *Home Healthcare Nurse* 6:6, 1992.

Feldman C et al: Decision making in case management of home healthcare clients, *Journal of Nursing Administration* 23:1, 1993.

Goldrick BA, Larson EL: Wound management in home care: an assessment, *Journal of Community Health Nursing* 10:1, 1993.

Goodwin DR: Critical pathways in home healthcare, *Journal of Nursing Administration* 22:2, 1992.

Haddad A et al: Teamwork in home infusion therapy: the relationship between nursing and pharmacy, *Home Health Care Nurse* 11:1, 1993.

Health care financing administration: *Health Insurance Manual-11,* Washington, DC, 1990, Government Printing Office.

Humphrey C, Milone-Nuzzo P: *Home care nursing: an orientation to practice,* East Norwalk, Conn, 1991, Appleton & Lange.

Jaffe M, Skidmore-Roth L: *Home health nursing care plans,* 2nd ed, St. Louis, 1993, Mosby Year Book.

Jewell M, Peters D: An assessment guide for community health nurses, *Home Healthcare Nurse* 7:5, 1989.

Mallory C, Hartshorn J: *Acute nursing care in the home: a holistic approach,* Philadelphia, 1989, JB Lippincott.

Marrelli TM: *The nurse manager's survival guide: practical answers to everyday problems,* St. Louis, 1993, Mosby Year Book.

Martin K, Scheet N: The Omaha system: providing a framework for assuring quality of home care, *Home Healthcare Nurse,* 6:3, 1988.

Maturen V, Zander K: Outcomes management in a prospective pay system, *Caring* 12:6, 1993.

Matz B, Gary G: Patient outcomes measure home health care accomplishments, *Nursing Management* 42:5, 1993.

504

Morgan K: National certification for home care RNs, *Nursing Management* 22:9, 1991.

Mueller R: Cancer pain: which drugs for which patient, *RN* 55:5, 1992.

Pearson M: The nurse, the elderly caregiver and stress, *Caring* 12(1), 1993.

Salsberry PJ et al: Home health care services for AIDS patients: one community's response, *Journal of Community Health Nursing* 10:1, 1993.

Sherry D: The incredible, F-L-E-X-I-B-L-E nurse, *Nursing 85* 15(12):72, 1985.

Shriver A: Creating a culture of excellence in home care, *Nursing Management* 24:5, 1992.

Skipper M: Launching an agency ethics committee, *Caring* 11:6, 1992.

Stanhope M, Knollmueller R: *Handbook of community and home health nursing,* St. Louis, 1992, Mosby Year Book.

Stein J et al: The emergence of the home care pharmacist, *Caring* 11:11, 1992.

Tonore M, Bivona B: The nutrition screening initiative, *Caring* 11:12, 1992.

Twardon C, Gartner M: A strategy for growth in home care the clinical nurse specialist, *Journal of Nursing Administration* 22:10, 1992.

Warling M: Legal aspects of the client's record: a guide for community health nurses, *Caring* October 1982, 14–17.

Williams M, Walker G: Managing swallowing problems in the home, *Caring* 11:12, 1992.

Yannaco T: Radiation therapy: implications for home care, *Caring* 12:2, 1993.

Young C: Tube feeding at home, *American Journal of Nursing* 92:4, 1992.

INDEX

508

Essentials for Practice

**HOME HEALTH NURSING CARE PLANS,
2nd Edition**
Marie Jaffe, RN, MS; Linda Skidmore-Roth, RN, MS
1993 (0-8016-6699-6)
- This compact, spiral-bound reference tool is essential for nurses who plan and implement nursing care in the home setting.
- Incorporates nursing diagnoses, short-term and long-term outcome criteria, nursing interventions, and client/family interventions in each care plan.

**THE NURSE MANAGER'S SURVIVAL GUIDE:
PRACTICAL ANSWERS TO EVERYDAY
PROBLEMS**
T. M. Marrelli, RN, BSN, MA
1993 (0-8016-6449-7)
- This book addresses crucial management activities, such as daily operations, time management, budgeting, and decision making.
- Covers key interpersonal management responsibilities, such as negotiating with others, handling patient and family complaints, delegating, motivating, and team building.

HANDBOOK OF HOME CARE IV THERAPY
Joanne C. LaRocca, RN, MN, CRNI
1993 (0-8016-6910-3)
- This handbook provides accessible, accurate, and concise information on major home infusion therapies, including IV line assessment and management.
- Covers important topics, including hydration therapy, antibiotic therapy, chemotherapy, hemotherapy, parenteral nutrition, and pain management.

**To order, ask your bookstore
manager or call toll-free 1-800-
426-4545. We look forward to
hearing from you soon.**